COMMUNITY-BASED PARTICIPATORY RESEARCH FOR HEALTH

Advancing Social and Health Equity

third edition

NINA WALLERSTEIN
BONNIE DURAN
JOHN G. OETZEL
MEREDITH MINKLER
Editors

JB JOSSEY-BASS™
A Wiley Brand

Published by Jossey-Bass
A Wiley Brand
One Montgomery Street, Suite 1000, San Francisco, CA 94104-4594—www.josseybass.com

Edition History
John Wiley and Sons, Inc. (2e, 2008; 1e, 2003)

Jossey-Bass books and products are available through most bookstores. To contact Jossey-Bass directly call our Customer Care Department within the U.S. at 800-956-7739, outside the U.S. at 317-572-3986, or fax 317-572-4002.

Wiley publishes in a variety of print and electronic formats and by print-on-demand. Some material included with standard print versions of this book may not be included in e-books or in print-on-demand. If this book refers to media such as a CD or DVD that is not included in the version you purchased, you may download this material at http://booksupport.wiley.com. For more information about Wiley products, visit www.wiley.com.

Library of Congress Cataloging-in-Publication Data

Names: Wallerstein, Nina, 1953- editor.
Title: Community-based participatory research for health: advancing social and health equity / edited by Nina Wallerstein, Dr.P.H, Professor of Public Health, College of Population Health Director, Center for Participatory Research, University of New Mexico (UNM), Bonnie Duran, Dr.P.H., Associate Professor, University of Washington School of Social Work, Director of the Center for Indigenous Health Research, Indigenous Wellness Research Institute, John G. Oetzel, Professor, Waikato Management School, University of Waikato, Meredith Minkler, Dr.P.H., MPH, Professor, Graduate School, Community Health Sciences, University of California, Berkeley, Professor Emerita, School of Public Health.
Description: Third edition. | Hoboken, NJ : Jossey-Bass & Pfeiffer Imprints, Wiley, [2017] | Includes bibliographical references. |
Identifiers: LCCN 2017018499 (print) | LCCN 2017021064 (ebook) | ISBN 9781119258865 (epdf) | ISBN 9781119258872 (epub) | ISBN 9781119258858 (paperback)
Subjects: LCSH: Public health—Research—Citizen participation. | Public health—Research—Methodology. | Community health services. | BISAC: MEDICAL / Public Health.
Classification: LCC RA440.85 (ebook) | LCC RA440.85 .C65 2017 (print) | DDC 362.1072—dc23
LC record available at https://lccn.loc.gov/2017018499

Cover design: Wiley
Cover image: © MAGNIFIER/Shutterstock

Printed in the United States of America
THIRD EDITION

PB Printing SKY10058753_102723

From Nina: To my late parents, Robert and Judith Wallerstein, who modeled for me values of justice and compassion.

From Bonnie: Gratitude to my parents, siblings, and community members for sharing their values, wisdom, and patience.

From John: To my children, Spencer and Ethan, who inspire me to make a positive contribution in the community.

From Meredith: To Roy and Fran Minkler, who as parents and human beings taught by example the power of deep concern with fairness, caring, keeping a sense of humor, and never giving up.

CONTENTS

PART SEVEN: PROMISING PRACTICES TO OUTCOMES: HEALTHY PUBLIC POLICY

THE EDITORS

NINA WALLERSTEIN, DrPH, professor of public health, College of Population Health, and director, Center for Participatory Research (cpr.unm.edu), University of New Mexico (UNM), has been developing CBPR and empowerment, Paulo Freire–based interventions for more than thirty years. She has written over 150 articles and chapters and seven books, including the Freirean *Problem-Posing at Work: A Popular Educator's Guide*. In 2016, she received the inaugural Community Engaged Research Lecture award from UNM. She's had a long-term CBPR research relationship with several New Mexican tribes to support intergenerational culture-centered family prevention programming with children, parents, and elders; and she has worked with the Healthy Native Community Partnership for more than ten years. Since 2006, she has worked to strengthen the science of CBPR and community-engaged research. She is currently principal investigator (PI) of Engage for Equity, an NINR-funded RO1 to assess promising partnering practices associated with outcomes and to develop partnership evaluation and reflection tools and resources. She has collaboratively produced with Latin American colleagues an empowerment, participatory research, and health promotion curriculum available in Spanish, Portuguese, and English (http://cpr.unm.edu/curricula-classes/empowerment-curriculum.html) and cosponsors an annual summer institute in CBPR for health at the University of New Mexico.

BONNIE DURAN, DrPH (mixed-race Opelousas and Coushatta) is professor in the School of Social Work at the University of Washington, and is also Director of the Center for Indigenous Health Research at the Indigenous Wellness Research Institute (www.iwri.org). Using Indigenous theories to guide her work, Bonnie's research includes intervention and prevalence studies of substance abuse and other mental disorders, violence, and treatment seeking in Native communities. Her overall aims are to work with communities to design interventions and descriptive studies that are empowering, culture-centered, sustainable, and that have maximum public health impact.

JOHN G. OETZEL is a professor in the Waikato Management School at the University of Waikato. He uses CBPR to collaboratively work with communities to address various health issues to improve health equity. His current work includes the collaborative development of interventions with two Māori health organizations in New Zealand related to pre-diabetes and positive aging. He is also a member of the Engage for Equity research team investigating promising practices for CBPR in the United States. He contributes expertise in research design and evaluation and believes in the importance of collaborative design to ensure that the research evaluation fits the context and needs of communities as well as to ensure interventions are culturally centered. He is author or coauthor of three books: *Managing Intercultural Communication Effectively* (with Stella Ting-Toomey, 2001, Sage); *Intercultural Communication: A Layered Approach* (2009, Pearson); and *Theories of Human Communication,* 11th ed. (with Stephen Littlejohn and Karen Foss, 2017, Waveland). He is coeditor of two other books: *The Sage*

Handbook of Conflict Communication (with Stella Ting-Toomey, 2006, Sage, and 2nd edition in 2013). In addition, he is also author of more than ninety articles and book chapters.

MEREDITH MINKLER, DrPH, MPH, is professor in the Graduate School, Community Health Sciences, University of California, Berkeley, and professor emerita in the School of Public Health. Founding director of the UC Berkeley Center on Aging, Minkler continues to work with community and other partners to help develop the evidence base for implementing healthy public policy in areas including healthy retail in low-income neighborhoods, environmental exposures, immigrant worker health and safety, criminal justice reform, and HIV/AIDS. A recent Fulbright specialist in South Africa in CBPR, she has offered trainings on community-engaged research in Hong Kong, Singapore, Australia, the United Kingdom, and in numerous states and provinces in the United States and Canada. Minkler has coauthored close to two hundred articles and coauthored or edited nine books, including *Community Organizing and Community Building for Health and Welfare* (Rutgers, 2012).

THE CONTRIBUTORS

MARGARITA ALEGRÍA, PhD, is the chief of the Disparities Research Unit at Massachusetts General Hospital and professor in the Departments of Medicine and Psychiatry at Harvard Medical School. Alegría has served as PI on more than fifteen federally funded research grants and has published more than two hundred professional publications on topics such as the improvement of health care services delivery for diverse racial and ethnic populations, conceptual and methodological issues with multicultural populations, and ways to bring the community's perspective into the design and implementation of health services.

ALEX J. ALLEN, III, MSA, is the president and CEO of the Chandler Park Conservancy. He collaborates with residents, stakeholders, local institutions, business, government, and the philanthropic community to transform Chandler Park into a campus with exceptional educational, recreational, and conservation opportunities for youth and families on Detroit's eastside and the region. He has effectively led organizations, collaborative initiatives, and has improved the quality of life for people who live, work, play, and visit communities in the United States. His experience includes managing grants for compliance and budget integrity, convening stakeholders for planning and project implementation, supervising and monitoring youth programs, fund-raising, reporting and evaluation, and CBPR.

JORGE ALONZO, JD, is a research associate at Wake Forest School of Medicine and is part of a team that specializes in HIV-prevention research using CBPR with immigrant Latinos. He has been involved in the design, implementation, and evaluation of HIV-prevention interventions for Latino gay and bisexual men and men who have sex with men (MSM) and Latina transgender women. He has also been involved in projects exploring the impact of immigration enforcement on access to and use of public health services among Latinos.

ANDREA AULT, PhD, MPA, is the senior director of the Mental Health Innovation Lab in the New York City Department of Health and Mental Hygiene. She was previously the associate director of the Health Equity Lab at Cambridge Health Alliance, where her research focused on racial-ethnic disparities in mental health care, dissemination and implementation research, and CBPR.

MAGDALENA AVILA, DrPH, MPH, MSW, is associate professor, community health education, Department of Health, Exercise and Sports Science, College of Education, University of New Mexico. She self-identifies as an activist scholar in community health and CBPR, in her partnering with Latino and other Indigenous communities of color, and in her use of a social justice framework. Her areas of research are environmental health, environmental racism, and community health impact assessments in working with rural and urban communities, and she has expanded her research capacity by incorporating digital story making into her CBPR work with Latino communities.

STEPHANIE BAKER, PhD, MS, PT, is assistant professor of public health at Elon University and a member of the Greensboro Health Disparities Collaborative. Her work is focused on social determinants of racial inequities in health, community organizing as a tool for public health change, antiracism pedagogy, and CBPR.

BARBARA BAQUERO, PhD, MPH, is assistant professor of community and behavioral health at the University of Iowa, College of Public Health. She is a founding member of the Healthy Equity Advancement Lab (HEAL), an academic-community research lab dedicated to advancing health equity through research and training. She serves as PI and deputy director of the University of Iowa, Prevention Research Center, funded by the CDC.

STEVEN BARNETT, MD, is associate professor of family medicine and public health sciences at the University of Rochester and director of the Rochester Prevention Research Center: National Center for Deaf Health Research. He is a sign language–skilled family physician researcher with a career focus on health care and collaborative health research with deaf sign language users and people with hearing loss, their families, and communities.

ADAM B. BECKER, PhD, MPH, is associate professor of pediatrics and preventive medicine in the Feinberg School of Medicine at Northwestern University. He is also executive director of the Consortium to Lower Obesity in Chicago Children (CLOCC) at Ann and Robert H. Lurie Children's Hospital of Chicago. He has used CBPR to examine and address the impact of stressful community conditions on the health of women raising children, youth violence prevention, and the impact of the social and physical environment on physical activity.

LORENDA BELONE, PhD, MPH, (Diné/Navajo) is assistant professor at the University of New Mexico (UNM) College of Education. She is a senior fellow with the Center for Participatory Research, a center that supports networks of research with community partners in New Mexico addressing health inequities, and a senior fellow with the UNM Center for Health Policy. Since 2000, she has been actively engaged in CBPR research that has involved southwest Native American communities. She currently is co-PI on a NIDA-funded RIO multi-tribal implementation and evaluation study (1R01DA037174-03).

EVAN BISSELL, MPH, MCP, is an artist based in the Bay Area. He teaches art and social change at UC Berkeley and is involved in participatory research and art projects in multiple settings across the country that support equitable systems and liberatory processes. His work has been exhibited in institutions and galleries across the country. He is the creator of knottedline.com and freedoms-ring.org.

KRISTIN BLACK, PhD, MPH, is a postdoctoral fellow in the Cancer Health Disparities Training Program in the Department of Health Behavior at the University of North Carolina at Chapel Hill. Her PhD is in maternal and child health, and her career commitment is to use CBPR approaches to understand and address race-specific inequities in cancer survivorship and reproductive health.

JULIA GREEN BRODY, PhD, is executive director and senior scientist at Silent Spring Institute, an independent research group founded in 1994 by breast cancer activists to create a "lab of their own" focused on environmental factors and prevention. Her research, supported by the National Institutes of Health, investigates everyday exposures to carcinogens and endocrine-disrupting chemicals from consumer products, workplaces, and pollution.

PHIL BROWN, PhD, is University Distinguished Professor of Sociology and Health Sciences at Northeastern, where he directs the Social Science Environmental Health Research Institute. His books include *No Safe Place: Toxic Waste, Leukemia, and Community Action*; *Toxic Exposures: Contested Illnesses and the Environmental Health Movement*; and *Contested Illnesses: Citizens, Science, and Health Social Movements*. He directs an NIEHS training program "Transdisciplinary Training at the Intersection of Environmental Health and Social Science."

LISA CACARI-STONE, PhD, MA, MS, is associate professor in the College of Population Health and assistant director with the RWJF Center for Health Policy at the University of New Mexico. Her scholarly interests focus on upstream determinants of health, including societal and political structures and relationships that differentially affect population health and policy interventions that influence health equity. Her community-engaged research with Latino and US-Mexico border communities encompass macro-level determinants (e.g., immigration policy, health reform); the community level (e.g., impact of neighborhood context and migration on substance use); and the interpersonal level (e.g., the role of promotores de salud in chronic disease management among Latinos). Cacari Stone is widely trusted for her work in translating and disseminating data for policy making with governments, community-based organizations, coalitions, and foundations.

CHARLOTTE YU-TING CHANG, DrPH, MPH, is coordinator of research to practice and evaluation and associate project scientist at the Labor Occupational Health Program, School of Public Health, University of California, Berkeley. Her work has focused on advancing the movement of research into practice in worker health and safety, with a particular interest in the role and processes of research partnerships with workers and community members. She has worked and written on a range of projects involving immigrant worker populations and communities as well as on research to practice lessons learned in construction health and safety.

VIVIAN CHÁVEZ, DrPH, is associate professor of health education at San Francisco State University. A storyteller by nature, she has collaborated with community-based organizations to disseminate their work. She coedited *Prevention Is Primary: Strategies in Community Well-Being,* coauthored *Drop That Knowledge: Youth Radio Stories,* translated Media Advocacy into Spanish, and made a film about cultural humility that is widely accessible. Her work integrates the language of the arts, culture, and the body for health and social change.

BOWEN CHUNG, MD, MSHS, is associate professor–in-residence of psychiatry at the UCLA David Geffen School of Medicine, an adjunct scientist at the RAND Corporation, and an attending physician at Harbor-UCLA Medical Center. He has been a PI and co-PI on ten federally funded research grants and is the author of more than thirty scientific publications. He has been working with the same community partners for nearly fifteen years.

VICKI COLLIE-AKERS, PhD, MPH, is associate director of health promotion research at the KU Center for Community Health and Development. She serves as an investigator on several projects promoting health equity and reduction in health disparities in the Kansas City metropolitan area. Additionally, she directs several evaluation projects that support partners who are working to promote health through their comprehensive initiatives. Her research primarily focuses on applying a CBPR orientation to understand how collaborative partnerships and coalitions can improve social determinants of health and equity and reduce disparities in health outcomes.

CHRIS M. COOMBE, PhD, MPH, is assistant research scientist in the Department of Health Behavior/Health Education at the University of Michigan School of Public Health and is affiliated with the Detroit Community-Academic Urban Research Center. She has extensive experience designing, implementing, and evaluating collaborative research and interventions using CBPR. Coombe's work focuses on understanding how urban social and physical environments contribute to racial and socioeconomic inequities and translating that knowledge into policy interventions to promote health and equity.

JASON CORBURN, PhD, MCP, is professor in the Department of City and Regional Planning and the School of Public Health, University of California, Berkeley. He directs the Institute of Urban and Regional Development and the Center for Global Healthy Cities. He is the author of a number of award-winning books on community-based action research for health equity, including *Street Science* (MIT Press, 2005), *Toward the Healthy City* (MIT Press, 2009), and *Slum Health* (University of California Press, 2016).

JANA CORDEIERO, MPH, is an independent public health and nonprofit consultant, strategist, and researcher with more than twenty-five years of experience working with universities, foundations, community-based organizations, and health departments to develop and evaluate effective public health policies and programs. She worked with other advocates in the Bay Area to successfully pass public health policies to prevent chronic diseases fueled by sugary drinks, including warning label legislation, sugary drink taxes on distributors, and resisting pouring rights contracts at universities.

JESSICA CUCULICK, PhD, is associate professor, Department of Liberal Studies, at the National Technical Institute for the Deaf, Rochester Institute of Technology. Cuculick coordinates the applied liberal arts associate degree program and is the professional development director for the Rochester bridges to the doctorate program (www.deafscientists.com). She is codirector for the Deaf Health Lab and the PI for the deaf health literacy research project. Cuculick has been involved with CBPR with the National Center for Deaf Health Research (NCDHR) at the University of Rochester, such as breastfeeding and cardiovascular health perspectives in the Deaf community.

SAMUEL CYKERT, MD, is a professor of medicine at UNC-CH in the Division of General Internal Medicine and Clinical Epidemiology. He also serves as the director of the UNC School of Medicine program on health and clinical informatics. Combining his research training and interest in health policy, he currently serves as a PI on multiple projects that address health disparities in cancer treatment and chronic care management.

GAIL DANA-SACCO, PhD, MPH, is on the faculty of the Center for American Indian Health at the Johns Hopkins University, where she works with tribal communities to research violence and injury and to develop and implement structural and behavioral strategies to improve health outcomes.

ROBIN DEAN, MPH, MA, is a public health consultant offering health advocacy and qualitative research services to clients working to create healthy, connected communities in which everyone has a voice. In 2014, she advocated through coordinating writers' media submissions for soda tax campaigns in San Francisco and Berkeley, and in 2016 she secured endorsements for Oakland's and San Francisco's winning soda tax measures. Robin has produced case studies and evaluations, including a Berkeley Media Studies Group issue brief on an Oregon affordable housing coalition's media advocacy effort and a case study of girls' education in Mali.

SANETA DEVUONO-POWELL, JD, MCP, is a city planner and attorney who works on community health. She is currently senior planner at Changelab Solutions and has written on incarceration and its impacts on families as well as on community-based participatory action research. Her current work is focused on racial disparities in health and the links between health disparities and housing.

LORI DEWINDT, MA, is health project coordinator, Rochester Prevention Research Center: National Center for Deaf Health Research (RPRC/NCDHR), University of Rochester Medical Center. DeWindt has worked in the field of Deaf community health as a RPRC/NCDHR research coordinator and as a psychotherapist at the Deaf Wellness Center at the University of Rochester.

PAULA DOMINGO DE GARCIA is a resident of the South Valley and one of the main promotoras of the S.V.P.E.J. research team. She is an immigrant from the Indigenous community Nahua de Cuentepec in Temixco, Mexico. Before coming to New Mexico, she worked with the Independent Commission of Human Rights of Morelos to save her native language, Nahuatl, and with the National Council to Promote Education in the rural community of Tlatepetl, Tepoztlan. She currently works as a teaching assistant at Dolores Gonzales Elementary School and as a federal court interpreter translating from Nahuatl to Spanish. She is currently studying for her AA in Early Childhood Multicultural Education.

AILEEN ALFONSO DULDULAO, PhD, MSW, is the maternal, child, and family health epidemiologist for the Multnomah County Health Department in Portland, Oregon. She has held research fellowships from the National Institute of Mental Health, the National Institute of Minority Health and Health Disparities, and the University of Washington Institute for Translational Health Sciences. Her social work background includes extensive experience in direct social service provision with immigrant and refugee communities experiencing domestic violence, sexual assault, mental illness, poverty, and employment discrimination.

ALEXEI DUNAWAY is the executive director of Ongoza, an accelerator for youth-led social businesses in Nairobi, Kenya. Previously he contributed to several human rights trials in Spain, the United States, and El Salvador; conducted research for Human Rights Watch and the Council on Foreign Relations; and helped coordinate the world pilot of a youth-led community mapping initiative at the Centro de Promoção da Saúde (CEDAPS) in Rio de Janeiro, Brazil. He also served as a Fulbright research scholar in Mozambique.

EUGENIA ENG, MPH, DrPH, is professor of health behavior at the Gillings School of Global Public Health, University of North Carolina at Chapel Hill. She has more than thirty years of CBPR experience, including field studies conducted with rural communities of the US South, Sub-Saharan Africa, and Southeast Asia to address socially stigmatizing health problems such as pesticide poisoning, cancer, and STI-HIV. Her CBPR projects include the NCI-funded Accountability for Cancer Care through Undoing Racism and Equity, the CDC-funded Men As Navigators for Health, the NCI-funded Cancer Care and Racial Equity Study, the NHLBI-funded CVD Black Church: Are We Our Brother's Keeper? In addition to her coedited book, *Methods for Community-Based Participatory Research for Health,* she has more than 115 publications on the lay health advisor intervention model, the concepts of community competence and natural helping, and community assessment procedures.

JESSICA ESTRADA is a health program coordinator at the San Francisco Department of Public Health Community Health Equity & Promotion Branch, and formerly co-coordinator of the Tenderloin Healthy Corner Store Coalition. She received her bachelor of science from the University of California, Davis, and has worked in public health, youth development, and community organizing, with a passion for health equity, since 2006.

JENNIFER FALBE, ScD, MPH, is an assistant professor of nutrition and human development at the University of California, Davis. Her research focuses on evaluating policies and programs to reduce health disparities and improve diet quality, such as soda taxes, healthy retail programs, and primary care and community interventions.

STEPHEN FAWCETT, PhD, is senior advisor in KU Center for Community Health and Development, and codirector of the World Health Organization Collaborating Centre for Community Health and Development at the University of Kansas. Author of nearly two hundred publications and cofounder of the Community Tool Box, his research examines how collaborative action affects improvements in population health and equity.

SARAH FLICKER, PhD, is associate professor in the Faculty of Environmental Studies at York University in Toronto, Canada. Her program of research focuses on youth environmental, sexual, and reproductive justice issues. Her research has informed policy at the municipal, provincial, and federal levels. Flicker and her teams have won a number of prestigious awards for youth engagement in health research.

VINCENT FRANCISCO, PhD, is Kansas Health Foundation Professor of Community Leadership and senior scientist with the Schiefelbusch Institute for Life Span Studies. He is codirector of the KU Center for Community Health and Development, a World Health Organization Collaborating Centre at the University of Kansas.

NICHOLAS FREUDENBERG, DrPH, is Distinguished Professor of Public Health at the City University of New York Graduate School of Public Health and Health Policy, where he also directs the CUNY Urban Food Policy Institute. For the past thirty years, he has developed, implemented, and evaluated community health policies and programs designed to improve the health and reduce health inequalities facing vulnerable urban populations.

CATALINA GARZÓN, PhD, has coordinated CBPR, leadership development, action planning, and curriculum development partnerships with environmental and social justice organizations and coalitions for more than twenty years. Her recent collaborations include a photo-novella on alternatives to the criminalization of youth with Communities United for Restorative Youth Justice and a Health Impact Assessment of freight transport planning with the Ditching Dirty Diesel Collaborative. Garzón is a recipient of the Thomas I. Yamashita Prize honoring outstanding social change activists who serve as a bridge between academia and the community.

LAWRENCE W. GREEN, DrPH ScD (Hon), emeritus professor of epidemiology and biostatistics at the University of California at San Francisco, served as director of the US Office of Health Information and Health Promotion under the Carter Administration and director of the Office of Science and Extramural Research at CDC. He has been on the full-time faculties of UC Berkeley, Johns Hopkins University, Harvard, the University of Texas, and the University of British Columbia. He headed a Canadian team in producing the first study of participatory research in health promotion for the Royal Society of Canada.

DEREK M. GRIFFITH, PhD, is associate professor of medicine, health, and society and founder and director of the Center for Research on Men's Health at Vanderbilt University. In November 2013, Griffith was presented with the Tom Bruce Award by the Community-Based Public Health Caucus of the American Public Health Association in recognition of his leadership in community-based public health and for his research on "eliminating health disparities that vary by race, ethnicity, and gender."

ADRIAN GUTA, MSW, PhD, is assistant professor at the School of Social Work, University of Windsor, Canada. His research examines the social, cultural, and ethical dimensions of HIV prevention, treatment, and care; related clinical and social service programing; and public health interventions through a combination of critical theoretical work and applied CBPR.

J. RICARDO GUZMAN, MSW, MPH, served as CEO for the Community Health and Social Services Center (CHASS), a federally qualified health center, in Detroit from 1982 through 2016. During his tenure, he increased funding for the uninsured and underinsured residents of Detroit, focusing on African American and Latino communities, and broadened services to include domestic violence and sexual assault programs and CBPR efforts to address underlying causes of health disparities in minority populations. He has received national and local awards for his role in expanding access to culturally and linguistically appropriate health services.

Guzman currently serves as chairperson of the board of directors for the National Association of Community Health Centers in Washington, DC.

BUDD HALL, PhD, is professor of community development at the University of Victoria and UNESCO co-chair in community-based research and social responsibility in higher education. He has been working within a participatory research framework since 1973.

SUSANA HENNESSEY LAVERY, MPH, is health educator with the San Francisco Department of Public Health, Community Health Equity and Promotion Branch (1992 to present). She codesigns and implements the CAM (community action model) for policy development with San Francisco's diverse communities. She played a lead role in development of healthy retail efforts, is the SFDPH staff member for the HealthyRetailSF program, and sits on the steering committee of the Tenderloin Healthy Corner Store Coalition. For more than a decade, she has participated on the Bay Area committee of Vision y Compromiso, a statewide community health worker network. She is coauthor of numerous professional publications.

CHRISTINA HOLT serves as the associate director for Community Tool Box services at the KU Center for Health Promotion and Community Development, where she directs the Community Tool Box, a free global resource that offers seven thousand pages of practical guidance for creating change and improvement. She has served as a speaker and technical consultant for groups including the World Health Organization, World Bank, United Nations, Peace Corps, and Institute of Medicine.

CHERYL HYDE, MSW, PhD, is associate professor at Temple University, School of Social Work. Her primary areas of scholarship and teaching are organizational and community capacity building, multicultural education, feminist praxis, social movements and collective action, and socioeconomic class issues. She is a past president of the Association for Community Organization and Social Administration, former editor of the *Journal of Progressive Human Services,* and a member of several social science and social work editorial boards and has practice experience in feminist, labor, and anti-oppression movements.

NADIA ISLAM, PhD, is an assistant professor in the Department of Population Health at NYU School of Medicine. She is deputy director of the NYU Center for the Study of Asian American Health and the research director for the NYU-CUNY Prevention Research Center. She serves as PI on numerous federally funded initiatives evaluating the impact of culturally adapted community-clinical linkages strategies on improving health outcomes in racial and ethnic minority communities. Islam's work has been featured in *Diabetes Care,* the *American Journal of Public Health,* and other peer-reviewed journals.

BARBARA A. ISRAEL, DrPH, MPH, is professor of health behavior and health education, School of Public Health, University of Michigan. She has published widely and is actively involved in a number of CBPR partnerships examining and addressing, for example, the social and physical environmental determinants of health inequities in cardiovascular disease and childhood asthma and capacity building for and translating research findings into policy change.

JUSTIN JAGOSH, PhD, is honorary research associate, Institute for Psychology, Health and Society, University of Liverpool, and director for the Centre for Advancement in Realist Evaluation and Synthesis (www.liv.ac.uk/cares). He was coinvestigator on a comprehensive realist review and evaluation of the CBPR. He runs regular training workshops in realist methodology, including an annual summer school and a biennial international realist methodology conference. See his website at www.realistmethodology-cares.org.

CAMARA PHYLLIS JONES, MD, MPH, PhD, a family physician and social epidemiologist, focuses on naming, measuring, and addressing the impacts of racism on the health and well-being of the nation. Her allegories on race and racism illuminate topics that are otherwise difficult for many Americans to understand or discuss. She is past president of the American Public Health Association and a senior fellow at the Satcher Health Leadership Institute and Cardiovascular Research Institute at the Morehouse School of Medicine. She was previously an assistant professor, Harvard School of Public Health (1994 to 2000), and a medical officer at the Centers for Disease Control and Prevention (2000 to 2014).

NORA JONES, MS, is executive director of the Partnership Project and the founding president of Sisters Network Greensboro, a national breast cancer survivorship organization for African American women. Currently, she is the lead community coinvestigator for the ACCURE (Accountability for Cancer Care Through Undoing Racism and Equity) Research Study.

MIRIA KANO, PhD, research investigator, Department of Family and Community Medicine, University of New Mexico, is the director of regional coordination for the geographic management of cancer health disparities program region 3. She served as PI on the Patient-Centered Outcomes Research Institute Pipeline to Proposal Award (highlighted in Appendix 2). Kano has been a coinvestigator and research team member on four federally funded research grants, as well as senior program manager for the New Mexico Center for the Advancement of Research, Engagement and Science on Health Disparities, a P-20 center funded through the National Institute for Minority Health and Health Disparities.

SARAH L. KASTELIC, PhD, MSW, is executive director of the National Indian Child Welfare Association, where she serves as PI on several federally funded projects addressing the well-being of American Indian and Alaska Native children. She is a citizen of the Native village of Ouzinkie near Kodiak, Alaska, and the founding director of the Policy Research Center at the National Congress of American Indians.

DMITRY KHODYAKOV, PhD, is senior behavioral-social scientist at RAND and core faculty member at Pardee RAND Graduate School. He specializes in methods of stakeholder and patient engagement, expert elicitation, and intervention evaluation. Khodyakov is the author of more than forty-five peer-reviewed publications and has served as PI or co-PI on research projects funded by PCORI, NIEHS, and CMS, among others.

LAURA C. LEVITON, PhD, is senior advisor for evaluation at the Robert Wood Johnson Foundation in Princeton, New Jersey, having overseen more than 120 national, state, and local evaluations and a wide variety of other social research related to health. Leviton has coauthored three books: *Foundations of Program Evaluation* (Sage, 1991), *Confronting Public Health Risks* (Sage, 1997), and *Managing Applied Social Research* (Wiley, 2017).

RICHARD LICHTENSTEIN, PhD, recently retired as S. J. Axelrod Collegiate Professor of Health Management and Policy at the University of Michigan School of Public Health, where he taught for more than forty years. His research interests include CBPR, racial and ethnic disparities in health, barriers to health insurance coverage for low-income children, and efforts to increase diversity in the health workforce.

ALEXANDRA LIGHTFOOT, EdD, is research assistant professor in the Department of Health Behavior in the Gillings School of Global Public Health at the University of North Carolina at Chapel Hill. She also directs the Community Engagement, Partnerships and Technical Assistance Core at the Center for Health Promotion and Disease Prevention, a CDC-sponsored prevention research center. She conducts research using the CBPR approach in collaboration with communities across North Carolina and provides training and technical assistance to build and strengthen community-academic research partnerships.

ALISA LINCOLN, MPH, PhD, is interdisciplinary professor of Sociology and Health Sciences and the director of the Institute on Urban Health Research and Practice at Northeastern University. Lincoln's research examines the way that social exclusion and marginalization contribute to and are a consequence of poor mental health. She has led the way in developing innovative models by which we can increase the involvement of stakeholders and mental health service users in the process of research through her NIMH-funded CBPR projects.

JULIE E. LUCERO, MPH, PhD, is assistant professor in the School of Community Health Sciences at the University of Nevada, Reno. She is a mixed-methods researcher who uses CBPR to promote social justice and health equity. She researches trust in community-academic partnerships, social determinants, diversity and inclusion, and research ethics.

MAYA MAGARATI, PhD, is a sociologist at the Indigenous Wellness Research Institute (IWRI) in the University of Washington's School of Social Work, where she serves as the associate director of the Community Engagement and Outreach Core. She has served as a coinvestigator in multiple federally funded participatory research studies to cocreate knowledge with Indigenous communities focused on culture-centered behavioral health protective factors.

JACK MAKAU is executive director of Shack/Slum Dwellers International–Kenya (SDI-Kenya). He has almost twenty years of experience with mapping and surveying informal settlements. He has worked in cities across Africa and advised the UN-Habitat, World Bank, and numerous organizations on participatory slum upgrading.

LILLI MANN, MPH, is research associate in the Department of Social Sciences and Health Policy at Wake Forest School of Medicine. She is involved in the development, implementation, and evaluation of CBPR studies, focusing on interventions promoting health services access, sexual and reproductive health, HIV prevention, HIV care linkage, and retention among racial and ethnic minority and sexual and gender-identity minority communities.

KELLY MATTHEWS, BSW, is outreach coordinator for the Rochester Prevention Research Center: National Center for Deaf Health Research. Matthews has worked in the Deaf community in the fields of HIV/AIDS, mental health, supported employment, obesity, and multiple public health initiatives.

ELI MOORE, MA, was cofounder of the Safe Return Project and has facilitated CBPR processes with environmental justice communities, farm workers, youth, and others over the last fifteen years. Eli is currently a program manager at the Haas Institute for a Fair and Inclusive Society at UC Berkeley.

RACHEL MORELLO-FROSCH, PhD, is an environmental health scientist and professor in the School of Public Health and the Department of Environmental Science, Policy and Management at the University of California, Berkeley. Her research examines social determinants of environmental health disparities among diverse communities in the United States with a focus on environmental chemicals, air pollution, and climate change.

THE MORRIS JUSTICE PROJECT (MJP) is a collaborative research team of neighborhood residents in the south Bronx and members of the Public Science Project, the CUNY Graduate Center, John Jay College, and Pace University Law Center. The project was founded in 2011 after a group of local mothers, whose sons had been harassed by police as a result of a stop-and-frisk policy disproportionately affecting African Americans and Latinos, decided to take action. MJP's research includes large community surveys and "sidewalk science," for example, temporary art installations in public spaces to gather and share data on residents' concerns. The collective has shared its research in numerous venues including the 2015 Citizen Science Forum at the White House.

MICHAEL MUHAMMAD, PhD, is the current Paul B. Cornely Postdoctoral Fellow in the University of Michigan's School of Public Health Center for Research on Ethnicity, Culture, and Health (CRECH). His work focuses on contemporary racism, eugenic ideology, structural inequality, and the evaluation of CBPR partnerships including the Detroit Community-Academic Urban Research Center University of Michigan.

JENNIFER NALL, MPH, is health-promotion disease-prevention director at the Forsyth County Health Department in Winston-Salem, North Carolina. She has worked in the field of HIV/STIs for more than fifteen years and has experience with HIV counseling and testing, community-based interventions, and program evaluation.

EMILY J. OZER, PhD, is clinical-community psychologist, professor of community health sciences at the UC Berkeley School of Public Health, and cofounder of the Innovations for Youth (I4Y) Center. She has authored more than sixty articles in participatory research, trauma and resilience, and school-based interventions (funded by NIDA, NICHD, William T. Grant

Foundation, and CDC). Learning experiences with participatory research in India and Latin America inspired her dual foci on youth-led participatory research and psychological resiliency in the face of stress and trauma. Ozer seeks equitable and sustained collaborations to challenge rigid notions of evidence and to highlight insider expertise in changing the conditions for positive development of marginalized adolescents and their communities.

LAURA CHANCHIEN PARAJÓN, MD, MPH, is the medical director and cofounder of the nonprofit organization AMOS Health and Hope. Based in Nicaragua, AMOS is dedicated to using community-based and empowering approaches to reduce health disparities in Nicaragua. She is passionate about applying CBPR frameworks in global health as well as training health professionals and community health workers in CBPR principles and practice.

EDITH A. PARKER, DrPH, MPH, is professor and chair of the Department of Community and Behavioral Health, University of Iowa College of Public Health, and was previously associate professor at University of Michigan School of Public Health. Her research focuses on community-engaged health promotion interventions. She has served as the PI or Co-PI on more than twenty federally funded grants.

MYRA PARKER, JD, PhD, is an enrolled member of the Mandan and Hidatsa tribes and serves as an assistant professor in the Center for the Study of Health and Risk Behavior in the University of Washington School of Medicine's Department of Psychiatry. Her research experience as a coinvestigator on public health research with American Indian and Alaska Native communities involves CBPR and disparities research funded through NIMHD, NIAAA, NIDA, and NIDDK.

CYNTHIA PEARSON, PhD, is the director of the research at the Indigenous Wellness Research Institute. She is the author of more than sixty scientific publications and has served as a principal and coinvestigator on more than thirty-two federally funded grants using an CBPR approach in developing ethical research training curriculum, conducting studies on epidemiology of HIV prevention and co-occurring mental and drug use disorders, and developing trauma-informed HIV-prevention interventions among American Indian and Alaska Natives.

AMBER AKEMI PIATT, MPH, works at PolicyLink with the Convergence Partnership, advising funders on strategies to advance health and equity through policy and practice changes. She also serves on the Innovations for Youth (I4Y) community advisory board, Alameda County Human Relations Commission, and the Sea Change Program's advisory board. She has worked on CBPR and YPAR projects since 2010 and sees participatory research as a critical way to democratize knowledge and build community power.

MICHELE POLACSEK, PhD, MHS, is associate professor of public health at the University of New England and recently served as PI on three grants examining school food and beverage marketing environments, including digital marketing. She also recently served as lead investigator on two studies evaluating innovative approaches to promote nutrition among low-income populations in a supermarket setting. Michele has taught CBPR online and worked to develop innovative teaching tools for this setting.

ABIGAIL REESE, CNM, MSN, is a doctoral candidate in health policy at the UNM College of Nursing, and a Robert Wood Johnson Foundation Nursing and Health Policy Collaborative Fellow. She is a certified nurse-midwife with extensive clinical and teaching experience in diverse practice settings. She currently serves as the program director for the New Mexico Perinatal Collaborative. Her research focuses on access to care for underserved women.

ANGELA REYES, MPH, is the founder and executive director of Detroit Hispanic Development Corporation, a nonprofit community-based organization that works to create individual-level change with youth and families and community systems–level change. She is also a founding board member of the Detroit Community-Academic Urban Research Center, established in 1995, which involves multiple funded collaborative research and intervention projects aimed at increasing knowledge and addressing factors associated with health disparities of residents in Detroit, Michigan.

SCOTT D. RHODES, PhD, MPH, FAAHB, is professor and chair of the Department of Social Science and Health Policy, Wake Forest School of Medicine in Winston-Salem, North Carolina. He is director of the Program in Community Engagement within the Wake Forest Clinical and Translational Science Institute. Rhodes currently has published more than 150 articles and thirty book chapters. His community-engaged and CBPR has been funded by the National Institutes of Health, the Centers for Disease Control and Prevention (CDC), Health Resources & Services Administration (HRSA), Robert Wood Johnson Foundation, amfAR: The American Foundation for AIDS Research, the Cone Health Foundation, and the Kate B. Reynolds Foundation.

AL RICHMOND, MSW, executive director of Community Campus Partnerships for Health (CCPH), has a career that has uniquely blended social work and public health to address racial and ethnic health disparities. As an international community health leader, Richmond advocates for transformative partnerships to address the most critical issues facing our society. He is adamant that "no meaningful and impactful change in our society is possible without partnerships. Partnerships are not an option, but an imperative."

LINDA ROBERTSON DrPH, RN, MSN, is associate director, health equity, education and advocacy at the University of Pittsburgh Cancer Institute (UPCI) and assistant professor of medicine at the University of Pittsburgh. She focuses her efforts and research on building community partnerships and addressing health equity issues along the cancer care continuum.

IVES ROCHA is a psychologist from Federal University of Rio de Janeiro and has worked with public health, health promotion, and grassroots development since 2007. He is program technical advisor of CEDAPS—The Centre for Health Promotion—and coordinator of youth-led digital mapping in Brazil, a global initiative of UNICEF. He develops and monitors participatory methodologies, especially with adolescents and young people. Ives is proficient in Construção Compartilhada de Soluções Locais social technology, consisting of participatory and local-based diagnostic, plans of action, monitoring, and evaluation of grassroots experiences.

PATRICIA RODRÍGUEZ ESPINOSA, MS, MPH, is a doctoral candidate in clinical psychology, University of New Mexico; a Robert Wood Johnson fellow, UNM Center for Health Policy; and a psychology intern with VA Palo Alto Health Care System, affiliated with Stanford. Her research centers on the health of Latino and other minorities in the U.S. with special attention to the role of cultural and social determinants of health in the development of health disparities. She is interested in the application of CBPR in multicultural psychology.

LETICIA RODRIGUEZ GARCIA, MPH, Community Health Worker (CHW) is a graduate research assistant at Portland State University. She has more than fifteen years of experience as a CHW. Her research interests include CBPR, the roles of CHWs, and health disparities among immigrant communities. She has presented at various local and national conferences on CHW research–related efforts.

CLEO SAMUEL, PhD, is assistant professor of health policy and management at the University of North Carolina at Chapel Hill. She is a health services researcher with expertise in cancer care disparities and health informatics.

VICTORIA SÁNCHEZ, DrPH, associate professor in the College of Population Health at the University of New Mexico, focuses her research on how people come together and build capacity to enhance health equity and community well-being.

SHANNON SANCHEZ-YOUNGMAN, PhD, is a research assistant professor and political scientist at the University of New Mexico. Her research focuses on the development and impact of health and social policy on women of color and children in the United States.

KELLEY P. SAWYER is a PhD candidate in anthropology at the University of New Mexico.

JENNIFER SCHAAL, MD, retired ob-gyn, is a founding member of the Greensboro Health Disparities Collaborative (GHDC) and an active antiracist organizer. She was a clinical investigator for hormone replacement research while in practice and has participated actively in the CBPR work of the GHDC. She has served on community research advisory boards for local and national research grants; has copresented multiple CBPR workshops, keynotes, and research presentations; and has coauthored peer-reviewed publications and book chapters.

JERRY SCHULTZ, PhD, is co-director of the KU Center for Community Health and Development at the University of Kansas. His work is focused on building the capacity of communities to solve local problems, understanding community and systems change, evaluating community health and development initiatives, and developing methodologies for community improvement. He has coauthored numerous articles on evaluation, empowerment, and community development. He has been a consultant to foundations, community coalitions, and state agencies. Schultz was given the Society for Community Research and Action Award for Distinguished Contribution to the Practice of Community Psychology in 2007 and is a fellow of the Society for Applied Anthropology.

AMY J. SCHULZ, PhD, MPH, is professor of health behavior and health education at the University of Michigan School of Public Health. She has served as PI for the Healthy Environments Partnership since 2000 and multi-PI for community action to promote healthy environments since 2014, both CBPR partnerships focused on environmental justice and health equity in Detroit. She has authored more than 130 professional publications and has served as PI on eleven federally funded research grants.

LAURO SILVA is a native-born New Mexican from the Capitan Mountains. As a grassroots organizer and legal professional, Lauro has worked for social justice for five decades with rural and urban communities in public policy, community organizing, and law, especially for poor Chicanos/as, Mexican immigrants, and Native Americans. He has worked with New Mexico's asylum refugees from Honduras, Guatemala, and El Salvador; with the Migrant Farmworker Councils and Clinics; and with the environmental civil rights health movement. Among many positions, he has been president of the Mountain View Neighborhood Association and community PI of the South Valley Partners for Environmental Justice in Albuquerque.

FLORENCE M. SIMÁN, MPH, is the director of health programs at El Pueblo, an organization based in Raleigh, North Carolina, whose mission is for Latinxs to achieve positive social change. Florence is a founding board member of El Pueblo. She has worked on several photovoice projects, some led by UNC students, and is passionate about using photos as a tool to encourage dialogue and to advocate for social justice.

BETH SMITH, RN, NE-BC, MSN, is the professional services practice manager at the Cone Health Cancer Center. She has served as the oncology navigator for the ACCURE Research Study.

ANDREW SUSSMAN, PhD, MCRP, is assistant professor in the Department of Family and Community Medicine at the University of New Mexico. He is the director of RIOS Net, a practice-based research network and has conducted research on a variety of primary care health disparities topics among medically underserved populations in New Mexico.

ERIKA SUTTER, MPH, is deputy director of the Rochester Prevention Research Center: National Center for Deaf Health Research at the University of Rochester Medical Center. She has worked with RPRC/NCDHR since 2004 and is skilled in American Sign Language (ASL). Her research experience includes the design, implementation, and dissemination of research studies and community-based initiatives in the areas of Deaf health, health disparities, community health and CBPR, adolescent health and mental health, adolescent access to care, and youth development.

RAJESH TANDON, PhD, is internationally acclaimed in participatory research, and founder and director of the Society for Participatory Research in Asia (PRIA), providing support to grassroots initiatives in South Asia. He has championed capacity building of the marginalized through their knowledge and empowerment and has authored more than one hundred articles, a dozen books, and training manuals on democratic governance, civic engagement, participatory research, and people-centered development. For his work on gender, he received the Government of India's

Social Justice award, 2007; is the first Indian inducted into the International Adult and Continuing Education Hall of Fame, 2011; and was appointed UNESCO co-chair on Community-Based Research and Social Responsibility in Higher Education (2012–2016 and 2016–2020).

AMANDA E. TANNER, PhD, MPH, is associate professor in the Department of Public Health Education at the University of North Carolina Greensboro. Her research focuses on sexual and reproductive health with specific areas of expertise including HIV and sexually transmitted disease prevention, HIV care, intervention science, and microbicide and contraceptive access and acceptability. She has served as PI or coinvestigator on multiple federally funded research grants and has more than fifty peer-reviewed publications.

PAM TAU LEE, BA, is a retired instructor at City College of San Francisco and a former project director at the Labor Occupational Health Center, School of Public Health, University of California, Berkeley. She also was a founding member of the Chinese Progressive Association, San Francisco, and the Asian Pacific Environmental Network. A long-time activist and practitioner of popular education, community organizing, and CBPR, she has made major contributions to improving the working conditions of immigrants and women.

KARI THATCHER, MPH, is the prevention specialist at the North Carolina Coalition Against Domestic Violence and began serving as cochair of the Greensboro Health Disparities Collaborative in January 2017. She takes a network-oriented approach to community and institutional organizing, driven by a belief in the importance of leadership and capacity building at the neighborhood level. She also works independently, training and consulting with organizations and communities working for racial equity.

RYAN THAYER, MA, is a community organizer and co-coordinator of the Tenderloin Healthy Corner Store Coalition. As a sixth-generation San Franciscan, he holds a BA in urban studies and planning from San Francisco State University and an MA in urban affairs from the University of San Francisco. Since 2010, Thayer has cultivated community leadership to participate in a food system that promotes equity and justice.

MAKANI N. THEMBA is chief strategist at Higher Ground Change Strategies based in Detroit, Michigan. A social justice innovator and pioneer in the field of change communications and narrative strategy, she has spent more than twenty years supporting organizations, coalitions, and philanthropic institutions in developing high-impact change initiatives. Higher Ground Change Strategies is her newest project, which she describes as "a place where change makers can get the support they need to take their work to the next level." Higher Ground helps partners integrate authentic engagement, systems analysis, and change communications and more for powerful, vision-based change.

ROBB TRAVERS, PhD, is associate professor and chair, Department of Health Sciences, Wilfrid Laurier University, Waterloo, Ontario. He is director of the Equity, Sexual Health and HIV Research Group at Laurier's Centre for Community Research, Learning and Action. His CBPR focuses on social exclusion and its impact on the health of gender and sexual minorities.

CHAU TRINH-SHEVRIN, DrPH, is associate professor of population health and medicine at the NYU School of Medicine and directs the Department of Population Health's Section for Health. Trinh-Shevrin is PI and founding director of the NIH NIMHD Center of Excellence, the Center for the Study of Asian American Health, and co-PI of a CDC-sponsored NYU-CUNY Prevention Research Center. She has more than ninety peer-review scientific and professional publications.

LAVERN VAUGHN is case manager for Catholic Charities of San Francisco and a founding member of The Safe Return Project in Richmond, California. The Safe Return Project is a participatory action research process involving formerly incarcerated residents in conducting research, engaging community members, and developing policy proposals to reduce recidivism and improve community health and safety. During her years with Safe Return, Vaughn and seven other Safe Return leaders conducted an extensive survey of recently released residents, interviewed more than six hundred community members, and researched and developed policies that have been adopted at the city, county, and state level. Vaughn is a lifelong Richmond resident, mother, grandmother, and passionate advocate for justice and her community.

AARON T. VISSMAN, PhD, MPH, is associate director of the Center for Health and Human Services Research at Talbert House in Cincinnati, Ohio. He has published mixed-methods research investigating correlates of antiretroviral adherence and the effectiveness of multilevel HIV/AIDS prevention interventions. He received the Ruth L. Kirschstein National Research Service Award (2013–2015). Ongoing studies investigate multilevel correlates of naloxone distribution and the effectiveness of opioid overdose and HCV prevention interventions.

TAMISHA WALKER is founder and executive director of Safe Return Project. Walker has been a Richmond-based community organizer and known advocate on issues related to mass incarceration and racial disparity in the criminal justice system since her release from incarceration in 2009. Tamisha shares a powerful personal story about the journey to healing and successful reentry. She has six years of community-organizing experience in a city affected by trauma and economic inequality, including her own personal experience with trauma and poverty growing up in Richmond, California. Her educational experience includes professional training in research and advocacy for the formerly incarcerated and their families, violence-prevention strategies, and conflict mediation to reduce urban gun violence.

PEI-RU WANG, PhD, is senior research and evaluation analyst at the Multnomah County Health Department Community Capacitation Center in Oregon. She leads a number of evaluation projects on community health worker and community leadership programs. She is also a seasonal facilitator and trainer using popular education, inspired by Paulo Freire. She has years of experience working in a nonprofit organization supporting CHWs in the Asian Pacific Islander, African, and Slavic communities.

JOMELLA WATSON-THOMPSON, PhD, is associate professor of applied behavioral science and associate director for the KU Center for Community Health and Development at the University of Kansas. She leads participatory research and evaluation efforts in the areas of adolescent substance abuse prevention, community and youth violence prevention, and positive youth development.

KENNETH B. WELLS, MD, MPH, is affiliated adjunct staff at RAND and David Weil Endowed Professor of Psychiatry and Biobehavioral Sciences at UCLA David Geffen School of Medicine and of Health Policy and Management at UCLA Fielding School of Public Health. He is director of the Semel Institute Center for Health Services and Society and codirector of the California Behavioral Health Center of Excellence and Robert Wood Johnson Clinical Scholars Program at UCLA. His research focuses on improving mental health outcomes, particularly depression, through a community-partnered, participatory research approach.

WEST OAKLAND ENVIRONMENTAL INDICATORS PROJECT (WOEIP) is a nonprofit dedicated to working with neighborhood organizations, physicians, researchers, and public officials to ensure West Oakland residents have a clean environment, safe neighborhoods, and access to economic opportunity. It is codirected by Brian Beveridge, and Margaret Gordon, who has received multiple city, county, and Bay Area honors for her environmental justice work.

NOELLE WIGGINS, EdD, MSPH, is director of Capacity Building and Collaboration, Whole Person Care Program, LA County Dept. of Health Services. Previously, director at Multnomah County Community Capacitation Center Portland, Oregon, she has more than thirty years training and supervising community health workers (CHWs). Publications and presentation topics include CHWs, popular education, participatory research and evaluation, and empowerment theory and measurement.

CATHLEEN E. WILLGING, PhD, is center director and senior research scientist at Behavioral Health Research of the Southwest, Pacific Institute for Research and Evaluation. As a medical anthropologist, her research focuses on public mental health and substance use services in the United States, health care reform, implementation science, and the advancement of culturally and contextually relevant programs to support populations affected by health and health care disparities.

KATHRINE E. WRIGHT, MPH, is a public health doctoral student at the University of Nevada, Reno, specializing in social and behavioral health. She received her master of public health degree at Michigan State University, where she specialized in public health nutrition. Her research interests include using CBPR to address the causes and impacts of food insecurity and hunger to promote health equity in marginalized populations.

MICHAEL T. WRIGHT, LICSW, MS, has been involved in community-based health initiatives since 1984 in the United States and Germany, having served as a psychotherapist, program manager, clinical supervisor, researcher, and consultant. Wright was formerly the director of international relations at the Deutsche AIDS-Hilfe, the national German AIDS organization. He is currently professor for research methods, Catholic University of Applied Sciences, Berlin, and heads the central office of the International Collaboration for Participatory Health Research. He is coordinator of PartKommPlus, a national research consortium in Germany applying participatory health research to examine integrated municipal strategies for health promotion.

PREFACE

Health equity is assurance of the conditions for optimal health for all people. Achieving health equity requires valuing all individuals and populations equally, recognizing and rectifying historical injustices, and providing resources according to need. Health disparities will be eliminated when health equity is achieved.

CAMARA PHYLLIS JONES

This third edition of *Community-Based Participatory Research for Health: Advancing Social and Health Equity* shows the long-standing importance of doing research and interventions *with* communities rather than *to* communities or only *in* communities. Community-originated research questions, borne from lived experience, guide the work. Community-designed program evaluations, whose results will provide important bases for action, are prioritized. Academics, or other professionally trained research partners, collaborate on research in service of the community rather than pursuing questions that only scratch the tickle of their own intellectual curiosity.

In this book, community-based participatory research (CBPR) practitioners share their experiences, models, tools, and lessons learned about the enriching work of academically trained researchers and community members who join together in partnership. They partner to identify and answer urgent scientific questions. They partner to design, conduct, and evaluate relevant interventions. They partner to acknowledge and address the impacts of systems and structures on human health, pushing beyond our society's dominant and narrow focus on the individual. They partner not only to acknowledge the importance of context on health but also to intervene on those contexts. And they partner to address the systems of structured inequity that determine the range of contexts in our society and the differential distribution of populations into those contexts.

CBPR is the research operationalization of health equity. Operationalizing health equity involves answering three questions: What is health equity? How do we get there? And how is health equity related to health disparities (Jones, 2014)?

1. *What is health equity?* Health equity is assurance of the conditions for optimal health for all people. *Assurance* is a process, not an outcome, and *assurance of the conditions for optimal health* requires making sustained, long-term investments in communities. It requires going beyond a narrow focus on individual genes and individual behaviors to address the contexts of people's lives, the social determinants of health (including poverty and adverse neighborhood conditions). As an important theoretical and well-illustrated addition to this third edition, CBPR acknowledges the importance of context and sees context as a major and legitimate focus for intervention.

But assurance of the conditions for optimal health *for all people* also requires intervention on the social determinants of equity (including racism and other systems of structured inequity). These social determinants are the systems of power that determine the range of contexts in a given place and time, as well as who lives in which context. Their mechanisms are embodied in our structures, policies, practices, norms, and values, which, in turn, are the elements of decision making. Structures are the who, what, when, and where of decision making, including who is at the table and who is not and what is on the agenda and what is not. As illustrated particularly in the final section of this book, policies are the written how of decision making. Practices and norms are the unwritten how of decision making, and values are the why. By connecting the power bases of academia, community, progressive policy makers, and other key stakeholders, CBPR enables a more concerted effort to shape structures, change policies, reveal practices, influence norms, and challenge those values that are antithetical to health and social equity.

2. *How do we get there?* Achieving health equity requires (a) valuing all individuals and populations equally, (b) recognizing and rectifying historical injustices, and (c) providing resources according to need. Academically trained CBPR researchers value community members by honoring all they bring to the work. This means honoring, first, their lived experience as the basis for identifying important research questions and their expertise in creating solutions as the basis for promising interventions. But it also means honoring their wisdom by bringing unrepresented voices to research and policy decision-making tables, their time through equitable resource sharing, their talent through investment and training, and their treasure in people and organizations. Community members involved in CBPR value academics and other outside research partners by honoring their expertise in refining research questions and evaluation strategies and honoring their good will, a necessary element for an authentic, empowering, and sustained partnership.

Recognizing and rectifying historical injustices requires researching the history of each "problem" to be solved in order to gain insights into effective solutions. As theorized and illustrated throughout this book, the context of CBPR acknowledges the possibility of previous academic research efforts in communities that were not predicated on equal partnership, were not sustained over time, did not invest in community knowledge or resources, or did not return findings and other resources for reflection and action to the community.

Providing resources according to need requires agreement on metrics of need, followed by a fearlessness in making sustained unequal investments that are based on need. Within the context of CBPR, it is reflected in the investment of research expertise, money, and infrastructure in those communities with the highest burdens, not in communities of convenience. And it respects community prioritization of need in terms of problem identification.

3. *How is health equity related to health disparities?* Health disparities will be eliminated when health equity is achieved. Health disparities are differences in outcomes, whereas health equity is all about opportunity structures and societal valuation. To operationalize this notion, researchers and non-researchers alike need to invest in opportunities, measure impacts on opportunities, and patiently await outcomes in a generation. We should make long-term investments in communities and develop deep intergenerational partnerships. This includes research funding for CBPR, which continues to go disproportionately to academic and other non-community partners.

CBPR moves the research enterprise from indulging the intellectual curiosity of academics in the ivory tower to unearthing and addressing questions of high relevance to partner communities. It can bridge resources between those who currently have the power to decide, the power to act, and the control of resources with those whose lives are currently undervalued and whose opportunities are currently constrained.

Health equity, the assurance of the conditions for optimal health for all people, is an active process requiring all hands on deck. CBPR offers one potent mechanism for engaging in the work of achieving health equity. Indeed, the very act of partnership between academically trained researchers and community members can be a revolutionary first step. Whether you are currently positioned in academia, a health or social services department, a city or regional planning office, or in a community, open these pages and learn from the history of others to become inspired and better equipped for your part in this journey.

REFERENCE

Jones, C. P. (2014). Systems of power, axes of inequity: Parallels, intersections, braiding the strands, *Medical Care, 52,* S71–S75.

CAMARA PHYLLIS JONES, MD, MPH, PhD
August 2017

ACKNOWLEDGMENTS

The burgeoning growth across the world of community-based participatory research (CBPR), community-engaged research, action research, and other participatory approaches to health, education, and social justice has made this book a challenge and a gift to produce almost a decade after the second edition. We owe many thanks to the countless academic, practitioner, and community colleagues who have built on the legacy of participatory pioneers and global histories of struggle to re-form and re-create research as a place for knowledge democracy and social and health equity. We have learned so much from others' narratives, personal stories, and the many theoretical frameworks, scientific and cultural analyses, ethical dilemmas faced in practice, and other insights, which have enriched this book, and *us*, immeasurably. Although too numerous to mention by name, their contributions are cited throughout the book, and they are deserving of special recognition.

Many people in specific helped us to make this book a reality, and we are grateful to the many coauthors whose hard work and belief in the power and potential of CBPR are reflected in the following pages. Each of them writes with commitment and passion, whether as a community partner, practitioner, clinician, or academic for whom conducting participatory action-oriented research *with,* rather than *on* or *in,* communities is a continuing goal.

Each of us also is supported and inspired by our colleagues, students, and community partners working with the University of New Mexico, University of Washington, University of Waikato, New Zealand, and the University of California, Berkeley. We owe thanks to the W.K. Kellogg Foundation, the California Endowment, the Robert Wood Johnson Foundation (RWJF), PolicyLink, the Community-Campus Partnerships for Health, and the Community-Based Public Health Caucus of the American Public Health Association for their trail-blazing support and inspiration in CBPR on so many levels. We thank especially community members who have been our teachers, as well as our families and friends, because this book, similar to the first two editions, is in part due to their collective wisdom and support.

From Nina: great appreciation goes first to my colleagues as editors and authors on this book, who together have made this an almost completely new work. I am thrilled to see the strength of effort throughout the country and globally that these chapters represent. For me personally, I owe a great deal of thanks to the tribal research partners I have had the honor of working with, including education and health professionals, elders, youth, and others from the Pueblo of Jemez, the Ramah Band of Navajo, the Mescalero Apache Tribe, the Navajo Nation, and from the Healthy Native Community Partnership. I continue to appreciate colleagues and friends from public and community health throughout New Mexico, who have maintained a commitment to social justice these many years.

In a wider network, I have deep gratitude to partners in the Engage for Equity and Research for Improved Health studies, members of the national CBPR Think Tank, and to my participatory health research colleagues around the world, especially from Latin America, Brazil and Nicaragua, who keep opening my eyes to Freirean empowerment as a path to equity. I wouldn't be able to do this work without the co-learning community connected to UNM's College of Population Health and Center for Participatory Research: students, faculty, staff, doctoral RWJF and UNM

Health Policy fellows, as well as other community-engaged committed scholars across the UNM campus. Special thanks also to colleagues from San Francisco State University's Department of Health Education. My friends and family, siblings, parents, and especially now the younger generation of nieces and nephews have been deep sources of inspiration. Finally, I couldn't do this work without the love from my lifelong partner, David Dunaway, and our son, Alexei, whom I now have the pleasure of seeing create his own equity-based work.

From Bonnie: a deep bow of gratitude to Meredith Minkler for my doctorate—I wouldn't have it without her faith in me and encouragement; to Nina for her brilliant, kind, and stern mentorship and partnership over many years; and to John for applying his remarkable skills and values in our work together. I'd like to thank all the tribal communities who have taught me the fundamental meaning of participatory research, self-determination, and decolonization and who have generously shared Indigenous epistemologies and healing modalities. A special thanks to the Tribal College and university presidents and community, including AIHEC, the Navajo, and Lummi Nation IRBs, for their truth-telling, insistence on tribal benefit, and use of Indigenous theories of etiology and change. Deep gratitude bows to my Buddhist teachers and colleagues at the Insight Meditation Society and Spirit Rock Meditation Center for the wisdom, compassion, and refuge. And special thanks and love to Stan Kondo for his warmth, patience, support, and partnership.

From John: I want to thank Nina and Meredith for including me as a coeditor of this edition and to Nina and Bonnie for being long-time collaborators. I look forward to our continued work together. I also want to thank my community and academic partners on the He Pikinga Waiora and Kaumātua Mana Motuhake projects for their inspiration, passion, collaboration, and inclusiveness (Tihei Mauri Ora!). It is such a pleasure to work with you. Further, I want to thank a few people whom I collaborate with outside of work. To my mates at the Raglan Volunteer Fire Brigade (EAD), thanks for being great teachers and practitioners of collaboration and helping me do something positive for the community. And last and most important, to my family, Spencer, Ethan, and Keri: I appreciate your love and support always.

From Meredith: my sincere thanks to friends and coeditors Bonnie Duran, John Oetzel, and our visionary lead, Nina Wallerstein, who remains a dear friend and role model and one who never lets overcommitment keep her (or me) from taking on exciting, new collaborative efforts, such as this book. My deepest gratitude goes as well to my community teachers and partners, including the Tenderloin Healthy Corner Store Coalition, the Chinese Progressive Association, the Richmond (California) Safe Return Project, and the California Senior Leaders Alliance. I also remain indebted from afar to the men and women of Concerned Citizens of Tillery, North Carolina, their visionary leaders Gary Grant and Naeema Muhammad, and their lead academic research partner, the late Steve Wing, who together exemplified a standard of CBPR and community organizing to which I can only aspire.

Among my family and friends, my late father was my inspiration, guide, and shining light, even in his last days, and the greatest teacher I have ever known. My late mother showed in her long struggle with Alzheimer's the same gifts of love, concern for others, and optimism that characterized the whole of her life. My siblings Donna, Jay, Chris, and Joan are each among my closest friends and a source of pride in the separate paths they have taken and the values they share. I am grateful, as well, to extended family members Betsy Minkler, Rose Marie Springer, Joyce Lashof, and to dear friends whose deep caring and support make my own work possible. My husband, Jerry Peters, and our sons, Jason Peters and Marquis Parks, have been the source of much love, pride, support, and humor, and I owe them my deepest gratitude.

COMMUNITY-BASED PARTICIPATORY RESEARCH FOR HEALTH

PART 1

INTRODUCTION: HISTORY AND PRINCIPLES

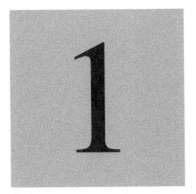

CHAPTER 1

ON COMMUNITY-BASED PARTICIPATORY RESEARCH

NINA WALLERSTEIN, BONNIE DURAN, JOHN G. OETZEL, AND MEREDITH MINKLER

COMMUNITY-BASED PARTICIPATORY RESEARCH (CBPR) has established itself as a valued research approach for its contributions to increasing health equity through an orientation that is *community-based,* and often *community-directed,* rather than merely *community placed.* Increasing demand by communities, tribal nations, governmental and philanthropic funders, and committed academics have altered much of the landscape of research and its production of knowledge by integrating community leaders and members as key partners throughout a community-engaged research process. The W.K. Kellogg Foundation's Community Health Scholars Program (2001) defined *community-based participatory research* in the health field as "a collaborative approach to research that equitably involves all partners in the research process and recognizes the unique strengths that each brings. CBPR begins with a research topic of importance to the community with the aim of combining knowledge and action for social change to improve community health and eliminate health disparities" (p. 2).

Reflecting the growing application of CBPR principles and strategies in community development, program design and implementation, and evaluation, we propose a broader definition that still incorporates the use of research and data. "CBPR embraces collaborative efforts among community, academic, and other stakeholders who gather and use research and data to build on the strengths and priorities of the community for multilevel strategies to improve health and social equity."

Together with many related action, participatory, and community-engaged research traditions, CBPR turns upside down the more traditional applied research paradigm, in which the outside researcher largely has determined the questions asked, the research tools employed, the interventions developed, and the kinds of outcomes documented and valued (Gaventa & Cornwall, 2015). In their new edited book, Budd Hall and Rajesh Tandon, two of the early founders of global participatory research, reiterate the call for knowledge democracy to reclaim the "expertise residing in the world of practice, beyond academia" (Hall, Tandon, &Tremblay, 2015, p. 26).

Although often and erroneously referred to as *research methods,* CBPR and other collaborative approaches are not methods at all but an *orientation or a fundamentally different approach to research.* As Cornwall and Jewkes (1995) classically pointed out, what is distinctive about this approach "is not the methods but the methodological contexts of their application; the attitudes of researchers, which in turn determine how, by and for whom research is conceptualized and conducted," and "the corresponding location of *power* at every stage of the research process" [italics added, p. 1667].

Central to CBPR and related approaches is a commitment to consciously change the power relationship between researcher and researched, seeking to eradicate the distinction between who does the studying and who gets studied (or decides what gets studied). CBPR, as an overall approach, has been used with every kind of research method (Israel, Eng, Schulz, & Parker, 2013): from qualitative focus groups or ethnographic inquiry, to neighborhood mapping or use of geographical information systems, to epidemiology, and to survey methods. What matters is "the experience and partnership of those we are normally content simply to measure" (Schwab & Syme, 1997, p. 2050) and the creation of a "mutually reinforcing partnership" (Cargo & Mercer, 2008, p. 327).

NEW AND CONTINUING CHALLENGES AND OPPORTUNITIES

In the decade since the publication of the second edition of this book (Minkler & Wallerstein, 2008), CBPR has grown as a field in its effectiveness in creating culture-centered research (Dutta, Anaele, & Jones, 2013), improving external validity and attention to implementation contexts (Yano et al., 2012), honoring practice-based and community evidence (Green, 2006), strengthening reflexive practice (Muhammad et al., 2015), and solidifying connections to communities of color and other marginalized communities to challenge health inequities (Wallerstein & Duran, 2010). However, CBPR faces continuing and new challenges.

Key among these is the stark contextual realities within which we work. Health and social inequities continue to rise to untenable levels, across the United States and globally (Bor, Cohen, Galea, 2017; Marmot & Bell, 2012). Within the United States, structural racism within institutions, such as the criminal justice system, and conscious and unconscious bias still pervade our national consciousness and contribute to the suffering of real people and communities. As this book goes to press, a new and troubling political context in the United States, with grave threats to vulnerable groups, including to undocumented immigrants, the devaluation of science and inquiry, and the threatened withdrawal of federal funding in a wide range of areas, portend real threats to CBPR partnerships and health and social equity. These conditions affect all of us and our capacities to recognize and redress power and privilege differences across academia and communities and agencies.

The research institution is not immune from this context, with historical and current abuse or misuse all too often having fostered mistrust of research within communities who have faced "helicopter" or "drive-by" research when data is solicited, taken, and not returned to the community. "Evidence-based" approaches, those that have received sufficient funding to be systematically evaluated and published in the academic literature, still dominate the acceptable choices for research interventions and privilege internal validity over external validity, or relevance of findings to "real-world" contexts. Such approaches are sometimes unacceptable or non-translatable to other diverse communities. Further, the "evidence-based" approaches that "count" in traditional academic and other research settings often ignore, discount, or erase the "community evidence" and local knowledge necessary to create culturally effective and sustainable interventions. Growing calls for translational research, whose findings can more quickly and effectively be incorporated into practice, programs, and policies, have been critical in beginning to redress such imbalances (Cytron et al., 2014). Yet often, translation is thought to be unidirectional, that is, a one-way or top-down approach to move research results from the academy to the community, rather than as bidirectional, mutual-learning processes.

Despite these challenges, there has been increased visibility of and support for CBPR and community-engaged research (CEnR) in multiple sectors. The Centers for Disease Control and Prevention (CDC) launched its Prevention Research Centers in 1986 with community participation a central part of their mission. The first of the National Institutes of Health (NIH) to fund CBPR was the National Institute of Environmental Health Science (NIEHS), supporting environmental justice research in 1995. NIEHS was followed by multiple other institutes, most notably the National Institute of Minority Health and Health Disparities and the Native American Research Centers for Health, a partnership between the Indian Health Service and NIH.

Since the mid-2000s, there has been additional growth in federal and foundation funding opportunities for CBPR (see Appendix 5). These have included community engagement components within Clinical Translational Science Awards (CTSAs); the Patient Centered Outcomes Research Institute (PCORI), inviting patient, family, and patient advocate engagement; NIH transdisciplinary team science centers that include community partner involvement; as well as leading foundations sponsorship of CBPR training programs (see Chapter 19 and Appendix 5).

Support has become evident through new federal publications, with a recent Institute of Medicine (IOM) call to educate health professionals about social determinants through forming community partnerships for transformational learning (IOM, 2016). This builds on an Office of Behavioral and Social Science Research (OBSSR) report, calling for working with communities to understand the complexities of culture (Kagawa-Singer, Dressler, George, & Elwood, 2015) and a previous IOM call for leveraging community involvement and culture for improved health interventions (IOM, 2012). In 2015, the North American Primary Care Group updated their 1988 policy on responsible participatory research in primary care settings and called for even greater patient and community involvement in research (Allen et al., 2017).

CBPR and CEnR publications have grown across multiple health, clinical, education, and social science disciplines, with top-ranked academic journals offering special issues on CEnR, CBPR, and Action Research in addition to multiple new books (Abma et al., 2018, Blumenthal, DiClemente, Braithwaite, & Smith, 2013; Bradbury, 2015; Hacker, 2013; Hall et al., 2015; Israel et al., 2013; Rowell, Bruce, Shosh, & Riel, 2017; Stringer, 2014; Wright & Kongats, 2018). Finally, many new resources, training programs, and guides are proliferating, and can often be found through the Community Campus Partnerships for Health and CES4 Health websites, as well as on individual program sites (see, for example, Parry, Salsberg, & Macaulay, 2017; see Appendix 10 for resources specifically on measures of engagement).

Although these increased opportunities, especially in the acceptance of CEnR and CBPR, have been welcome, they also have brought new challenges. The first of these is definitional, with the question of whether we have fallen into the trap of believing that any community engagement is a good thing (Draper, Hewitt, & Rifkin, 2010). Trickett (2011) has raised concerns about utilitarian usage of CBPR by researchers, for example, seeking engagement to facilitate recruitment of minorities into "our" research trials, versus a broader worldview that seeks a range of community capacity, health, and social justice outcomes.

A second challenge is the need for more rigorous and mixed-method evaluation of whether and how participatory practices contribute to outcomes, with a complementary inquiry to identify metrics or measures to assess engagement practices and outcomes. A plethora of reviews within the last several years have begun to identify multilevel health outcomes from CBPR and related research, with several analyzing the ingredients of participatory practices that make a difference (Drahota et al., 2016; O'Mara-Eaves et al., 2015; Rifkin, 2014; Salimi et al., 2012). Although many of us are part of this effort to identify emerging "best" or promising practices, the most important questions may be (1) under what conditions and contexts do partnerships choose which practices are "best" or promising in their experience; and (2) how will our chosen practices affect research designs and interventions to produce our desired (and also possibly unintended) outcomes within communities and the academy, including, most importantly, improvement of health equity?

Further, some still question the scientific rigor of the field, for example, regarding the challenge of how to maintain community decision-making after starting a randomized control trial protocol (Buchanan, Miller, & Wallerstein, 2007; Coghlan, 2004; Northridge et al., 2000; Salimi et al., 2012). Greater interest in complexity science, adaptive designs, and social network analyses, however, have enabled a broader discussion of methodologies for evaluating community participation and interventions (Franco et al., 2015; Hawe, 2015; Trickett et al., 2011) and for incorporating strategies that promote a broader bandwidth of validity (Bradbury, 2015). Decolonizing research methodologies (Denzin, Lincoln, & Tuhiwai Smith, 2008; Tuhiwai Smith, 2012) have called for Indigenous and community knowledge and use of mixed methodologies for ascertaining partnership effectiveness to reach broad goals of knowledge democracy and justice.

AGENDA FOR THE NEW EDITION

With this backdrop of challenges and opportunities, this is an almost completely new edition of *Community-Based Participatory Research for Health,* offering a twofold agenda. First, we wish to celebrate the recognition of CBPR and CEnR as solid, community-driven, and shared leadership enterprises and their importance for making inroads toward health equity. Second, we wish to tackle head on the challenges frequently encountered in this work through interweaving theory, methods, and case studies with thoughtful exploration of core issues of trust, racism, cultural humility, power and privilege, self-reflective practice, and ethics, with emphasis on practices that contribute to outcomes.

We invite you, as students, academics, and community practitioners in fields such as public health, social welfare, nursing, medicine, communication, community and regional planning, public policy, education, social sciences, and other fields, to enter these explorations with us and become more inspired by and proficient in applying CBPR approaches in your own work. The new edition has been reframed to follow the CBPR conceptual model first presented in the second edition (Wallerstein et al., 2008). Use of this revised model (see Chapter 6) enables us to more deeply present cases that address the contextual settings for research, the partnership relationships and practices, the ethics and choice of research and evaluation methods, and a commitment to individual and community health, equity, and social justice outcomes. All of our case studies are new, many of which tackle core issues of our time, such as institutional racism and its contributions to inequities and suffering. We look to CBPR as one strategy for promoting healing within communities and for advocating for desperately needed policy and societal change.

In this chapter, we now situate CBPR principles within a brief history of other traditions and provide an overview of current reviews of CBPR and community engagement effectiveness. We end the chapter with an outline of the book and a hope that the conceptual frameworks, case studies, and practical tools presented through the chapters and appendices are useful as you reflect on and strengthen your own partnering practices.

CORE PRINCIPLES OF CBPR WITHIN A CONTINUUM OF COMMUNITY ENGAGEMENT

Over the last several decades, the term *community-based participatory research* has moved solidly into US and global health discourse and practice. Numerous variations of the term exist, however; key among them are *action research* (widely used in the education field and within the United Kingdom, Australia, and New Zealand); *collaborative action research* (used in Australia); *community-based research* (term in Canada); *participatory action research* and *participatory research* (widely used in Latin America, the Global South, and for youth); *collaborative inquiry; reflexive practice, feminist participatory research; community-partnered participatory research; tribal participatory research; street and citizen science;* and *participatory health research,* the term of the International Collaboration for Participatory Health Research (see Appendix 3).

These terms have largely come from two historical traditions: the Northern, more pragmatic tradition (with social psychologist Kurt Lewin originally proposing *action research* in the 1940s as a cycle of fact-finding, action, and reflection) and the Southern emancipatory tradition (with the terms *participatory research* and *participatory action research* emerging from the roots of Brazilian educator Paulo Freire's (1970, 1973) popular education and the liberatory movements in the 1970s in Asia, Africa, and Latin America). (See Chapter 2 for discussion of these traditions.)

Adherents to these different terms continue to engage in lively debate over which one best captures the principles and ideological commitments espoused. We argue, however, that although these different approaches often vary in goals and in change theories, they also share a set of core principles, summarized by Israel and her colleagues (see Chapter 3), who say the following of CBPR:

- It is participatory.
- It is cooperative, engaging community members and researchers in a joint process in which both contribute equally.

- It is a co-learning process.
- It involves systems development and local community capacity building.
- It is an empowering process through which participants can increase control over their lives.
- It achieves a balance between research and action.

Building on the work of scholars of color, Indigenous, and feminist participatory researchers, we add to these principles an additional one, recognizing the importance of intersectional power and privilege, i.e., how race-ethnicity, racism, immigrant status, gender, sexual orientation, social class, and culture affect the research process (Minkler, Garcia, Rubin, & Wallerstein, 2012). As discussed in Chapter 4, such realities underscore the need for academics to adopt cultural humility (see Appendix 4) and its task of lifelong learning, being open to reflecting on one's biases and positions of power and privilege.

Indigenous researchers have added other principles grounded in tribal sovereignty, recognizing the authority of tribal communities to control research processes, demand that data be shared and returned to tribes, and approve all publications, in addition to deepening the recognition of core values of respect and relevance (Noe et al., 2006; Walters et al., 2009). Tribal institutional review and research review boards have added the principle of returning benefit to the communities (Becenti-Pigman et al., 2008) as part of their authority (Chapter 14), and so have emerging numbers of community ethics boards and review processes (see Chapters 15 and 16).

The growth in the use of the term *community-engaged research* in the 2000s was spawned, in part, by the extensive investment in CTSA translational research infrastructures in academic health centers. A CTSA published continuum of engagement (in English and Spanish) ranges from community outreach at one end, through coordination and collaboration, to shared leadership at the other (McCloskey et al., 2011). Although recognizing that community engagement can shift over time, the inclusion of outreach, unfortunately, may reinforce a unidirectional, rather than bidirectional, perspective. The continuum, "on-in-with," from the Community Engagement Core of the University of New Mexico NM-CARES Health Disparities Center clearly shows the difference of research that takes place *on* targeted communities, versus *in* community settings, versus research *with* community partners. It is the *with* perspective that reflects the CBPR definition of equity and strengths of all partners.[1]

Community development advocates and public health professionals, however, have long warned against the cooptation or manipulation of communities through language and methods that purport to foster participation and engagement, while in fact using local communities to the advantage of the researchers (Arnstein, 1969; Cooke & Kothari, 2001; Draper et al., 2010). Although an extreme example, the four-decade-long Tuskegee study of untreated syphilis in Black males, which continued to withhold treatment long after penicillin was available, to study the long-term effects of the disease (Reverby, 2009), provides a deeply disturbing example. As Thomas and Quinn (2001) point out,

> the study included culturally-appropriate and grassroots approaches to ensure the involvement and continued participation of [Black physicians and prisoners] . . . The Public Health Service was extremely successful in enlisting Black church leaders, elders in the community and plantation owners to encourage participation. (p. 1499)

The underlying racism inherent in this study remains an indelible reminder of the human costs of unethical scientific research and the ways in which "community participation," can, and sometimes has, been used to for horrific and unjust ends.

To ensure the inclusion of CBPR values and principles, in a recent review of the accelerating extent of community-engaged and partnered research awards within the US Environmental Protection Agency, Yuen, Park, Seifer, and Payne-Sturges (2015) added a "community-driven" column to the CTSA continuum, beyond shared leadership, which mirrors the CBPR definition that research should be based on community priorities, strengths, and actions. Balazs and Morello-Frosch (2013) have gone further in constructing an explanatory continuum that shows the evolution from community members being research subjects to becoming research partners, depending on their level of participation. Focus groups to elicit community opinions, for example, are not in themselves CBPR. CBPR requires structures for participation such as community advisory boards or equitable partnership teams that have decision-making authority. As Balazs and Morello-Frosch (2013) further assert, integrating community members as full research partners enables science to be rigorous and relevant, with greater reach, by working deeply with communities (see Chapter 15).

Ultimately, these continua remind us of the importance of reflecting on our own values and commitment to confront power dynamics within research processes to benefit communities. To live up to the espoused principles of CBPR for health—principles accenting true partnerships among researchers, communities, clinical providers, patients, and other stakeholders and achieving a balance between research and action toward health equity—is the emancipatory end of the continuum that should serve as a gold standard for CBPR practice. Particularly for professionals in fields such as public health, social welfare, and community planning, among others, with their roots in concerns for social justice, CBPR in this sense provides an important goal for which to strive in our collaborative work with communities.

EFFECTIVENESS OF CBPR AND COMMUNITY-ENGAGED RESEARCH

The first systematic review of CBPR, by the Agency of Health Care Research and Quality in 2004, spanned the years 1975–2003 and found sixty CBPR studies, with thirty identified as interventions and thirteen with a policy focus. Few of these studies had rigorous designs and only twelve documented outcomes (Viswanathan et al., 2004). Within Britain, corollary interest in assessing the impact of community engagement within research and population health initiatives spawned multiple reports (Popay et al., 2007; Staley, 2009).

Since that time, and especially since 2009, when CBPR became a medical subject heading (MESH) in the Library of Medicine, there has been a significant growth of systematic reviews and meta-analyses that have found compelling evidence of positive impacts on health outcomes (Anderson et al., 2015; Carter, Tregear, & Lachance, 2015; Cook, 2008; Cyril, Smith, Possamai-Inesedy, & Andre, 2015; de las Nueces, Hacker, DiGirolamo, & Hicks, 2012; Drahota et al., 2016; Milton et al., 2012; O'Mara-Eves et al., 2015; Yuen et al., 2015).

In a systematic review of impacts of community engagement among disadvantaged populations, Cyril and colleagues (2015) found that 88 percent of twenty-four studies had positive outcomes, with defined CBPR studies showing higher community involvement throughout research processes. A meta-analysis of 131 CEnR articles, including randomized and non-randomized designs, found positive impacts on health behavior, health consequences, self-efficacy, and perceived social support (O'Mara-Eves et al., 2015). de Las Nueces et al. (2012), in a systematic review of CBPR clinical trials with racial-ethnic minorities, found 89 percent of their nineteen articles to have behavioral and clinical outcomes and high success in retaining minority participants.

Thompson et al. (2016) identified NIH-funded population health and disparities centers that focused on CBPR projects to empower communities toward health equity. Salimi and colleagues (2012) sought to review community empowerment by assessing community participation in all the stages of research. They found that more studies involved community members in selecting research questions (42 percent), with only 8 percent having community members involved in proposal writing or with financial responsibilities. Involving community members throughout research processes has been validated as a promising practice that is associated with outcomes of shared power relations in research and community transformation (see Chapters 6 and 17). Drahota and colleagues (2016), in their systematic review across multiple disciplines, identified fifty community-academic partnership studies, documenting 78 percent with proximal outcomes, such as synergy or knowledge exchange, with one-third reporting capacity and system outcomes, such as improved community care, sustainable partnerships, or changed community context.

Some studies have sought to identify the type of participatory engagement, such as communities identifying health needs and mobilizing, communities collaborating on design, communities consulting on intervention design, and community members collaborating or leading intervention delivery, such as using lay health workers (Brunton, O'Mara-Eves, & Thomas, 2014; O'Mara-Eves et al., 2015). Lay-delivered interventions had the largest effect sizes in a recent Cochrane Review of collaborations, which found limited other impacts on ethnic-racial minority health (Anderson et al., 2015).

The growing number and positive outcomes of these reviews help document the power of CBPR and CEnR in contributing to intermediate outcomes such as community capacities and longer-term health outcomes. Recent NIH-funded experimental trials, based in long-time culturally-grounded CBPR partnerships, are producing more evidence of outcomes (Dickerson et al., in press). For meta-studies, however, the Cochran criteria of comparison trials or health-specific outcomes are too limited.

A growing literature exists, for example, in CBPR policy studies, which don't show up in comparison designs but that document substantial health impacts from policy changes (Minkler et al., 2012). Because they often affect the health and social environments of large numbers of people, such studies (see Chapters 20 to 23) also should be included in systemic reviews.

Increasing evidence of impacts from participatory processes document that they are highly complex and not controllable as defined intervention impacts (Abma et al., 2017; Rifkin, 2014; South & Phillips, 2014; Trickett et al., 2011). Empowerment strategies in CBPR, for example, based on Paulo Freire's (1970) dialogical methods, are not predictable interventions but rather dynamic processes within dynamic contexts. Evaluation of such efforts needs to include context as much as processes and outcomes. Jagosh and colleagues (2012) have found that broader goals of joint policy advocacy and capacity-building may be equally important to perceived partnership success, in addition to specific grant outcomes. Calls for CBPR as a liberatory social movement further challenge us to critically analyze how we can best achieve improved health equity for all (Devia et al., 2016; Tremblay, Martin, Macaulay, & Pluye, 2017).

In sum, CBPR should not be seen simply as an instrumental strategy but rather as grounded by its commitment to community priorities and decision making. Although we are pleased by the growing evidence of specific outcomes, we also seek broader intermediate and long-term outcomes, such as changed power dynamics, cultural revitalization, community empowerment, and improved health and social equity (see Chapters 17 and 18).

ORGANIZATION OF THIS BOOK

In this third edition, we build on our core values of health equity and social justice as we present new diverse case studies that represent ongoing frontiers of CBPR and CEnR. With the addition of two new editors, we have made major changes in our framing, following the domains of the CBPR conceptual model (see Chapter 6), first introduced in the second edition. Although much cutting-edge participatory research continues outside the United States, our purpose is to focus primarily on CBPR in the contemporary United States, in part so that we can carefully attend to the geopolitical and sociohistorical contexts so central to this work. However, we frequently draw on the wisdom of leading participatory research, action research, participatory action research, and participatory health research scholars and practitioners in the Global South from Latin America, Asia, and Africa, and from Canada, Europe, the United Kingdom, Australia, New Zealand, and elsewhere, and we believe that many of the skills and conceptual and ethical issues raised will have relevance beyond the United States. (See global issues in Chapters 7, 18, 23; Appendices 3, 6; and the Afterword.)

Part 1 begins with this chapter introducing the field, with Chapter 2 presenting its historical and theoretical antecedents and new concepts of cognitive justice and knowledge democracy from the Global South. Chapter 3 describes and illustrates the classic, as well as evolving principles of CBPR.

In Part 2, Chapter 4 examines race, racism, power and privilege; Chapter 5 discusses the dynamics of trust in partnerships.

Part 3 begins the new framing by introducing the CBPR conceptual model with its four domains, with case studies focusing on the first domain, "Context," and the second domain, "Partnering Processes." Chapter 6 first introduces the history and domains of the CBPR conceptual model. Chapter 7 discusses CBPR within a youth context. Chapter 8 provides a randomized control trial to transform structural racism and bias within the context of cancer health care. Chapter 9 discusses the challenges of alignment and misalignment among academic and community partners.

Part 4 continues to the third domain of the model, "Research and Interventions," with case studies on how partnering processes contribute to the promising practices of culturally and locally appropriate research design and implementation. Chapter 10 explores community-engaged methods within health care system research projects. Chapter 11 speaks to the creation of culture-centered interventions within the Deaf and hearing impaired community. Chapter 12 challenges us to integrate CBPR principles into interventions with highly diverse Asian populations. Chapter 13 presents a developmental process for engaging Latino communities in every step of research design and implementation.

In Part 5, we extend our research methods into core ethical promising practices. We learn the importance of culture and governance within tribal contexts (Chapter 14) and unpack ethical issues within (Chapter 15) and beyond (Chapter 16) institutional review boards (IRBs) and research review boards.

Part 6 then continues to the fourth "Outcomes" domain of the model, with Chapter 17 providing evidence, from testing the CBPR model, of promising partnering practices associated with a range of intermediate and long-term outcomes. Chapter 18 showcases US and Nicaraguan case studies of participatory evaluation outcomes with lay health advisors. Chapter 19 shares personal stories and outcomes for faculty members of color who have benefited from CBPR pipeline programs.

In Part 7, we deepen the focus on policy outcomes, with Chapter 20 providing an overview and an adapted CBPR policy model. We incorporate powerful examples of policy environmental changes within food security and healthy retail (Chapter 21), criminal justice reform (Chapter 22), and youth mapping of their living conditions within Kenyan and Brazilian slums (Chapter 23).

We conclude with appendices designed to provide tools and applications so partnerships can put some of the messages central to this book into practice in their own CBPR efforts. The afterword by long-time participatory research international scholars brings us back to knowledge democracy in the global context.

CONCLUSION

Although the United States continues to have profound health and social inequities based on race, ethnicity, class, gender, age, ability-disability, sexual orientation, and gender identity, the fight for equity can be won only if vulnerable and oppressed communities can be fully engaged as partners in taking action to address the health and social problems about which they—not "outsider experts"—know most deeply. With communities now more directly under siege, the need for CBPR visibility and sustainability is even more pronounced.

Our primary goal in this book is to provide a highly accessible text that will stimulate practitioners, students, and academics in health and related fields, as well as community partners and researchers, as they engage—intellectually and in practice—in collaborative inquiry for action. We hope that those with substantial experience and newcomers will find themselves challenged by the theory, methods, and case studies.

We end this chapter with a quote from Pia Moriarty (1993), who in her work with the Commission on Social Justice for the San Francisco Archdiocese wrote about the visceral nature of deep learning and its importance for us, as we seek to create equitable partnerships and knowledge for personal and societal transformation:

> Deep learning involves the whole body, blood and bone, not just the theoretical or cataloguing of insightful facts and analyses. Deep learning moves the feet to walk in a new way, moves the eyes to see from the new perspective won by that walking, and moves the hands to fashion the tangible world into a new image envisioned by the new seeing. (p. 1)

QUESTIONS FOR DISCUSSION

1. Cornwall and Jewkes (1995) argue that CBPR is not a research method but an "orientation to research" that reflects a different stance from traditional research. How would you describe this alternative paradigm to a friend or colleague who's never heard of CBPR?

2. CBPR is described as a promising approach for health equity research. What CBPR characteristics do you think are most important for the study of health inequities *with* marginalized communities?
3. Community engagement is described as a continuum from outreach to shared leadership and community-driven approaches. The more emancipatory forms of CBPR are presented as a "gold standard" for which professionals might strive. Do you agree with this? Why or why not?

NOTE

1. http://hsc.unm.edu/programs/nmcareshd/cec.shtml

REFERENCES

Abma, T., Cook, T., Ramgard, M., Kleba, E., Harris, J., & Wallerstein, N. (2017). Social impact of participatory health research: Collaborative non-linear processes of knowledge mobilization. *Journal of Action Research*. www.tandfonline.com/doi/full/10.1080/09650792.2017.1329092

Abma, T., Banks, S., Cook, T., Dias, S., Madsen, W., Springett, J., & Wright, M. (2018). *Participatory research for health and social well-being*. New York: Springer Basic.

Allen, M. L., Salsberg, J., Knot, M., LeMaster, J. W., Felzien, M., Westfall, J. M., Herbert, C. P., Vickery, K., Culhane-Pera, K. A., Ramsden, V. R., Zittleman, L., Martin, R. E., & Macaulay, A. C. (2017). Engaging with communities, engaging with patients: Amendment to the NAPCRG 1998 policy statement on responsible research with communities. *Family Practice, 34*(3), 313–321.

Anderson, L. M., Adeney, K. L., Shinn, C., Safranek, S., Buckner-Brown, J., & Krause, L. K. (2015). Community coalition-driven interventions to reduce health disparities among racial and ethnic minority populations. *Cochrane Database of Systematic Reviews, 6*(CD009905). doi:10.1002/14651858.CD009905.pub2

Arnstein, S. R. (1969). A ladder of citizen participation. *Journal of American Instructional Planners, 35*, 216–224.

Balazs, C. L., & Morello-Frosch, R. (2013). The three Rs: How community-based participatory research strengthens the rigor, relevance, and reach of science. *Environmental Justice, 6*(1), 9–16.

Becenti-Pigman, B., White, K., Bowman, B., Palmenteer-Holder, N. L., & Duran, B. (2008). Research policies, processes and protocol: The Navajo Nation Human Research Review Board. In M. Minkler & N. Wallerstein, *Community-based participatory research for health: Processes and outcomes* (2nd ed., pp. 441–446). San Francisco, CA: Jossey-Bass.

Blumenthal, D., DiClemente, R., Braithwaite, R., & Smith, S. (2013). *Community-based participatory health research: Issues, methods and translation to practice* (2nd ed.). New York: Springer.

Bradbury, H. (Ed.). (2015). *The Sage handbook of action research* (3rd ed.). Thousand Oaks, CA: Sage.

Bor, J., Cohen, G. H., & Galea, S. (2017). Population health in an era of rising income inequality: USA, 1980–2015, *Lancet, 389*(10077), 1475–1490.

Brunton, G., O'Mara-Eves, A., & Thomas, J. (2014). The "active ingredients" for successful community engagement with disadvantaged expectant and new mothers: A qualitative comparative analysis. *Journal of Advanced Nursing, 70*, 2847–2860.

Buchanan, D. R., Miller, F. G., & Wallerstein, N. (2007). Ethical issues in community-based participatory research: Balancing rigorous research with community participation in community intervention studies. *Progress in Community Health Partnerships: Research, Education, and Action, 1*, 153–160.

Cargo, M., & Mercer, S. L. (2008). The value and challenges of participatory research: Strengthening its practice. *Annual Review of Public Health, 29*, 325–350.

Carter, M. W., Tregear, M. L., & Lachance, C. R. (2015). Community engagement in family planning in the U.S.: A systematic review. *American Journal of Preventive Medicine, 49*(2 Suppl 1), S116.

Coghlan, D. (2004). Action research in the academy: Why and whither? Reflections on the changing nature of research. *Irish Journal of Management, 25*(2), 1–10.

Cook, W. K. (2008). Integrating research and action: A systematic review of community-based participatory research to address health disparities in environmental and occupational health in the USA. *Journal of Epidemiology and Community Health, 62*(8), 668–676.

Cooke, B., & Kothari, U. (2001). Participation: The new tyranny? New York, NY: Zed Books.

Cornwall, A., & Jewkes, R. (1995). What is participatory research? *Social Science & Medicine, 41,* 1667–1676.

Cyril, S., Smith, B. J., Possamai-Inesedy, A., & Andre, M.N.R. (2015). Exploring the role of community engagement in improving the health of disadvantaged populations: A systematic review. *Global Health Action, 8,* 1–12.

Cytron, N., Pettit, K. L., Kingsley, G. T., Erickson, D. J., & Seidman, E. S. (Eds.). (2014). *What counts: Harnessing data for America's communities.* San Francisco, CA: Federal Reserve Bank of San Francisco and Washington, DC: Urban Institute. Retrieved from www.whatcountsforamerica.org

de las Nueces, D., Hacker, K., DiGirolamo, A., & Hicks, L. S. (2012). A systematic review of community-based participatory research to enhance clinical trials in racial and ethnic minority groups. *Health Services Research, 47,* 1363–1386.

Denzin, N. K., Lincoln, Y. S., & Tuhiwai Smith, L. (2008). *Handbook of critical and indigenous methodologies.* Thousand Oaks, CA: Sage.

Devia, C., Baker, E., Sanchez-Youngman, S., Barnidge, E., Golub, M., Motton, F., Muhammad, M., Ruddock, C., Vicuña, B., & Wallerstein, N. (2017). CBPR to advance social and racial equity: Urban and rural partnerships in Black and Latino communities. *BMC International Journal of Health Equity, 16,* 17. doi:10.1186/s12939-016-0509-3

Dickerson, D. L., Baldwin, J., Belcourt, A., Belone, L., Gittelsohn, J., Kaholokula, J. K., Lowe, J., Patten, C., & Wallersteinl, N. (in press). Encompassing cultural contexts within scientific research methodologies in the development of health promotion interventions. *Prevention Science. Special Issue: Innovations in intervention research with indigenous populations in the U.S.*

Drahota, A., Meza, R., Brikho, B., Naaf, M., Estabillo, J. A., Gomez, E., Vejnoska, S., Sufek, S., Stahmer, A., & Aarons, G. (2016). Community-academic partnerships: A systematic review of the state of the literature and recommendations for future research. *Milbank Quarterly, 94*(1), 163–214.

Draper, A. K., Hewitt, G., & Rifkin, S. (2010). Chasing the dragon: Developing indicators for the assessment of community participation in health programmes. *Social Science & Medicine, 71,* 1102–1109.

Dutta, M. J., Anaele, A., & Jones, C. (2013). Voices of hunger: Addressing health disparities through the culture-centered approach. *Journal of Communication, 63,* 159–180.

Franco, Z. E., Ahmed, S. M., Maurana, C. A., DeFino, M. C., & Brewer, D. D. (2015). A social network analysis of 140 community-academic partnerships for health: Examining the Healthier Wisconsin Partnership Program. *Clinical and Translational Science, 8,* 311–319.

Freire, P. (1970). *Pedagogy of the oppressed.* New York, NY: Seabury Press.

Freire, P. (1973). *Education for critical consciousness.* New York, NY: Seabury Press.

Gaventa, J., & Cornwall, A. (2015). Power and knowledge. In H. Bradbury (Ed.), *The Sage handbook of action research: Participative inquiry and practice.* (3rd ed.). Thousand Oaks, CA: Sage.

Green, L. W. (2006). Public health asks of systems science: To advance our evidence-based practice, can you help us get more practice-based evidence? *American Journal of Public Health, 96,* 406–409.

Hacker, K. (2013). *Community-based participatory research.* Thousand Oaks, CA: Sage.

Hall, B., Tandon, R., & Tremblay, C. (Eds.). (2015). *Strengthening community-university research partnerships: Global perspectives.* Victoria, BC, Canada: University of Victoria.

Hawe, P. (2015). Lessons from complex interventions to improve health. *Annual Review of Public Health, 36,* 307–323.

Institute of Medicine (IOM). (2012). *An integrated framework for assessing the value of community-based prevention.* Washington, DC: National Academies Press.

IOM. (2016). *A framework for educating health professionals to address the social determinants of health.* Washington, DC: National Academy of Sciences.

Israel, B. A., Eng, E., Schulz, A. J., & Parker, E. A. (Eds.). (2013). *Methods in community-based participatory research for health* (2nd ed.). San Francisco, CA: Jossey-Bass.

Jagosh, J., Macaulay, A. C., Pluye, P., Salsberg, J., Bush, P. L., Henderson, J., Sirett, E., Wong, G., Cargo, M., Herbert, C. P., Seifer, S. D., Green, L. W., & Greenhalgh, T. (2012). Uncovering the benefits of participatory research: Implications of a realist review for health research and practice. *Milbank Quarterly, 90*(2), 311–346.

Kagawa-Singer, M., Dressler, W. W., George, S. M., & Elwood, W. N. (2015). *The cultural framework for health: An integrative approach for research and program design and evaluation.* Bethesda, MD: Office of Behavioral and Social Sciences Research.

Lewin, K. (1946). Action research and minority problems. *Journal of Social Issues, 2,* 34–46.

Marmot, M., & Bell, R. (2012). Fair society, healthy lives. *Public Health, 126,* S4–S10.

McCloskey, D. J., et al. (2011), *Principles of community engagement* (2nd ed.). NIH Publication No. 11-7782, Clinical and Translational Science Awards Community Engagement Key Function Committee Task Force on the Principles of Community Engagement. Bethesda, MD: National Institutes of Health. Retrieved May 15, 2017, from www.atsdr.cdc.gov/communityengagement/pdf/PCE_Report_508_FINAL.pdf; see: https://ncats.nih.gov/ctsa/community.

Milton, B., Attree, P., French, B., Povall, S., Whitehead, M., & Popay, J. (2012). The impact of community engagement on health and social outcomes: A systematic review. *Community Development Journal, 47,* 316–334.

Minkler, M., Garcia, A., Rubin, V., & Wallerstein, N. (2012). *Community-based participatory research: A strategy for building healthy communities and promoting health through policy change.* Retrieved from www.policylink.org/sites/default/files/CBPR.pdf

Minkler, M., & Wallerstein, N. (2008). *Community-based participatory research for health: Processes and outcomes* (2nd ed.). San Francisco, CA: Jossey-Bass.

Moriarty, P. (1993). *Deep learning for earthquake country. Future of prophetic Christianity: Essays in honor of Robert McAfee Brown.* New York, NY: Orbis Books.

Muhammad, M., Wallerstein, N., Sussman, A. L., Avila, M., Belone, L., & Duran. B. (2015). Reflections on researcher identity and power: The impact of positionality on community-based participatory research (CBPR) processes and outcomes. *Critical Sociology, 41*(7–8), 1045–1063.

Noe, T. D., Manson, S. M., Croy, C., McGough, H., Henderson, J. A., & Buchwald, D. S. (2006). The influence of community-based participatory research principles on the likelihood of participation in health research in American Indian communities. *Ethnicity & Disease, 17*(1 Suppl 1), S6–S14.

Northridge, M. E., Vallone, D., Merzel, C., Greene, D., Shepherd, P., Cohall, A. T., et al. (2000). The adolescent years: An academic-community partnership in Harlem comes of age. *Journal of Public Health Management and Practice, 6*(1), 53–60.

O'Mara-Eves, A., Brunton, G., Oliver, S., Kavanagh, J., Jamal, F., & Thomas, J. (2015). The effectiveness of community engagement in public health interventions for disadvantaged groups: A meta-analysis. *BMC Public Health, 15*(1), 1352.

Parry, D., Salsberg, J., & Macaulay, A. C. (2017). *Guide to researcher and knowledge-user collaboration in health research.* Retrieved May 2017 from www.cihr-irsc.gc.ca/e/documents/Guide_to_Researcher_and_KU_Collaboration.pdf

Popay, J., Attree, P., Hornby, D., Milton, B., et al. (2007), *Community engagement in initiatives addressing the wider social determinants of health: A rapid review of evidence on impact, experience and process.* London, UK: National Collaborating Center of Community Engagement, National Institute for Health and Health Care Excellence.

Reverby, S. M. (2009). *Tuskegee's truths: Rethinking the Tuskegee syphilis study.* Ann Arbor, NC: UNC Press Books.

Rifkin, S. (2014). Examining the links between community participation and health outcomes: A review of the literature. *Health Policy and Planning, 29,* ii98–ii106.

Rowell, L., Bruce, C., Shosh, J., & Riel, M. (Eds.). (2017). *Palgrave international handbook of action research.* New York, NY: Springer Nature.

Salimi, Y., Shahandeh, K., Malekafzali, H., Loori, N., Kheiltash, A., Jamshidi, E., Frouzan, A. S., & Majdzadeh, R. (2012). Is community-based participatory research (CBPR) useful? A systematic review on papers in a decade. *International Journal of Preventive Medicine, 3*(6), 386–393.

Schwab, M., & Syme, S. L. (1997). On paradigms, community participation, and the future of public health. *American Journal of Public Health, 87,* 2049–2052.

South, J., & Phillips, G. (2014). Evaluating community engagement as part of the public health system. *Journal of Epidemiology and Community Health, 68,* 692–696.

Staley, K. (2009). *Exploring impact: Public involvement in NHS, public health and social care research.* Eastleigh, UK: INVOLVE.

Stringer, E. (2014). *Action research* (4th ed.). Thousand Oaks, CA: Sage.

Thomas, S. B., & Quinn, S. C. (2001). Light on the shadow of the syphilis study at Tuskegee. *Health Promotion Practice, 1,* 234–237.

Thompson, B., Molina, Y., Viswanath, K., Warnecke, R., & Prelip, M. (2016). Strategies to empower communities to reduce health disparities. *Health Affairs, 35,* 1424–1428.

Tremblay, M. C., Martin, D. H., Macaulay, A. C., & Pluye, P. (2017). Can we build on social movement theories to develop and improve community-based participatory research? A framework synthesis review. *American Journal of Community Psychology.* doi:10.1002/ajcp.12142

Trickett, E. J. (2011). Community-based participatory research as worldview or instrumental strategy: Is it lost in translation(al) research? *American Journal of Public Health, 101*(8), 1353–1355.

Trickett, E. J., Beehler, S., Deutsch, C., Green, L. W., Hawe, P., McLeroy, K., Miller, R., Rapkin, B., Schensul, J., Schulz, A., & Trimble, J. (2011). Advancing the science of community-level interventions. *American Journal of Public Health, 101,* 1410–1419.

Tuhiwai Smith, L. (2012). *Decolonizing methodologies: Research and Indigenous peoples* (2nd ed.). New York, NY: Zed Books.

Viswanathan, M., Ammerman, A., Eng, E., Gartlehner, G., Lohr, K. N., Griffith, D., et al. (2004). *Community-based participatory research: Assessing the evidence* (Evidence Report/Technology Assessment No. 99; Prepared by RTI International–University of North Carolina). Rockville, MD: Agency for Healthcare Research and Quality.

Wallerstein, N., & Duran, B. (2010). Community-based participatory research contributions to intervention research: The intersection of science and practice to improve health equity. *American Journal of Public Health, 100*(Suppl 1), S40.

Wallerstein, N., Oetzel, J., Duran, B., Tafoya, G., Belone, L., & Rae, R. (2008). What predicts outcomes in CBPR? In M. Minkler & N. Wallerstein (Eds.). *Community-based participatory research for health: Processes and outcomes* (2nd ed., pp. 371–392). San Francisco, CA: Jossey-Bass.

Walters, K., Stately, A., Evans-Campbell, T., Simoni, J., Duran, B., Schultz, K., Stanley, E., Charles, C., & Guerrero, D. (2009). "Indigenist" collaborative research efforts in Native American communities. In A. R. Stiffman (Ed.), *The field research survival guide* (pp. 146–173). New York, NY: Oxford University Press.

W.K. Kellogg Foundation Community Health Scholars Program. (2001). *Stories of impact [brochure].* Ann Arbor: University of Michigan, School of Public Health, Community Health Scholars Program, National Program Office.

Wright, M., & Kongats, K. (Eds.). (2018). *Participatory health research: International perspectives.* New York: Springer.

Yano, E. M., Green, L. W., Glanz, K., Ayanian, J. Z., Mittman, B. S., Chollette, V., & Rubenstein, L. V. (2012). Implementation and spread of interventions into the multilevel context of routine practice and policy: Implications for the cancer care continuum. *Monographs: Journal of the National Cancer Institute, 2012*(44), 86.

Yuen, T., Park, A. N., Seifer, S. D., & Payne-Sturges, D. (2015). A systematic review of community engagement in the US Environmental Protection Agency's extramural research solicitations: Implications for research funders. *American Journal of Public Health, 105*(12), e44–e52.

CHAPTER 2

THEORETICAL, HISTORICAL, AND PRACTICE ROOTS OF CBPR

NINA WALLERSTEIN AND BONNIE DURAN

The next few years comprise a key moment in which social science must up its game to address and challenge inequality, in alliance with other actors who are already raising their voices. The time is now.

ISSC

IN THIS HISTORICAL moment, the presuppositions of the academy, research, and health and social interventions cannot assert neutrality. Insights into the nature of science, language, and subjectivity outlined in history and critical social theory alert us to the operation of power in familiar discourses that have tended to disguise or neutralize it. Social and clinical research and practice benefit from this investigation, which provides an opportunity for professional, collective, and personal *reflexivity* on how and where research produces change. Health and social interventions benefit from agents (ourselves as researchers, practitioners, providers) who acknowledge how we embody histories, theories, values, and political stances, which may include documenting historical and current resistances to research. As CBPR and community-engaged researchers and practitioners, we can also benefit from the values and contributions of "knowledge systems of the South" (de Sousa Santos, 2013). The challenge for us is how to use our science to co-construct knowledge with those living with inequalities who may be best positioned to influence change in social and health practices, policies, and politics.

The forces promoting community-academic research partnerships come from government public policies, academic structures and incentives, and the pressures for engagement generated by civil society. Community and scientific leaders and workers and patients from many disenfranchised groups have begun to demand that research show greater sensitivity to communities' perceptions, needs, and unique circumstances, bringing new attention to the meaning of relationships, codes of conduct, trust, and mutually beneficial partnerships (Anderson & Olson, 2013).

Health disparities research is increasingly conducted within the framework of participatory research approaches (see Chapter 1 for multiple complementary terms and approaches). These approaches have the advantage of providing greater external validity, challenging standardized research protocols, and promoting responsible research conduct (Wallerstein & Duran, 2010). We see more deeply how race and racism, ethnicity, socioeconomic status, nativity, gender identity, sexual orientation, ableism, and so on affect core values and communication that constitute our research practices, even within our research partnerships (Muhammad et al., 2015), with implications for mistrust within research and science itself (Oetzel et al., 2015).

By broadening and deepening the team of researchers to include those who are often simply "researched," we not only strengthen research processes but also contribute to more nuanced, complex, and authentic research outcomes. The results are not "alternative facts" of the sort put forward by the Trump administration in the United States. Rather, they are a deeper and richer understanding of the topic under study, which in turn can improve the science and the translation of research findings into actions to improve health and social equity.

The majority of participatory research approaches can be traced to one of two historical traditions that represent distinct approaches within a continuum of values. Collaborative utilization–focused research, with practical goals of systems improvement, is sometimes called the *Northern tradition.* This is juxtaposed against openly emancipatory research, challenging the historical colonizing practices of research and political domination of knowledge by the elites, which is often called the *Southern tradition*[1] (Hall, Tandon, & Tremblay, 2015).

This chapter will articulate the historical roots of these two traditions and briefly discuss theories of participation, knowledge democracy, power, and contributions from feminist, postcolonial, and post-structuralist perspectives to clarify points of convergence and difference. Although we articulate differences, both traditions have embraced four pillars of "engaged excellence": delivering high-quality research, co-constructing knowledge, mobilizing impact-oriented evidence, and building enduring partnerships (Oswald, Gaventa, & Leach, 2017).

This chapter ends with practical approaches for implementing Freirean dialogical education to address challenges in the field. Key among these challenges are how—and how much—transformative change can, in fact, occur at the local level given current complex external forces, including growing conservative forces advocating deep cuts in federal and other government support. Although such questions may have relevance for the Northern and Southern traditions, their deep intersections with knowledge democracy, power sharing, and other concepts central to the progressive Southern tradition make them particularly relevant to CBPR praxis embedded in this worldview.

Although the best of CBPR contains dimensions from multiple traditions, this chapter argues that the paramount public health goal of eliminating health and social inequities demands a research practice within the emancipatory perspective, a practice that fosters the democratic participation of community members to transform their communities as well as for academics to transform institutions of higher education. Any discussion of theories of research engagement must acknowledge the systemic processes that produce widespread suffering and therefore affirm liberation and processes of liberation (Dussel, 2013). As the 2016 *World Social Science Report* specifies, social science is under an ethical demand to respond critically to such suffering (ISSC/IDS, 2016). Inequality has become a global concern for citizens, activists, scholars, and policy makers, because it is inexorably linked to issues of planetary survival, health, gender justice, cultural and cognitive justice, knowledge democracy, and more. Society's future directions have to be based on universally accepted values of equity, justice, inclusion, peace, and sustainability.

TWO HISTORICAL TRADITIONS

As part of the genesis of the Northern collaborative utilization-focused research approach, in the 1940s German social psychologist Kurt Lewin coined the term *action research* (Bargal, 2008). Lewin challenged the gap between theory and practice and sought to solve practical problems through a research cycle involving planning, action, and investigating the results of the action (Lewin & Gold, 1999). He rejected the positivist belief that researchers study an objective world separate from the meanings understood by participants as they act in their world.

This tradition emanates most broadly from sociologist Talcott Parsons and his predecessors, who viewed social progress as based on rational decision making, applying ever-increasing scientific knowledge to real-world problems. With an emphasis on practitioners acting as coequals to academically trained researchers in their inquiry process, action science researchers have often worked in a consensus model, with institutional changes based on new knowledge and transformational leadership that inspires a self-reflective community of inquiry. In education, for example, teachers have joined academics as co-researchers in research-practice partnerships (Glassman, Erdem, & Bartholomew, 2013; Coburn & Penuel, 2016). Humanistic psychology strengthened cooperative inquiry within this tradition, adopting a belief in human agency through reflexive inquiry (Rowan, 2006).

In the early 1970s, a second Southern tradition of participatory research was born, with impetus from Marxist critiques of structural crises of underdevelopment, liberation theology, and the search for new practice by adult educators and community developers among populations vulnerable to globalization. An outflow of social science and education academics from universities to work with land movements and community-based organizations created an openness to knowledge from people's experience (Fals-Borda, 2006).

Exiled Brazilian philosopher Paulo Freire, whose writings were banned during Latin American dictatorships in the 1970s, helped transform the research relationship from communities as *objects of study* to community members *participating in the inquiry* (Freire, 1970, 1982). To Freire (1982), reality was not objective facts to be discovered but "includes the ways in which the people involved with facts perceive them. . . The concrete reality is the connection between subjectivity and objectivity, never objectivity isolated from subjectivity" (p. 29). Rather than viewing research as neutral, participatory researchers adopted commitments to social justice, with the ideology that people who are poor and oppressed can transform their conditions through their own actions based on their critical consciousness (Fals-Borda & Rahman, 1991). (See also Chapter 18 on Transformative-Participatory Evaluation.)

By mid-1970s, progressive institutions outside academia took the lead with the International Participatory Research Network, composed of the International Council for Adult Education, Toronto, and centers in India, Tanzania, Netherlands, and Latin America. Similar nodes have included the Collaborative Action Research Group in Australia (Kemmis et al., 2013) and the Highlander Research and Education Center, Tennessee, the oldest adult education and social change center in the United States (Horton & Freire, 1990). The first international symposium on participatory research was held in Cartagena, Colombia, in 1977; and the eighth in 1997 also in Cartagena, attracting two thousand delegates from sixty-one countries, based in social movements and the popular education of Paulo Freire (Fals-Borda, 2006). Forty years after the first conference, the Action Research Network of the Americas, formed in 2012, joined this international movement with a third conference in Cartagena, honoring the memory of Orlando Fals-Borda.

The interests of CBPR participants from US communities of color often resonate with the Southern approach because these participants have recognized the colonizing role of research, education, and religion (Said, 1994). With Indigenous peoples, public health and medical discourses have often "deauthorized" traditional ways of knowing for the purposes of controlling Native populations. As recently as the 1960s, top health journals were publishing "research" and medical characterizations of Indigenous peoples as primitive, lacking hygiene, having exotic mental disorders, or dying out (e.g., Bahl, 1961).

Placing the different participatory and action research terms used by various disciplines on a continuum between the problem-solving utilitarian approach and the emancipatory approach is difficult because actual research practice varies by local context, history, and ideology of stakeholders. The same term may even be used with opposite meanings. *Action research* (Bradbury, 2015) and *participatory action research (PAR),* for example, have been used to describe the emancipatory participatory research tradition (McTaggart, Nixon, & Kemmis, 2017) and the organizational development tradition (Argyris & Schön, 1996; Whyte, 1991). In an exhaustive monograph on the different paradigms of collaborative social inquiry, Trickett and Espino (2004) called for greater transparency of researchers on their own assumptions, practice, and desired outcomes.

In general, however, organizational action science and related traditions grounded in the Lewinian model are to be found at the end of the continuum focusing on pragmatic use of knowledge, with participatory and "PAR" approaches (Fals-Borda, 1998, pg.169) associated with Southern liberatory Freirian goals generally clustered at the other end. The term CBPR emerged from the language and history of "community-based" public health practice in the United States with the "participatory research" values of the Southern tradition. Understanding these issues within the core concepts of participation, knowledge democracy, power, and Freirian praxis will enable each of us to reflect on our own practice at different times along the continuum, including how we may embody different elements from each tradition.

PARTICIPATION

Habermas (1987) observed that "in the process of enlightenment, there can only be participants" (p. 40). If we adopt Habermas's succinct statement for CBPR, the core questions become, What do we mean by *participation*? Who is participating, for whom are we participating, in what spheres are we participating, to what ends are we participating, and perhaps most important of all, who or what is limiting participation in shaping our lives? In other words, where does the power lie (Gaventa & Cornwall, 2015)?

For CBPR, in particular, we need to ask, "If all research involves participation, what makes research participatory?" (Cornwall & Jewkes, 1995, p. 1668). Despite decades of a value-based rhetoric of participation from the World Health Organization or development studies, only relatively recently have researchers begun to question whether the reality of participation reflects the ideal. Some have questioned the authenticity of the participatory process (Tandon, 1988) or through NIH-funding have sought participation for a limited purpose, such as increasing minority recruitment into research trials.

Cooke and Kothari (2001) argue that communities are often viewed naively, concealing power relations and masking biases. They propose three tyrannies: when community member decision making is overridden by development experts (or researchers), when group dynamics may reinforce individuals already in power, and when research methods dictate only one level of inquiry, that is, seeking local data rather than identifying larger social policies that constrain local action. These issues remind us that CBPR is not "reified out there, but constructed by a cadre . . . of professionals, be they academics, practitioners or policymakers, whose ability to create this discourse is indicative of the power they possess" (Cooke & Kothari, 2001, p. 15).

The most important issue for community-based participatory researchers may be the relationship between academic researchers and community members. Habermas (1987) theorizes about two distinct modern worlds: the *systems* world of legal, economic, and political systems and the *life* world of families and cultural traditions in which individuals reproduce their identities and knowledge. As the life world has become dominated by the systems world, people increasingly see themselves as objects—clients and consumers—rather than subjects or democratic members of civil society. Within CBPR, outside researchers may unwittingly become part of this dynamic. Even within CBPR goals of authentic partnership, the actual practice between researchers and community members remains complex and involves making power and positionality transparent (see Chapter 4; Appendix 4; Muhammad et al., 2015). In a participatory study of healthy communities in New Mexico, for example, not recognizing power differences between communities and the evaluator inhibited equal collaboration and therefore use of research findings (Wallerstein, 1999).

Participation or lack of participation in research has been shaped by patterns of historical abuse, with communities increasingly demanding decision making to determine what research is done and who will do it. If CBPR practitioners fail to recognize these histories, they might be denied entry or have their research undermined through overt or hidden forms of resistance. At the same time, the contribution of CBPR researchers should not be undervalued. Academics often know of funding opportunities and have key expertise to offer about important health issues. Negotiation, therefore, of shared guidelines or formal agreements, and paying attention to ethical issues, which are both part of IRBs (Chapter 15) and extend beyond individual harm and benefit considerations (Chapters 16), can become critical for participatory partnerships. In working with tribal sovereign nations, in particular, codes of ethics and tribal IRBs often couple community and cultural benefit with permission to conduct research (see Chapter 14; Canadian Institutes of Health Research, 2007–2010).

Who represents the community remains a key issue in participation. Although service providers are asked to serve on community advisory boards, they may or may not represent their constituents (Jewkes & Murcott, 1998). CBPR takes the view that community members themselves should participate in ongoing collaborative advisory and decision-making structures that go beyond participating in focus groups or in a single step of the research process. As discussed in Chapter 17, the community engaged for research index (CERI) documents community involvement in all research steps, from problem identification through data analysis and dissemination. Community involvement, along with other promising practices, such as sharing budgets (or the community agency as the principal investigator with subcontracts to academics), can facilitate greater equality in participation in the partnership (see Chapter 17). As Rifkin (1996) indicates, participation should not be seen as a magic bullet but as a complex and iterative process, which can change, grow, or diminish, based on the unfolding of power relations and the historical and social context of the research project.

KNOWLEDGE DEMOCRACY

The creation and the use of knowledge are inherently the motivating forces behind all research; yet similar to participation, CBPR raises questions of by whom, about whom, and for what purpose this knowledge is defined (Hall et al., 2013). Although positivist research paradigms consider knowledge creation to be neutral and value-free, CBPR researchers have often drawn from reflexive and interpretative inquiry that explore the dialectic between researcher and what is being researched (Denzin & Lincoln, 2000) or from viewing knowledge as historically and socially constructed (McTaggart et al., 2017).

CBPR critiques of positivism have been pointed, stating that traditional inquiry discounts experiential knowledge, reinforces subjects' passivity, and obscures other voices (Gaventa & Cornwall, 2015). Not only is positivism, "not the only method for gaining valid knowledge, but it is a powerful ideology that thwarts the field's interests in alleviating suffering and promoting social justice" (Buchanan, 1998, p. 440). Indigenous researchers have posed this difference as knowledge for the sake of knowing (i.e., for categorizing objective reality) versus knowledge for decolonizing, healing, and mobilizing (Atalay, 2012; Tuhiwai Smith, 2012). Dutta (2008) proposes a culture-centered approach (CCA) for health research, challenging ways that dominant-culture communication (re)produces marginalization of disenfranchised populations and promoting community agency and knowledge for transforming inequitable conditions. CCA is increasingly being adopted within CBPR as a mechanism for knowledge democracy (Wallerstein et al., under review).

Fundamental to knowledge democracy is understanding that knowledge within universities, as published evidence-based science, for example, is a partial percentage of knowledge across the globe. The earliest universities created exclusionary walls and were part of sociopolitical processes that enabled the canonization of academic disciplines and what the Portuguese sociologist Boavenura has called *epistemicide,* or the killing of community knowledge systems (de Sousa Santos, 2007; Hall & Tandon, 2017).

Knowledge democracy practices, however, are embedded within CBPR and other participatory research approaches. Inherent to knowledge democracy is the recognition of multiple ways of knowing, especially from marginalized, excluded populations, of multiple expressions of knowing, such as narrative, songs, theater; of using knowledge as a tool for social action and democracy; and, finally, as shared through open-access venues. Knowledge democracy requires unpacking of universalist premises by identifying those processes of discrimination or racism (Chapter 4; Singh, 2016) that have prevented people's experiences from being seen as valid. Most important for CBPR practitioners, it involves our own reflections, as ongoing reflexive practice, about our positionalities of power, our own questions of how to best co-construct knowledge, and our own challenges in applying research knowledge for social and health equity.

POWER RELATIONS

Although knowledge is a major source of power and control, other structural power relations are also central. CBPR takes place not only in the context of personal and historical relationships among researchers, their universities, and communities but also in the broader societal context of power relations in which the research takes place, the origins of the research, and the purpose of the research itself. Gaventa and Cornwall (2015) identify four dimensions of power in CBPR, analyzing how power is exercised and who is excluded. The pluralist liberal view assumes that power is a product of an open system of equal competing agendas, with lack of participation, possibly in expressing views within a partnership, seen as a function of choice. The second view argues that there is a hidden face to power in which some actors and issues are kept from open discussion through a mobilization of bias by powerful social norms or organizations. CBPR researchers may unwittingly play into this bias in calling, for example, for evidence-based interventions (Green, 2006). The third, and more insidious, dimension of power is one that excludes grievances by preventing conflicts or community ideas from even surfacing. Internalized racism (see Chapter 4), for example, may contribute to a culture of community members not feeling their voices are as valued as when academics speak.

To Foucault (1980), these three dimensions represent repressive forms of power, exercised through direct control, microaggressions, or indirect language that shapes people's opportunities to participate fully. Emancipatory CBPR uncovers these mechanisms of control, biases, and internalized representations of reality as key strategies for change. Foucault articulates a fourth perspective of power as productive. Rather than seeing repressive monolithic power, he conceptualizes power as a web of discourses and practices found in institutions, communities, and families. These power relationships are inherently unstable and therefore open to challenge.

To Foucault, knowledge symbolizes power. Repressive power, for example, can be used in overly technical research language that may inhibit community response. As productive power, however, research knowledge can enable communities to challenge existing limits and advocate for change. As Deveaux (1999) has noted, "Where there is power, there is resistance" (p. 242).

In CBPR, relationships between researchers and communities require commitment and trust, which may ebb and flow over time depending on contexts, events, and power relations (see Chapter 5). When researchers walk into a community, they bring histories of the research institution and other researchers with them. Scott (1990) has outlined the importance of recognizing the dynamic nature of public and hidden discourse. *Public transcripts* contain information in official language and are often what is brought to the table initially. Yet *hidden transcripts,* what community members fully think, may remain outside the knowledge given to the outside research team. With trust, some hidden transcripts may become public over time. Academics, however, may never have full access to phenomena being studied, such as spiritual ceremonies, though openness to mutual learning and community knowledge can enrich all of our understandings of the world.

A key strategy for mutual learning is the practice of cultural humility (Appendix 4), in which all partners are reflexive about their positions of power, whether by race-ethnicity, education, or community status, and are willing to negotiate these dynamics. Diane Wolf (1996) has argued that research power can be challenged in three specific arenas: (1) the positionality between researcher and researched, (2) decision making during the research, and (3) voice and representation in writing and publishing. In Foucault's framework, positions of power can reverse, and initial power of researchers may give way to community knowledge and gatekeeper functions, with new reciprocity of shared power or community-driven leadership.

In CBPR, there is never a perfect equilibrium of power. All research efforts undergo cycles of participation and questioning by community members, bringing greater or lesser participation and ownership. This dialectic of collaboration and skepticism between academic and community partners is probably a healthy tension for all to acknowledge and work with, even as relationships strengthen and grow.

FEMINISM, POST-STRUCTURALISM, AND POSTCOLONIALISM

Feminist participatory researchers add critical dimensions to our understanding of the theory and practice of CBPR. In early critiques, feminist writing challenged the exclusion of women through the use of universal language of "the oppressed" and the lack of attention to gender differences in data collection and analysis (Maguire, 2006). Over the past fifty years, feminism has shifted from studying women as a universal construct to understanding gender culturally and historically, with shifting and intersectional identities of class, race and ethnicity, sexual orientation, and other differences (Collins, 2000; Maguire, 2006; Reid & Frisby, 2008). Arguing for a transnational feminist praxis of understanding one's historical and political locations, Swarr and Nagar (2010) propose that dialogical collaboration in knowledge production (as opposed to the individual scholar) offers transformational opportunities to rethink and reclaim feminist issues of voice, subalternity, and representation in scholarship and in social activism.

Post-structuralism focuses on the ways that language and narratives construct reality and our view of social institutions, such as academia, public health, or medicine, and how these constructions are resisted by communities. Postcolonialism takes this further by using race or ethnicity as a primary lens through which to understand European colonization of other peoples and lands (Said, 1994). To counter the dominant portrayals of the *other,* CBPR research within a postcolonial tradition seeks to honor and integrate into interventions the cultural and community narratives of people's lives (Duran & Duran, 1995; Whitesell, Stanley & Allen, 2018).

The role of the outside researcher in this context may therefore be largely to weaken the power of dominant culture explanations and create spaces for competing community ideas and practices to emerge, furthering goals of knowledge democracy. African American women, for example, in public spaces may conform to societal roles, yet in church or family contexts, adopt more powerful roles (Collins, 2000). In complex ways, they are not accepting stories of themselves as the other, but creating new stories based on their productive power as strong sisters, mothers, or advocates.

In CBPR, feminist, post-structuralist, and postcolonialist theory share certain methods and goals: analyzing personal lives in relation to the structures (overt and hidden) that might control people's lives; celebrating strengths and agency, not just victimization; working for goals of social justice; and undermining the notion of the objectivity of science by taking into account political, sociocultural contexts and knowledge of people living within those contexts. These literatures have challenged the right of researchers to overstate their interpretations and thereby unintentionally silence the community. Although data analysis is often seen as an academic exercise (with specialized skills needed), community participation in analytic discussions and interpretation of the data can be one of the most important for translation of findings into applied use (Cashman et al., 2008).

In a now-classic paper, Fine (1994) articulated three researcher stances in relation to community: (1) *ventriloquy,* when researchers describe the other as objective truth, never using the word *I* nor connecting themselves to their analysis; (2) *voices,* when researchers speak for the other, presenting quotes without a critical analysis of context or history of people's experience; and (3) *activist feminist research,* when researchers negotiate, are explicit about their identity, and create community dialogue for a context-based interpretation of knowledge. Fine and Sirin (2007) took this third stance further with a participatory action research project undertaken with a Muslim American youth advisory board to investigate hyphenated identities in a post-9-11 politically contentious and fear-generating world. They were able to explore public and hidden discourses, focusing on the Freirian praxis of resistance from these young people "working the hyphen" as they spoke out about their lives.

PAULO FREIRE AND PRAXIS

Brazilian educator Paulo Freire has been a major source of inspiration within the Southern emancipatory participatory research tradition. Freire's popular or empowerment educational approach is one of collective dialogue to facilitate *conscientização* (Portuguese for critical consciousness in becoming a social change agent) and *praxis,* or the continuous cycle of action-reflection-action to improve community conditions (1970, 1982).

To promote learners as the subjects of their own liberation, Freire proposes a listening-dialogue-action-reflection approach (Wallerstein & Auerbach, 2004). The first step is *listening* to problems and themes identified by community members as shared issues providing motivation to act. The next step is creating opportunities for *dialogue* to generate collective analyses of these issues within their sociocultural or political context and then identifying strategies for collective *actions*. *Reflection,* or evaluating the impact of the actions, leads back to the next cycle of listening, further dialogue, and actions.

Much of the creativity of the Freirian approach lies in the development of *codes,* or triggers, about the issues or themes, such as pictures, videos, role-plays—any form that helps participants "see" their reality with new eyes and develop alternative ways of thinking and acting. For research, these could include identifying issues through photo-documentary and photovoice (see Chapters 13 and 23), characterizing conditions through Augusto Boal's *theater of the oppressed,* creating digital stories to make research accessible for community action, and other forms of participatory practices for transformation (Ledwith & Springett, 2012).

Freire's writings reinforce a deep belief in humanity and people's role in making change and as such have critical importance to CBPR:

> To be a good [participatory researcher] means above all to have faith in people; to believe in the possibility that they can create and change things . . . Liberation begins to the extent that men [and women] reflect on themselves and their condition in the world—the world in which and with which they find themselves. To the extent that they are more conscientized, they insert themselves as subjects into their own history. (adapted from Freire, 1971, p. 61)

In a dialogue book with Ira Shor, Freire discusses the risks and fears of transformation, which for researchers could mean letting go of control, acknowledging that resistance may be real, "if you don't risk, you don't create anything. Without risking, for me, there is no possibility to exist" (Shor & Freire, 1987, p. 61). McTaggart and colleagues (2017) call for transcending single-dimension research for a complex research practice that draws on critical theory, applied problem-solving, and reflexive-dialectical practice, all of which promote our understandings of personal and collective agency under specific local and global historical conditions. Freirian methodologies can be helpful in pointing researchers and communities to the dialogical processes that facilitate these complex understandings and support personal transformations so that partners, as individuals and within the partnership, can see their roles in applying research for change.

CONCLUSION

Issues of participation, power, knowledge democracy, and praxis are not abstract phenomena but rather authentic tensions that are enacted in academia and in community settings. If we, as partners, are not honest and reflexive about our own power bases, there is little hope that we will be able to transform power dynamics. We need to understand how our personal biographies inform our ability to interpret the world in understanding the problems and in visioning community strengths.

A major challenge for those of us in the CBPR field lies in the potential limits of CBPR, given the realities of globalization, the imposition of Western cultural and economic structures on the rest of the world, and the difficulties for local communities in making meaningful change. *Scaling up* has become a buzzword in world institutions seeking to bring lessons from small communities to nation-states (Gaventa & Cornwall, 2015). Can CBPR be scaled up when so much depends on relationship building and commitment to collaborative work over time? Can realities be transformed at the local level in order to enhance health and contribute to a more equitable society? Although these questions are important, we must ensure that critiques and challenges of CBPR do not play into conservative strategies that dismiss the role of communities participating in change (or that, conversely, leave the work of change to local communities without adequate external or public sector support).

Ultimately, CBPR is about knowledge democracy, recognizing the interconnections between the personal and the social, life worlds and system worlds, and the barriers and facilitators of human actions that move toward research for social change. This can be a daunting and contradictory task but one full of promise and hope as academics and communities engage together to promote more just societies.

QUESTIONS FOR DISCUSSION

1. What are the contributions of different participatory research traditions (for example, feminist participatory research, Lewinian action research, Freire, etc.) to CBPR?
2. For self-reflection, what is your particular theoretical approach to CBPR, or what are the components from which you draw?
3. How are tensions embedded in the concepts of participation, knowledge democracy, power, and Freirian praxis expressed in your current work? In future work you hope to do?

NOTE

1. The Global South includes Africa, Latin America, and developing Asia, including the Middle East; countries formally referred to as *third world, developing,* or *low resource*. The Global North includes the United States, Canada, Western Europe, and developed parts of Asia, as well as Australia and New Zealand: highly industrialized and "democratic" countries.

REFERENCES

Anderson, K., & Olson, S. (2013). *Leveraging culture to address health inequalities: Examples from Native communities; Workshop summary.* Washington, DC: Roundtable on Promotion of Health Equity and the Elimination of Health Disparities, Institute of Medicine, National Academies Press.

Argyris, C., & Schön, D. A. (1996). *Organizational learning II.* Reading, MA: Addison-Wesley.

Atalay, S. (2012). *Community-based archeology: Research, with, by, and for Indigenous and local communities.* Berkeley, CA: UC Press.

Bahl, I. (1961). I couldn't have gotten along without Sam. *Nursing Outlook, 9*(6), 352–356.

Bargal, D. (2008). Action research: A paradigm for achieving social change. *Small Group Research, 39*(1), 17–27.

Bradbury, H. (Ed.). (2015). *The Sage handbook of action research* (3rd ed.). Thousand Oaks, CA: Sage.

Buchanan, D. (1998). Beyond positivism: Humanistic perspectives on theory and research in health education. *Health Education Research, 13,* 439–450.

Canadian Institutes of Health Research. (2007–2010). *CIHR guidelines for health research involving aboriginal people.* Retrieved February 2017 from www.cihr-irsc.gc.ca/e/29134.html

Cashman, S., Adeky, S., Allen, A., Corburn, J., Eng, E., Israel, B., Montaño, J., Rafelito, A., Rhodes, S. D., Swanston, S., & Wallerstein, N. (2008). The power . . . the promise: Working with communities to analyze and interpret data and get to outcomes. *American Journal of Public Health, 98,* 1407–1418.

Coburn, C. E., & Penuel, W. R. (2016). Research–practice partnerships in education: Outcomes, dynamics, and open questions. *Educational Researcher, 45*(1), 48–54.

Collins, P. H. (2000). *Black feminist thought: Knowledge, consciousness, and the politics of empowerment* (2nd ed.). New York, NY: Routledge.

Cooke, B., & Kothari, U. (Eds.). (2001). *Participation: The new tyranny?* London, UK: Zed Books.

Cornwall, A., & Jewkes, R. (1995). What is participatory research? *Social Science & Medicine, 41,* 1667–1676.

Denzin, N. K., & Lincoln, Y. S. (Eds.). (2000). *Handbook of qualitative research* (2nd ed.). Thousand Oaks, CA: Sage.

de Sousa Santos, B. (2007). Beyond abyssal thinking: From global lines to ecologies of knowledge. *Eurozine, 33,* 45–89.

de Sousa Santos, B. (2013). *Epistemologies of the south: Justice against epistemicide.* Boulder, CO: Paradigm Publishers.

Deveaux, M. (1999). Feminism and empowerment. In S. Hesse-Biber, C. Gilmartin, & R. Lydenberg (Eds.), *Feminist approaches to theory and methodology* (pp. 236–256). New York, NY: Oxford University Press.

Duran, E., & Duran, B. (1995). *Native American postcolonial psychology.* Albany, NY: State University of New York Press.

Dussel, E. (2013). *Ethics of liberation: In the age of globalization and exclusion.* Durham, NC: Duke University Press.

Dutta, M. J. (2008). *Communicating health: A culture-centered approach.* Malden, MA: Polity Press.

Fals-Borda, O., (1998). *People's participation: Challenges ahead.* New York. Apex Press.

Fals-Borda, O. (2006). Participatory (action) research in social theory: Origins and challenges. In P. Reason & H. Bradbury (Eds.), *Handbook of action research: Participative inquiry and practice* (Concise ed., pp. 27–37). Thousand Oaks, CA: Sage.

Fals-Borda, O., & Rahman, M. A. (Eds.). (1991). *Action and knowledge: Breaking the monopoly with participatory action research.* New York, NY: Apex Press.

Fine, M. (1994). Working the hyphens. In N. K. Denzin & Y. S. Lincoln (Eds.), *Handbook of qualitative research* (pp. 70–82). Thousand Oaks, CA: Sage.

Fine, M., & Sirin, S., (2007). Theorizing hyphenated selves: Researching youth development in and across contentious political contexts. *Social and Personality Psychology Compass, 1*(1),16–38.

Foucault, M. (1980). *Power/knowledge: Selected interviews and other writings, 1972–1977* (C. Gordon, Ed.). New York, NY: Pantheon Books.

Freire, P. (1970). *Pedagogy of the oppressed.* New York, NY: Seabury Press.

Freire, P. (1971). To the coordinator of the culture circle. *Convergence, 4*(1), 61–62.

Freire, P. (1982). Creating alternative research methods: Learning to do it by doing it. In B. L. Hall, A. Gillette, & R. Tandon (Eds.), *Creating knowledge: A monopoly? Participatory research in development* (pp. 29–37). New Delhi, India: Society for Participatory Research in Asia.

Gaventa, J., & Cornwall, A. (2015). Power and knowledge. In H. Bradbury (Ed.), *The Sage handbook of action research: Participative inquiry and practice* (3rd ed.). Thousand Oaks, CA: Sage.

Glassman, M., Erdem, G., & Bartholomew, M. (2013). Action research and its history as an adult education movement for social change. *Adult Education Quarterly, 63,* 272–288.

Green, L. W. (2006). Public health asks of systems science: To advance our evidence-based practice, can you help us get more practice-based evidence? *American Journal of Public Health, 96,* 406–409.

Habermas, J. (Ed.). (1987). *Lifeworld and system: A critique of functionalist reason.* Boston, MA: Beacon Press.

Hall, B., Tandon, R., & Tremblay, C. (2015). *Strengthening community university research partnerships: Global perspectives.* Victoria, Canada: University of Victoria and PRIA.

Hall, B. L., Jackson, E. T., Tandon, R., Fontan, J., & Lall, N. (2013). *Knowledge, democracy and action: Community-university research partnerships in global perspectives.* Manchester, UK: Manchester University Press.

Hall, B. L., & Tandon, R. (2017). Decolonization of knowledge, epistemicide, participatory research and higher education. *Research for All, 1*(1), 6–19.

Horton, M., & Freire, P. (1990). *We make the road by walking: Conversations on education and social change.* Edited by B. Bell, J. Gaventa, & J. Peters. Philadelphia, PA: Temple University Press.

ISSC/IDS. (2016). *Challenging inequalities: Pathways to a just world: World Social Science Report 2016.* Paris, France: UNESCO Publishing. Retrieved February 25, 2017, from http://en.unesco.org/wssr2016

Jewkes, R., & Murcott, A. (1998). Community representatives: Representing the "community"? *Social Science & Medicine, 46,* 843–858.

Kemmis, S., Wilkinson, J., Edwards-Groves, C., Hardy, I., Grootenboer, P., & Bristol, L. (2013). *Changing practices, changing education.* London, UK: Springer.

Ledwith, M., & Springett, J. (2012). *Participatory practice: Community-based action for transformative change.* Bristol, UK: Policy Press.

Lewin, K., & Gold, M. (1999). *The complete social scientist: A Kurt Lewin reader.* Washington, DC: American Psychological Association.

Maguire, P. (2006). Uneven ground: Feminisms and action research. In P. Reason & H. Bradbury (Eds.), *Handbook of action research: Participative inquiry and practice* (Concise ed., pp. 60–70). Thousand Oaks, CA: Sage.

McTaggart, R., Nixon, R., & Kemmis, S. (2017). Critical participatory action research. In L. Rowell, C. Bruce, J. Shosh, & M. Riel (Eds.), *Palgrave international handbook of action research* (pp. 21–36). New York, NY: Springer Nature.

Muhammad, M., Wallerstein, N., Sussman, A. L., Avila, M., Belone, L., & Duran, B. (2015). Reflections on researcher identity and power: The impact of positionality on community-based participatory research (CBPR) processes and outcomes. *Critical Sociology, 41,* 1045–1063.

Oetzel, J. G., Villegas, M., Zenone, H., White Hat, E. R., Wallerstein, N., & Duran, B. (2015). Enhancing stewardship of community-engaged research through governance. *American Journal Public Health, 105,* 1161–1167.

Oswald, K., Gaventa, J., & Leach, M. (2017). Introduction: Interrogating engaged excellence in research. *IDS Bulletin, 47*(6). Retrieved from http://bulletin.ids.ac.uk/idsbo/article/view/2827

Reid, C., & Frisby, W. (2008). Continuing the journey: Articulating dimensions of feminist participatory research. In P. Reason & H. Bradbury (Eds.), *The Sage handbook of action research: Participative inquiry and practice* (2nd ed., pp. 93–105). Thousand Oaks, CA: Sage.

Rifkin, S. (1996). Paradigms lost: Toward a new understanding of community participation in health programmes. *Acta Tropica, 61,* 79–92.

Rowan, J. (2006). The humanistic approach to action research. In P. Reason & H. Bradbury (Eds.), *Handbook of action research: Participative inquiry and practice* (concise ed., pp. 106–116). Thousand Oaks, CA: Sage.

Said, E. (1994). *Culture and imperialism.* New York, NY: Vintage Books.

Scott, J. (1990). *Domination and the arts of resistance: Hidden transcripts.* New Haven, CT: Yale University Press.

Shor, I., & Freire, P. (1987). *A pedagogy for liberation: Dialogues on transforming education.* Westport, CT: Bergin & Garvey.

Singh, J. (2016). Cultivating an anti-racist position in post-race society. In People's Knowledge Editorial Collective (Eds.), *People's knowledge and participatory action research: Escaping the white-walled labyrinth* (pp. 45–52). Warwickshire, UK: Practical Action Publishing.

Swarr, A., & Nagar, R. (2010). *Critical transnational feminist praxis.* Albany, NY: State University of New York Press.

Tandon, R. (1988). Social transformation and participatory research. *Convergence, 21*(2), 5–18.

Trickett, E. J., & Espino, S.L.R. (2004). Collaboration and social inquiry: Multiple meanings of a construct and its role in creating useful and valid knowledge. *American Journal of Community Psychology, 34*(1–2), 1–69.

Tuhiwai Smith, L. (2012). *Decolonizing methodologies: Research and Indigenous peoples* (2nd ed.). New York, NY: Zed Books.

Wallerstein, N. (1999). Power between evaluator and community: Research relationships within New Mexico's healthier communities. *Social Science & Medicine, 49,* 39–53.

Wallerstein, N., & Auerbach, E. (2004). *Problem-posing at work: A popular educator's guide.* Edmonton, AB, Canada: Grassroots Press.

Wallerstein, N., & Duran, B. (2010). Community-based participatory research contributions to intervention research: The intersection of science and practice to improve health equity. *American Journal Public Health, 100*(Suppl 1), S40–S46.

Wallerstein, N., Oetzel, J., Duran, B., Magarati, M., Pearson, C., Belone, L., Davis, J., Dewindt, L., Lucero, J., Ruddock, C., Sutter, E., Villegas, M., & Dutta., M. (under review). Conceptualizing and measuring the culture-centered approach in community based participatory research. *Social Science & Medicine.*

Whitesell, N., Stanley, L., Allen, J. (2018). *Prevention Science. Special Issue: Innovations in intervention research with indigenous populations in the U.S.*

Whyte, W. (Ed.). (1991). *Participatory action research.* Thousand Oaks, CA: Sage.

Wolf, D. (Ed.). (1996). *Feminist dilemmas in fieldwork.* Boulder, CO: Westview Press.

CHAPTER 3

CRITICAL ISSUES IN DEVELOPING AND FOLLOWING CBPR PRINCIPLES

BARBARA A. ISRAEL, AMY J. SCHULZ, EDITH A. PARKER, ADAM B. BECKER, ALEX J. ALLEN, III, J. RICARDO GUZMAN, AND RICHARD LICHTENSTEIN

RESEARCHERS HAVE SOUGHT to address the disproportionate and growing burden of morbidity and mortality in recent decades in low social and economic resource communities and in communities of color. Yet, the history of research abuse and frequent absence of benefit to the communities most affected have understandably made community members skeptical of research. These challenges, as well as systematic exclusion of non-researchers from influence over the research process, have made it important for researchers to address fundamental questions such as, What is the purpose of research? Who benefits from research? How are the results of research used? How can research contribute to reducing health inequities? And what role does research play in community change and knowledge generation?

Community-based participatory research (CBPR), with its growing influence in addressing health inequities (Braun et al., 2015; Israel, Eng, Schulz, & Parker, 2013b; Jones & Wells, 2007; Minkler, Garcia, Rubin, & Wallerstein, 2012), has embraced the importance of these questions. A set of CBPR principles, first proposed in 1998 (Israel, Schulz, Parker, & Becker, 1998), has offered guidelines to encourage researchers to think about their own assumptions in conducting research with communities and to adopt an approach toward equitable community engagement.

Recognizing that each setting and research partnership is unique, local issues need to be considered when adhering to or adapting CBPR principles for distinct contexts. This chapter presents principles derived from the literature and the collective experiences of the authors and then uses case examples from the Detroit Community-Academic Urban Research Center (Detroit URC) and its affiliated partnerships[1] to illustrate them. Throughout the chapter, we emphasize the importance of flexibility, reflection, and critical analysis in applying and adapting these principles in different contexts.

CBPR DEFINITION AND KEY PRINCIPLES

The following ten principles capture key elements of CBPR as currently understood; the first nine of which were initially identified in 1998 by Israel and colleagues.[2] They are presented with the recognition that they will continue to evolve as further work is conducted and evaluated and that the extent to which any research endeavor achieves any combination of these principles will vary depending on the context, purpose, and participants involved. Most of the principles are located on a continuum, with the principles as described here representing an ideal goal toward which to strive. Finally, although each is presented here as a distinct principle, ultimately CBPR is an integration of them all.

CBPR Recognizes Community as a Unit of Identity

The concept of community as an aspect of collective and individual identity is central to CBPR. Units of identity—for example, membership in a family, friendship network, or geographical neighborhood—are socially constructed, created, and re-created through social interactions (Hatch et al., 1993; Steuart, 1993). Community is characterized by identification with and emotional connection to other members, common symbol systems, shared values and norms, mutual (although not necessarily equal) influence, collective interests, and joint commitment to meeting shared needs (Israel, Checkoway, Schulz, & Zimmerman, 1994). Communities of identity may exist within defined geographical boundaries or be made up of members of a dispersed group with acknowledged commonalities (e.g., shared racial, ethnic, gender, or ability-related identities). Community-based participatory approaches to research attempt to work with existing communities of identity and to strengthen a sense of community through collective engagement (Israel et al., 1994). Communities of identity contain many individual and organizational resources but may also benefit from skills and resources available outside of the community.

CBPR Builds on Strengths and Resources within the Community

CBPR seeks to identify and build on strengths, resources, and relationships that exist within communities of identity to address members' communal health concerns (Steuart, 1993). These may include individuals' skills and assets; networks of relationships characterized by trust, cooperation, and mutual commitment; and mediating structures such as churches and other organizations where members come together. CBPR explicitly recognizes and seeks to support or expand social structures and processes that contribute to the ability of community members to work together to improve health.

CBPR Facilitates Collaborative, Equitable Partnership in All Research Phases and Involves an Empowering and Power-Sharing Process That Attends to Social Inequalities

In CBPR all parties participate in and share control, as desired, over all phases of the research process, including problem definition, data collection, interpretation of results, and application of results to address community concerns (Israel et al., 1998; Stringer, 2007). CBPR partnerships focus on issues identified by community members (Israel, Eng, Schulz, & Parker, 2013a) and create processes that enable equitable engagement in the research. Recognizing that marginalized communities often have limited power to name or define their own experience and that inequalities among community members shape participation and influence in collective research and action, researchers involved with CBPR acknowledge inequalities between themselves and community participants. Attempts to address these inequalities involve explicit attention to the knowledge and expertise of community members and an emphasis on empowering processes that include sharing information, decision-making power, resources, and support among members of the partnership (Israel et al., 1994; Jones & Wells, 2007; Wallerstein, 2006).

CBPR Promotes Co-learning and Capacity Building among All Partners

CBPR is a co-learning process that facilitates the reciprocal transfer of knowledge, skills, and capacity (Corbie-Smith et al., 2015). For example, researchers can learn from community members' management and leadership skills and understandings about the community and broader social context, and community members can acquire further research skills. The emphasis here is on enhancing the capacity of all partners, improving the effectiveness of the CBPR effort, and increasing capacity that can be applied to members' other endeavors.

CBPR Integrates and Achieves a Balance between Research and Action for the Mutual Benefit of All Partners

CBPR seeks to build a broad body of knowledge about health while using the knowledge generated to support community and social change efforts that address concerns of the involved community (Corbie-Smith et al., 2015). Information is gathered to inform action, and new understandings emerge as participants reflect on actions taken. CBPR incorporates a commitment to the translation and integration of research results with community change efforts for the benefit of all partners.

CBPR Emphasizes Public Health Problems of Local Relevance and Ecological Perspectives That Attend to the Multiple Determinants of Health and Disease

CBPR addresses public health problems of concern to the community and considers the concept of health from a multidimensional perspective that emphasizes physical, mental, and social well-being. It also emphasizes an ecological model of health (Sallis & Owen, 2015) that considers and encompasses the individual, his or her immediate contexts (e.g., family, social network), and the larger social spheres or institutions in which they are embedded. Such approaches recognize and attend to biomedical, social, economic, cultural, and physical environmental factors as determinants of health and disease. Given these foci, CBPR efforts strive to achieve broadscale social changes intended to eliminate health inequities.

CBPR Involves Systems Development through a Cyclical and Iterative Process

CBPR involves systems development, so that a system (e.g., a partnership) develops the competencies to engage in a cyclical, iterative process that includes multiple phases. These include partnership development and maintenance; community assessment; problem definition, development of research methodology; data collection and analysis; interpretation of data; determination of action and policy implications; dissemination of results; action taking (as appropriate); and establishment of mechanisms for sustainability (Israel et al., 1994; Stringer, 2007).

CBPR Disseminates Findings and Knowledge Gained to All Partners and Involves All Partners in the Dissemination Process

CBPR disseminates findings and knowledge gained to all partners involved, in language that is understandable and respectful, and "where ownership of knowledge is acknowledged" (Bishop, 1994, p. 186; see also Hall, Tandon, & Tremblay, 2015). The ongoing feedback of data and use of results to inform action are integral to this approach (Baker, Mutton, Barnidge, & Rose, 2013; Schulz et al., 2011). This principle also calls for opportunities for all partners to engage in dissemination activities, for example, as coauthors or copresenters (Parker et al., 2013).

CBPR Requires a Long-term Process and Commitment to Sustainability

Given the negative experiences many communities have with research and the time and effort needed to rigorously follow the principles described here, CBPR requires a long-term process and commitment to sustainability on the part of all partners (Hatch et al., 1993; Israel et al., 2013a; Jones & Wells, 2007). To establish and maintain the trust required to conduct CBPR successfully and to accomplish the aim of reducing health inequities, this commitment must extend beyond a single research project or funding period and include a willingness to continue the partnership even without funding. Although there is no set time frame for the "long term," the emphasis is placed on development of relationships and commitments that extend beyond any one project. Some goals, for example, reducing environmental risks in a local community, may take decades to realize. Although a specific partnership may at some point decide not to continue, commitment to the relationships among partners or their organizations and to continued collaboration and support as needed and desired are critical characteristics of CBPR.

CBPR Addresses Issues of Race, Ethnicity, Racism, and Social Class and Embraces "Cultural Humility"

CBPR partnerships frequently involve community partners from historically marginalized groups and "outside" researchers and other institutional partners from more privileged backgrounds (Minkler, Garcia, et al., 2012). CBPR partners must strive to achieve what Tervalon and Murray-Garcia (1998) refer to as "cultural humility," recognizing that no one can fully master another's culture (Israel et al., 2013a; Minkler, Garcia, et al., 2012) (see Appendix 4). Cultural humility means a commitment to self-critique and self-reflection, including examining one's own racism and classism, addressing power imbalances, and establishing and maintaining authentic partnerships. One aspect of cultural humility in the research process is an understanding of the ways that questions of research validity may fail to reflect validity and relevance to diverse engaged communities (i.e., external validity). Thus, in addition to recognizing the need for traditional research validity, to develop sound and useful knowledge for policy and social change, CBPR partnerships must also encompass critical reflection regarding the ways that racism, classism, sexism, and other isms operate to delegitimize community knowledge. A commitment to cultural humility and to addressing these power imbalances can support partnerships' efforts to develop a more complete and less biased understanding of social processes, enhancing the "rigor, relevance, and reach" of the science produced in the process (Balazs & Morello-Frosch, 2013) (See also Appendix 1).

ISSUES IN DEVELOPING AND FOLLOWING CBPR PRINCIPLES

A number of critical issues can arise that need to be addressed when adopting or adapting guidelines such as those previously described. Several examples are discussed in the following sections.

No One Set of CBPR Principles Is Applicable to All Partnerships

Although our partnerships strongly support and work to apply the described CBPR principles, we recommend equally strongly that this particular set of principles not be adopted as is and imposed on other partnerships. Although some core values *underlying* the principles may be applicable in most situations, not all of the principles will be applicable in all settings and communities. Other principles, with complementary values, have been published, for example, for tribes (LaVeaux & Christopher, 2009; Walters et al., 2009); health care partnerships (Jones & Wells, 2007); HIV/AIDS partnerships in and with marginalized communities (Udoh et al., 2013); or they are written as ethical guidelines (also see Chapters 14–16 and Appendices 2, 3, 8, and 9). In keeping with the CBPR approach, principles must be *owned* by the partners involved and therefore need to be adapted to the local context of each partnership. The process of jointly developing principles provides an opportunity for dialogue and sharing of perspectives that helps build trust and establish relationships among partners (Udoh et al., 2013). (See Appendix 2 for development of LGBTQ+ principles and referral to Latino border principles and Appendix 3 for a set of international participatory health research principles.)

Developing our initial set of CBPR principles took nearly two years and involved numerous negotiations and revisions before adoption by the original partners (Schulz, Israel, Selig, & Bayer, 1998). Several years later, when the Detroit URC partnership was established, these principles were distributed, discussed, and adapted over a much shorter time frame. It took the partnership longer to internalize and own the principles through experiences gained over time. As particular decision points were faced, partners' interpretations of the meaning of some principles deepened. A set of CBPR principles therefore needs to develop and change within the dynamics of a specific partnership, ultimately viewed as a fluid and evolving process.

Each CBPR Partnership Must Define Its "Community"

CBPR principles will vary across partnerships, in part depending on how the "community" is defined and who represents that community. Recognizing that no single definition is applicable in all situations, an emerging CBPR partnership needs to discuss critical questions such as the following:

- Who is or represents the community?
- Who has influence, and how, if at all, are they involved?
- Who decides who the community partners will be in a CBPR effort?
- Are the community partners involved as individuals or as representatives of community-based organizations (CBOs)?
- If as individuals, do community members have a constituency that they represent and to whom are they accountable?
- If as a CBO, what is the connection or link between the CBO and the residents of the community in which it works?
- How do the participants involved in the partnership compare to members of the community in terms of income, education, gender, race or ethnicity, and other identities?
- Who has the time, resources, skills, and flexibility to serve on committees, attend meetings, or review documents as necessary?

The Detroit URC and affiliated partnerships initially involved two geographically bounded communities of identity: predominantly African American East Side Detroit and southwest Detroit, with Detroit's largest percentage of Latinos. During the formation phase, academic and health department partners who established the Detroit URC invited community partners as organizational representatives from CBOs highly respected by the community (Israel et al., 2001). To the extent possible, individuals who held or were appointed by those who held leadership positions within a CBO were selected to serve on the Detroit URC board (Israel et al., 2001).

Members of the board, even those who reside within the community, can be somewhat different from community members at large, often in education and income. But such differences do not mean that they are not community members, and partners from academia and health agencies need to be careful not to impose a definition of what it means to be "from the community." Indeed, in marginalized communities, it is often those with more formal education and income who are best situated to participate in CBPR but at the same time having an inside view of life in the community (Steuart, 1993). Critical reflections by individuals and the collective are central to these conversations about who represents the community and the accountability of the partnership to the community.

All Partners Must Decide What It Means to Have a "Collaborative, Equitable Partnership" and How to Make That Happen

Perhaps one of the most critical principles of CBPR is the emphasis on shared control in decision making. As an ideal to strive for, this is a core value of CBPR, but how is equity and shared influence and control ensured? Every partnership needs to ask itself whether members are *partners* or just *part* of the *partnership*—in other words, are all partners ready and able to share power? This requires considerable time and attention to the partnership process from all involved, which may be frustrating for some, particularly if it is perceived to draw time and energy away from accomplishing specific objectives (Israel, Lantz, et al., 2013).

The Detroit URC has engaged in a number of strategies to define and try to achieve a collaborative, equitable partnership (Israel et al., 2001). In one group exercise, each member identified the characteristics of effective groups that they had belonged to and then used them to create operating norms for working together (e.g., mutual respect, everyone's opinion is valued, agree to disagree) (Israel et al., 2001). These norms were distributed at a board meeting, used as key indicators in the partnership evaluation, and reviewed and revised as deemed necessary by the board.

Another procedure is the board's use of consensus rather than majority rule in decision making. Although substantial evidence shows that consensus results in improved decisions on complex issues and enhanced commitment to the decision, it can take considerable time and may hamper some decision making (Johnson & Johnson, 2014). The Detroit URC board employs a slight variation, referred to as the 70 percent rule, which requires that each partner be at least 70 percent in favor of a given decision. This approach has enabled board members to thoroughly examine issues and consider multiple perspectives prior to making a decision, giving everyone the opportunity to express opinions, influence the decisions made, and develop support for decisions reached without the expectation that everyone will be in complete agreement on all decisions (Becker, Israel, & Allen, 2013; Israel et al., 2001).

The Detroit URC also works toward equitable distribution of resources for involved partners, including direct and indirect costs associated with grants (Lantz et al., 2001). Recent evidence shows that sharing resources is associated with improved partnership outcomes (Oetzel et al., 2015). Although core Detroit URC funding and some affiliated partnership's project funds go primarily to the university involved, several arrangements contribute to more equitable distribution. These include (1) board and steering committee review of core funding and influence in budget-related decisions, (2) CBOs serving as fiduciary and lead organizations on some grants, (3) CBOs subcontracting for specific work, and (4) CBOs always receiving modest compensation. The distribution of resources has the potential to create conflicts in a partnership and requires ongoing consideration (Jones & Wells, 2007). Not all partner organizations may have an interest in or capability for managing large-scale projects, and this may be an area in which to focus capacity-building efforts. In addition, other ways to distribute the benefits and rewards of participating in CBPR projects need to be explored by a partnership (for example, attendance and presentations at professional meetings) (Brakefield Caldwell et al., 2015).

Although, for the most part, the Detroit URC and affiliated partnerships have used a highly participatory, informal, and somewhat fluid approach to achieve equity, there has also been attention to more formal, structural approaches, such as establishing memoranda of understanding (MOUs) and developing partnership bylaws (Oetzel et al., 2015; Yonas et al., 2013). Although these may be helpful for partnership success, in other situations, the very formality of such structures may negatively affect trust and power sharing. Here again, partnerships should discuss and select strategies that are most appropriate based on their history, norms, and preferences.

Although shared influence and equity are goals of CBPR, some inequities among partners are difficult to erase, especially when they involve race, gender, and class. Acknowledging and discussing these inequities may reduce the impact they may have on the relationships and the work of the partnership (Udoh et al., 2013).

Not Everyone Will Be Involved in the Same Way in All Activities

Another core value of CBPR is that all partners participate in all phases of the research process. Here again, CBPR partnerships need to determine what that means for them, realizing that not everyone may be involved in the same way in all activities. For example, in the East Side Village

Health Worker Partnership and the Healthy Environments Partnership (Detroit URC–affiliated partnerships), the steering committees played major roles in developing a conceptual framework, designing a survey, interpreting results, and applying them to implement intervention strategies (Schulz et al., 2011, 2015). By their own choice, the steering committees were not involved in survey data entry or statistical analysis. Given time demands and technical aspects, different levels of involvement may be appropriate for different partners, and partners are also given opportunities to enhance their skills, as desired. Finally, and regardless of decisions made about data entry and analysis, it is crucial that results be fed back to partners in ways that are understandable and useful and that all partners engage in the interpretation process, which might include requesting additional statistical analyses.

Establish Procedures for Dissemination

Questions related to the dissemination of findings include the following:

- Who will be the coauthors of publications and copresenters at professional meetings?
- How are these decisions made?
- What are their roles and responsibilities?
- What happens when only one partner is invited to present or submit an article?
- How is a balance reached between providing feedback to the community and writing publications?

Here again, there is no one answer to these questions that will work for all partnerships. Rather, a partnership needs to develop procedures to ensure that the dissemination principle is followed.

The Detroit URC–affiliated Community Action Against Asthma (CAAA) steering committee established a dissemination subcommittee, made up of an equal number of university and community partners, which met over several months to draft dissemination procedures (also see Appendix 9). These procedures, subsequently modified by the full steering committee, spell out selection processes and roles for coauthors and copresenters (Parker et al., 2013). Although we recommend that written dissemination procedures be established, flexibility is important in order to accommodate requests that may not fit within the specified parameters.

Recognize and Value Priorities Identified by the Community

Although CBPR emphasizes the importance of addressing social determinants of health at multiple levels of practice, researchers need to be careful not to impose that approach on the partnership. Understandably, community partners may initially be interested in addressing issues that seem more amenable to change than trying to address policies associated with social determinants of health. Indeed, community-organizing literature indicates that effective organizing is built on winning tangible, small-scale changes in a relatively short period of time (Minkler & Wallerstein, 2012). As noted by Minkler, Pies, and Hyde (2012), one of the key ethical precepts of community organizing and, we would add, of CBPR partnerships, is self-determination. A CBPR effort may begin by addressing priority issues identified by the community, evolve over time as partners engage in dialogue about the impact of social determinants on their priority issues, and eventually develop strategies to affect those determinants.

The East Side Village Health Worker Partnership used a stress process model as a conceptual framework for addressing the social determinants of health on Detroit's East Side (Parker, Schulz, Israel, & Hollis, 1998). Although the general model was included in the proposal written by members of the researcher team, a more specific, locally defined stress process model was developed by the steering committee (Parker et al., 1998). Based on this model and subsequent in-depth interviews and surveys with community members, village health workers prioritized the issues they wanted to address, such as enhancing relationships with the police, safety for children, and fostering environments that support diabetes management and prevention. Although each of these issues has underlying social determinants, the partnership's initial strategies emphasized short-term activities (Halloween parties for children or participating in a "Police Week"). These successful events led to an increased sense of community, and through ongoing conversations, some participants also began to engage in broader-scale policy and social changes.

Work with the Cultural Diversity of the Partners Involved

CBPR partnerships are likely to involve partners who differ in ethnicity and race, gender, social class, sexual orientation, ability-disability, community or academic role, academic discipline, and more. The multiple perspectives represented require development of a common language, trust, and mutual respect; understanding of the various cultures; and recognition that different participants may have different goals, agendas, and degrees of commitment to CBPR. Participants will also contend with conflicting loyalties and multiple demands on their time and will vary in what they can contribute to the CBPR effort. As noted, each CBPR partnership also has to consider how structural inequities contribute to the cultural differences that exist within it.

The Community Action Against Asthma project was the first Detroit URC–affiliated project to involve participants from East Side and southwest Detroit as well as researchers from environmental health and behavioral sciences. Initially, some researchers who had less experience with CBPR were perceived by community partners as being somewhat aloof and interested only in their research findings and not in the community members themselves. In addition, some Latino community partners interpreted some comments from African American partners as discriminatory toward Latinos. Undoing Racism training, small-group meetings, conflict resolution, and other strategies may be effective means of ensuring that partner diversity is respected and celebrated (Becker et al., 2013; Yonas et al., 2006, 2013; also see Chapters 4 and 8).

Differences also occur across research disciplines. On several occasions, for example, environmental and social scientists in CAAA have used the same words with different meanings. The term *qualitative data,* for example, was used by environmental scientists to mean any data not calibrated by a machine; thus, the results of a closed-ended survey were considered qualitative. In the social sciences, however, *qualitative data* involves open-ended data collection approaches. The recognition of these language differences has contributed some humor to our conversations but also a commitment to ongoing work to develop mutually understandable language.

Partnership Size Must Be Decided by and Appropriate for the Community

A frequently asked question is, What is the most appropriate or effective number of partners to include in a CBPR effort? No firm answer can be found in the literature; rather, the specific context and goals have to be considered, and the initial partners involved have to decide what is most appropriate in their particular situation. Our own experience suggests that a CBPR partnership start small, beginning with partner organizations from only one or two communities of identity. Such an approach has the advantage of building on existing relationships and the likelihood of identifying mutually agreed-on goals. It is further supported by evidence that the most effective size for problem-solving groups is eight to twelve individuals (Johnson & Johnson, 2014). If there are preestablished, long-standing relationships in the community of identity, a partnership might be effective with a somewhat larger initial number of partners. There also may be limits to skills and resources in smaller groups, such that a slightly larger core group (ideally not more than twelve to sixteen partner organizations) may be needed.

In our own work, we often use a Venn diagram approach to participation. At the center of a series of overlapping circles is a core group of project partners who make up the partnership decision-making core. Specific work groups or action teams may consist of other individuals or organizations invited to participate as members of an outer, nonoverlapping circle, along with members of the core group. Another approach that we use could more closely be represented using a concentric circle diagram, in which the core partners in the CBPR effort are represented in the center circle, and other organizations are invited to participate in a more limited way (outer circle). For example, the Detroit URC board, which is the core governance body, has established a Community-Academic Research Network involving more than one hundred academic researchers and fifty CBOs (www.detroiturc.org/expertise-programs/community-academic-research-network.html). In general we recommend that the core group remain fairly small, recognizing that there are multiple approaches to expanding to include others as needed. It is helpful to develop a set of criteria for new membership and for the existing partners to discuss and agree on the needs of the partnership and the expectations and responsibilities of new members. Spelling out criteria more formally (see, for example, Detroit URC criteria for membership: www.detroiturc.org/resources/urc-cbpr-tools.html) can be useful, while retaining flexibility in implementation to retain the strength of a community-driven participatory process.

Recognize That CBPR Principles Alone Do Not Dictate Research Design

Some confusion in the field is manifested in the suggestion that CBPR, by definition, dictates the types of research design and methods that are appropriate. CBPR is an approach to conducting research, rather than a method, and no one design or method is appropriate for all CBPR efforts (see Chapter 1). Instead, each partnership must decide what works best for its research question and community context. In our East Side Village Health Worker Partnership, in addition to conducting in-depth group dialogues and interviews on the stress process, we conducted a random sample survey with community residents to assess beliefs, opinions, and experiences more broadly (Parker et al., 1998).

In addition, although we suggest that research designs that involve the use of a control group that receives no direct benefit from the research are neither appropriate nor ethical in the context of CBPR, there are other viable designs. For example, the Healthy Environments Partnership implemented a lagged study design in which half of the participants in any cohort were randomly selected to receive the intervention and the lagged "control group" waited eight weeks before they began the intervention, a fairly standard design (Schulz et al., 2015).

Continually Evaluate How Well CBPR Principles Are Followed

To develop and maintain an effective CBPR partnership and to enhance participants' understanding of the factors that contribute to this effectiveness, it is necessary to conduct an ongoing evaluation of the extent to which, and in what ways, the CBPR principles are being implemented (Israel et al., 2001; Israel, Lantz, et al., 2013). Increasingly, partnerships are seeking methods and metrics to reflect on their own development and to assess their effectiveness over time (Israel et al., 2013; Oetzel et al., 2015) (see also Appendix 10).

Since its founding, the Detroit URC has conducted evaluations to assess board members' perceptions and experiences of the board's activities, processes, and progress, including accomplishments, adherence to CBPR principles, challenges, and facilitating factors (Israel et al., 2001; Israel, Lantz, et al., 2013). An evaluation subcommittee of the board initially guided this assessment, which included multiple data collection methods (e.g., in-depth interviews, closed-ended survey questionnaires). Evaluation results have been fed back and discussed at board meetings. This process has enhanced members' understanding of the CBPR principles adopted and contributed to modifications in board processes to more effectively follow them (Israel et al., 2001; Israel, Lantz, et al., 2013).

CONCLUSION

Researchers, practitioners, and community members committed to addressing social and economic inequities in health status need more equitable approaches to research that involve action and knowledge generation beneficial to, and reflective of, the communities involved. CBPR is one approach that engages diverse partners in strategies aimed at obtaining multiple perspectives in order to address community-identified concerns. Our CBPR principles may be used as guidelines by those interested in this approach. We reiterate that no one set of existing principles is appropriate for all communities and all situations. Similarly, there is not just one approach to CBPR. As partnerships consider the issues raised here, each will develop its own approach to inquiry and change, along with principles that are appropriate for its own partners working together in their specific context. What is crucial is the long-term commitment to reducing fundamental inequalities that exist throughout the systems in which we live and work.

QUESTIONS FOR DISCUSSION

1. In what ways do the principles discussed in this chapter add to our understanding of CBPR's theoretical base? How do they reflect this theory?
2. The chapter authors state that "no one set of CBPR principles is applicable to all partnerships." Think of a partnership you are familiar with or that you have read about. Are there principles you might modify to better meet the needs of this partnership? Is there a new principle you would propose?
3. The Detroit URC made a conscious decision to include as partners community-based organizations rather than less formal, grassroots groups or individuals. What might be a benefit or downside of this approach?

NOTES

1. The Detroit Community-Academic Urban Research Center, established in 1995, fosters and supports the development, implementation, and evaluation of interdisciplinary, collaborative, community-based participatory research projects that aim to eliminate health inequities in Detroit (www.detroiturc.org). The authors thank Katie Abdou and Julia Weinert for their valuable assistance in the preparation of this manuscript.
2. This discussion includes excerpts and revised portions from a set of CBPR principles originally presented by Israel et al. (1998, pp. 177–180), with permission from the publisher.

REFERENCES

Baker, E. A., Mutton, F., Barnidge, E., & Rose, F. (2013). Collaborative data collection, interpretation, and action planning in a rural African American community: Men on the move. In B. A. Israel, E. Eng, A. J. Schulz, & E. A. Parker (Eds.), *Methods in community-based participatory research for health* (2nd ed., pp. 435–462). San Francisco, CA: Jossey-Bass.

Balazs, C. L., & Morello-Frosch, R. (2013). The three R's: How community-based participatory research strengthens the rigor, relevance and reach of science. *Environmental Justice, 6*(1). doi:10.1089/env.2012.0017

Becker, A. B., Israel, B. A., & Allen, A. (2013). Strategies and techniques for effective group process in CBPR partnerships. In B. A. Israel, E. Eng, A. J. Schulz, & E. A. Parker (Eds.), *Methods in community-based participatory research for health* (2nd ed., pp. 69–96). San Francisco, CA: Jossey-Bass.

Bishop, R. (1994). Initiating empowering research? *New Zealand Journal of Educational Studies, 29,* 175–188.

Brakefield Caldwell, W., Reyes, A. G., Rowe, Z., Weinert, J., & Israel, B. A. (2015). Community partner perspectives on benefits, challenges, facilitating factors, and lessons learned from community-based participatory research partnerships in Detroit. *Progress in Community Health Partnerships: Research, Education, and Action, 9*(2), 299–311.

Braun, K. L., Stewart, S., Baquet, C., Berry-Bobovski, L., Blumenthal, D., Brandt, H. M., et al. (2015). The National Cancer Institute's community networks program initiative to reduce cancer health disparities: Outcomes and lessons learned. *Progress in Community Health Partnerships* (Suppl. 9), 21–32.

Corbie-Smith, G., Bryant, A. R., Walker, D. J., Blumenthal, C., Council, B., Courtney, D., & Adimora, A. (2015). Building capacity in community-based participatory research partnerships through a focus on process and multiculturalism. *Progress in Community Health Partnerships: Research, Education, and Action, 9*(2), 261–273.

Hall, B., Tandon, R., & Tremblay, C. (Eds.). (2015). *Strengthening community-university research partnerships: Global perspectives*. Victoria, BC, Canada: University of Victoria.

Hatch, J., Moss, N., Saran, A., Presley-Cantrell, L., & Mallory, C. (1993). Community research: Partnership in Black communities. *American Journal of Preventive Medicine, 9*(6), 27–31.

Israel, B. A., Checkoway, B., Schulz, A. J., & Zimmerman, M. A. (1994). Health education and community empowerment: Conceptualizing and measuring perceptions of individual, organizational, and community control. *Health Education Quarterly, 21,* 149–170.

Israel, B. A., Eng, E., Schulz, A. J., & Parker, E. A. (2013a). Introduction. In B. A. Israel, E. Eng, A. J. Schulz, & E. Parker (Eds.), *Methods for community-based participatory research for health* (2nd ed., pp. 3–37). San Francisco, CA: Jossey-Bass.

Israel, B. A., Eng, E., Schulz, A. J., & Parker, E. A. (Eds.). (2013b). *Methods for community-based participatory research for health* (2nd ed.). San Francisco, CA: Jossey-Bass.

Israel, B. A., Lantz, P. M., McGranaghan, R., Guzman, J. R., Lichtenstein, R., & Rowe, Z. (2013). Documentation and evaluation of community-based participatory research partnerships: The use of in-depth interviews and closed-ended questionnaires. In B. A. Israel, E. Eng, A. J. Schulz, & E. A. Parker (Eds.), *Methods for community-based participatory research for health* (2nd ed., pp. 369–397). San Francisco, CA: Jossey-Bass.

Israel, B. A., Lichtenstein, R., Lantz, P. M., McGranaghan, R. J., Allen, A., Guzman, J. R., et al. (2001). The Detroit Community-Academic Urban Research Center: Lessons learned in the development, implementation, and evaluation of a community-based participatory research partnership. *Journal of Public Health Management and Practice, 7*(5), 1–19.

Israel, B. A., Schulz, A. J., Parker, E. A., & Becker, A. B. (1998). Review of community-based research: Assessing partnership approaches to improve public health. *Annual Review of Public Health, 19,* 173–202.

Johnson, D. W., & Johnson, F. P. (2014). *Joining together: Group theory and group skills* (11th ed.). Boston, MA: Allyn & Bacon.

Jones, L., & Wells, K. (2007). Strategies for academic and clinician engagement in community-partnered participatory research. *Journal of the American Medical Association, 297,* 407–410.

Lantz, P. M., Viruell-Fuentes, E., Israel, B. A., Softley, D., & Guzman, J. R. (2001). Can communities and academia work together on public health research? Evaluation results from a community-based participatory research partnership in Detroit. *Journal of Urban Health, 78,* 495–507.

LaVeaux, D., & Christopher, S. (2009). Contextualizing CBPR: Key principles of CBPR meet the Indigenous research context. *Pimatisiwin: A Journal of Aboriginal and Indigenous Community Health, 7*(1), 1–25.

Minkler, M., Garcia, A. P., Rubin, V., & Wallerstein, N. (2012). *Community-based participatory research: A strategy for building health communities and promoting health through policy change.* Oakland, CA: PolicyLink.

Minkler, M., Pies, C., & Hyde, C. A. (2012). Ethical issues in community organization and community participation. In M. Minkler, *Community organizing and community building for health and welfare* (3rd ed., pp. 110–129). New Brunswick, NJ: Rutgers University Press.

Minkler, M., & Wallerstein, N. (2012). Improving health through community organization and community building: Perspectives from health education and social work. In M. Minkler, *Community organizing and community building for health and welfare* (3rd ed., pp. 37–58). New Brunswick, NJ: Rutgers University Press.

Oetzel, J. G., Villegas, M., Zenone, H., White Hat, E., Wallerstein, N., & Duran, B. (2015). Enhancing stewardship of community-engage research through governance. *American Journal of Public Health, 105*(6), 1161–1167.

Parker, E. A., Robins, T. G., Israel, B. A., Brakefield, C. W., Edgren, K., & Wilkins, D. J. (2013). Developing and implementing guidelines for dissemination: The experience of the Community Action Against Asthma Project. In B. A. Israel, E. Eng, A. J. Schulz, & E. A. Parker (Eds.), *Methods for community-based participatory research for health* (2nd ed., pp. 405–433, 639–643). San Francisco, CA: Jossey-Bass.

Parker, E. A., Schulz, A. J., Israel, B. A., & Hollis, R. (1998). Detroit's East Side Village Health Worker Partnership: Community-based lay health advisor intervention in an urban area. *Health Education & Behavior, 25*(1), 24–45.

Sallis, J. F., & Owen, N. (2015). Ecological models of health behavior. In K. Glanz, B. K. Rimer, & K. Viswanath (Eds.), *Health behavior: Theory, research and practice* (5th ed., pp. 43–64). San Francisco, CA: Jossey-Bass.

Schulz, A. J., Israel, B. A., Coombe, C., Gaines, C., Reyes, A., Rowe, Z., et al. (2011). A community-based participatory planning process and multilevel intervention design: Toward eliminating cardiovascular health inequities. *Health Promotion Practice, 12*(6), 900–912.

Schulz, A. J., Israel, B. A., Mentz, G. B., Bernal, C., Caver, D., DeMajo, R., et al. (2015). Effectiveness of a walking group intervention to promote physical activity and cardiovascular health in predominantly non-Hispanic Black and Hispanic urban neighborhoods: Findings from the Walk Your Heart to Health Intervention. *Health Education & Behavior, 42*(3), 380–392.

Schulz, A. J., Israel, B. A., Selig, S. M., & Bayer, I. S. (1998). Development and implementation of principles for community-based research in public health. In R. H. MacNair (Ed.), *Research strategies for community practice* (pp. 83–110). New York, NY: Haworth Press.

Steuart, G. W. (1993). Social and cultural perspectives: Community intervention and mental health. *Health Education Quarterly* (Suppl 1), S99–S111.

Stringer, E. T. (2007). *Action research* (3rd ed.). Thousand Oaks, CA: Sage.

Tervalon, M., & Murray-Garcia, J. (1998). Cultural humility versus cultural competence: A critical distinction in defining physician training outcomes in multicultural education. *Journal of Healthcare for the Poor and Underserved, 9*(2), 117–125.

Udoh, I., Minkler, M., Dillard Smith, C., Chopel, A., Walton, S., Grijalva, C., et al. (2013). Developing and using a partnership covenant to guide a study of late stage HIV diagnosis. *Progress in Community Health Partnerships: Research, Education, and Action, 7*(4), 403–411.

Wallerstein, N. (2006). *Evidence of effectiveness of empowerment interventions to reduce health disparities and social exclusion.* Copenhagen, DK: Health Evidence Network, Regional Office, World Health Organization. Retrieved from www.euro.who.int/__data/assets/pdf_file/0010/74656/E88086.pdf

Walters, K., Stately, A., Evans-Campbell, T., Simoni, J., Duran, B., Schultz, K., et al. (2009). "Indigenist" collaborative research efforts in Native American communities. In A. R. Stiffman (Ed.), *The field research survival guide* (pp. 146–173). New York, NY: Oxford University Press.

Yonas, M., Aronson, R., Coad, N., Eng, E., Petteway, R., Schaal, J., & Webb, L. (2013). Infrastruture for equitable decision making in research. In B. A. Israel, E. Eng, A. J. Schulz, & E. A. Parker (Eds.), *Methods for community-based participatory research for health* (2nd ed., pp. 97–126). San Francisco, CA: Jossey-Bass.

Yonas, M. A., Jones, N., Eng, E., Vines, A. I., Aronson, R., Griffith, D. M., White, B., & DuBose, M. (2006). The art and science of integrating undoing racism with CBPR: Challenges of pursuing NIH funding to investigate cancer care and racial equity. *Journal of Urban Health, 83*(6), 1004–1012.

PART 2

POWER, TRUST, AND DIALOGUE: WORKING WITH DIVERSE COMMUNITIES

Well-documented and complex health and social inequities continue to challenge all nations across the globe and contribute to an immeasurable amount of suffering for living beings. These inequities are associated, in part, with historic and current-day power imbalances that often lead to loss of cultural and language identity, the discounting of traditional and place-based knowledge systems, and the pathologizing of ways of being. CBPR or community-engaged research (CEnR) is one response to health and social disparities among communities underserved by large national institutions such as economic systems, higher education, health and medicine, and social services and policy.

Consequently, most if not all CBPR and CEnR takes place among groups of people with varying types and degrees of diversity: race, cultural, language, economic, education, geographic, ability, and so on. Key elements of engagement success, therefore, are related to the ability of mainstream research institutions and community and other partners to acquire the skills and abilities to work across difference with trust and competence.

The two chapters in Part Two provide expert history, theory, and guidance about the need for trust, cultural and racial competence, and skill building when working across differences for equity. In Chapter 4, Michael Muhammad and colleagues adopt a critical perspective to explain how the intersecting dimensions of racism, power, and privilege can be reinscribed through the white normalcy found in everyday research practices, even among groups with similar values, ethnicities, and histories. The pernicious resistance to dismantling covert exploitive social structures (e.g., race and gender, education, economic privilege, etc.) is played out in CBPR through language: microaggressions, invalidations, and insults that affect trust and expose conflicted commitment, knowledge, and skills. The chapter illustrates problems and solutions through two case studies that highlight intersecting oppressions and power structures in research: pressures to conform to institutional research process that privileges dominant group values and communication styles and that devalue others. The chapter ends with recommendations for disrupting business as usual and creating equity in research partnerships. (Chapter 8 also provides concrete measures to undo racism in CBPR projects.)

In Chapter 5, Julie E. Lucero and colleagues review the strengths and challenges of the current literature and research on trust and its conceptualization and use in partnership research. Early literature on the topic often considered trust only from the academic partners' perspective and characterized trust as an "outcome" and dichotomous variable, present or absent. Lucero outlines the problems with these conceptualizations and provides qualitative and quantitative evidence from multiple partner perspectives for a multidimensional trust typology. The comprehensive and multisector perspectives of the typology provide important process variables for partnership to consider when assessing partnership relational dynamics and provide guidance on the ground for working with integrity across difference. Further issues of relationship processes are outlined in the descriptions of the CBPR model and partnership evaluation methods in Chapters 6 and 17.

CHAPTER 4

UNDERSTANDING CONTEMPORARY RACISM, POWER, AND PRIVILEGE AND THEIR IMPACTS ON CBPR

MICHAEL MUHAMMAD, CATALINA GARZÓN, ANGELA REYES, AND THE WEST OAKLAND ENVIRONMENTAL INDICATORS PROJECT

RACISM IS AN inescapable structural social determinant in the United States and globally, with deep and broad impact on health inequities in communities of color, and therefore with significant implications for the practice and outcomes of CBPR partnerships. The distribution of health inequities reflects the extensive structural inequalities prevalent within society intersecting across racial, ethnic, gender, sexual orientation, and socioeconomic class designations. Social attitudes and opinions also affect health for marginalized populations through knowledge produced that further constrain their ability to access resources providing health benefits.

Because of the cumulative effect of racism, which leads to widespread negative health outcomes, this chapter focuses on the complexities of racism. Structural inequality and institutional racism, most notably the residue of political and legal disenfranchisement and discrimination of American Indians, Asians, Blacks, and Latinos, has contributed to significant inequities in health for people of color (Gee & Ford, 2011; King, Smith, & Gracey, 2009; Williams, 2012). Cultural beliefs about the inherent differences between racialized social groups rationalize differential access to health-promoting resources through stereotypes, stigmatization, and implicitly held bias (Smedley, 2012). The multiple vulnerabilities produced by racism are further complicated through the intersection of positionality and power inequality.

This chapter adopts a critical perspective for how the intersecting dimensions of racism, power, and privilege can be reinscribed while conducting CBPR, even when participants share a common identity as people of color. In comprehending how whites benefit from a system of racialized oppression and privilege, CBPR practitioners will be positioned to better understand the systemic organization of modern racism, making overt acts of prejudice and discrimination obsolete, and understand how hegemonic reinforcement of existing racialized social relations can be consciously or *unconsciously* reproduced by any person, regardless of racial or ethnic identity. Readers also will become more familiar with the various forms that power and privilege can take in our work, within and beyond racism. Our goal is to build on these understandings and strengthen existing CBPR approaches for disrupting the reproduction of racial inequality and other hierarchies of power and privilege to promote sustainable, equitable partnering processes within diverse academic-community partnerships.

We offer two examples of how academics and community leaders can engage in ongoing strategies to conduct antiracist and power-equalizing interventions to deepen CBPR partnerships and increase the impact of research endeavors. In an environmental justice (EJ) case study from West Oakland, California, we illustrate how an African American community leader in the EJ movement and her academically trained research partner, a Latina who shared her deep commitment to addressing environmental racism, collaborated to colead an effective CBPR effort for action and change while also increasing honest dialogue within the partnership about power and privilege. Second, we offer the reflections of a multiracial, multicultural, interdisciplinary team at the University of New Mexico in confronting their own opportunities and limitations in seeking to create equitable research partnerships with communities of color who have faced long histories of racism.

CBPR AND THE EXPLORATION OF RACISM

More than twenty-five years of evidence demonstrate the role of CBPR in seeking to create equitable research environments in the pursuit of shared goals of health equity and environmental and social justice. However, far less attention has been placed on integrating the conceptual frames developed from antiracism research as a component of participatory partnering processes. This is especially important for confronting contemporary racism in the conduct of CBPR. Here is the *uncomfortable* part: all "whites" derive some degree of benefit (often including economic) from racism in the United States. A major challenge, therefore, concerning the practice of authentic CBPR is the need to train practitioners to perceive the covert mechanisms by which racism is reproduced within social relations and to maintain a self-awareness for how attention to equitable partnering processes is essential to disrupting the perpetuation of systemic racism.

Some CBPR scholars have employed theoretical, interpretive, and conceptual frameworks that aid researchers in clarifying how racial inequality undermines a genuine commitment to equitable partnering practices (Chavez et al., 2008). Popular approaches for antiracism work within CBPR coalesce around social justice, white privilege, cultural humility, and postcolonial epistemologies (Wallerstein & Duran, 2006). Jones's (2000) insightful allegory, the gardener's tale, has been used to deconstruct the differences among structural, interpersonal, and internalized racism. Each of these frameworks offers unique strengths, perspectives, and analytical techniques useful for studying the impact of racism in diverse CBPR partnerships. We add to these paradigms three cutting-edge theoretical and analytical approaches of antiracism scholarship—systemic racism, covert racism, and linguistic racial accommodation (LRA)—which are more specifically attuned to the task of clarifying the often obfuscated and subtle nature of contemporary racism.

UNDERSTANDING RACISM AND ANTIRACISM FRAMEWORKS

A major obstacle confronting those engaged in antiracism research, activism, and scholarship working from diverse backgrounds and across major disciplines is the lack of consensus in clearly defining the terms *race, racist,* and *racism.* Although social construction of identity has gained credibility over biological classifications of superior and inferior races (Smedley & Smedley, 2005), the addition of bi- and multiracial classifications along with the conflation of *race* with *ethnicity* increases the potential for confusion, miscommunication, and lack of conceptual clarity for antiracism CBPR work.

Three-Tiered Racism Framework

Jones (2000) has developed a framework for understanding racism as institutionalized, personally mediated, and internalized. Institutionalized racism manifests itself in material conditions and access to power, such as differential access to quality education, gainful employment, appropriate medical facilities, and clean environments. With regard to power, institutionalized racism includes differential access to information, including one's own history, resources, and voice, and differential representation in government and the media. Personally mediated racism refers to prejudice, discrimination, and judgments based on assumptions about others according to their race. As Jones (2000) notes, this "is what most people think of when they hear the word *racism* . . . It manifests as lack of respect, suspicion, devaluation, scapegoating, and dehumanization" (p. 300). Internalized racism does not need an outside judge of character. It is characterized by people's own belief in the negative messages they receive about their race or ethnicity. The core of this perspective is that "an oppressive society re-creates itself in its victims' hearts" (Sherover-Marcuse, 1986, p. 4). Internalized oppression addresses subjectivity, questions of power, and the part each person plays in the evolution of his or her own life story. It acknowledges that oppression does not *only* come from an external intersection of multiple systems of inequality; the enemy is also within.

Systemic Racism

Systemic racism adds a conceptual and interpretative scheme of structured relations with interdependent features that Feagin (2006) refers to as the *white racial frame.* This frame comprises a web of interrelated social practices, policies, attitudes, norms, and stereotypes that serve to reinforce social relations perpetuating white racial dominance. This interplay of social forces and institutional practices has created privileges and advantages for whites as a direct result of denying the same for people of color. Racial oppression has lasted for several centuries and has become well entrenched and pervasive across all major US institutions because of a "social inertia" that resists change. The white racial frame rationalizes and justifies racial and socioeconomic inequality according to a belief system that conveniently omits the violent oppression of people of color, including decades of legal discrimination as fundamental tenets of white privilege and status. Concurrently, a continuously shifting narrative lauding work ethic, intelligence, and cultural superiority is socially reproduced explaining white racial dominance.

Systemic racism will remain intact until the social processes reproducing the multilevel structures of racial hierarchy and power inequity are disrupted. What this implies is that whites must acknowledge the unearned privileges and benefits accruing from the ongoing oppression of American Indians, Asians, Blacks, and Latinos and become actively engaged in deconstructing embedded racist beliefs, practices, and policies throughout society.

Covert Racism and Microaggression

In contemporary society, overt expressions of racial prejudice and discriminatory practices are most often no longer publicly acceptable and, in some cases, illegal. However, resistance to dismantling inegalitarian social structures and relations is often encountered indirectly. Covert racism is subtle and allows for informal mechanisms of reward, prestige, or privilege not based on the rule of law (Coates, 2011). Covert racism can be language interwoven with racially coded meaning to induce racial animus and practices that serve to reinforce white privilege. Covert racist practices are skillfully employed to avoid open criticism of being racially motivated or clearly recognized as prejudice or discrimination. Covert racism is often expressed through microlevel interactions as *microaggressions,* meaning "commonplace verbal or behavioral indignities, whether intentional or unintentional, which communicate hostile, derogatory, or negative racial slights and insults" (Sue et al., 2007, p. 278). These can be *micro-insults,* expressed as unconscious remarks or actions that convey rudeness, such as a white county planning commissioner's openly snickering while Latino community residents offer testimony during public hearings, or *micro-invalidation,* often unconscious verbal comments or actions that exclude or negate the feelings or lived experiences of a person of color, such as holding an important community meeting in a Latino community with a large non-English-speaking population without Spanish language translators.

Racism is often subsumed within the dimensions of positionality and power inequity. In community-academic CBPR partnerships, power (e.g., positionality, education, income, and privilege) usually resides with academic researchers who are often white and live outside the communities they partner with. "Outside" experts can be faced with the dilemma of reinterpreting "insider" knowledge. The predilection to impose dominant group interpretive frames on local knowledge through re-articulation into more technical language may result in (unintentional) micro-invalidations that undermine mutual respect, co-learning, and devalues community partner contributions.

Linguistic Racial Accommodation (LRA)

A recent LRA framework and repertoire of analytical tools was developed by Cazenave (2016) for explicating "language-centered evenness and denial practices" that have become prevalent in mainstream discourses on race and racism. Cazenave calls the social reproduction of systemic racism through language, the ignorance, privilege, arrogance syndrome, a condition that occurs when dominant group members fail to recognize the oppression of subordinated groups: "that is the ignorance of not knowing, the privilege of not needing to know, and the arrogance of not wanting to know" (p. 17). Benign, abstract, and inconsequential language is often elicited to evade a serious critique of how whites continue to benefit from racism. For example, the terms *disadvantaged, at risk, or marginalized* are often used to describe communities of color. What is seldom mentioned is how these communities arrived in such condition, to what extent is racism responsible, and how whites as a dominant group derive benefit from impoverished and unstable communities of color. LRA conceptualizes how asymmetric power relations captivate the production of knowledge about racism with words and concepts that align with attitudes and behaviors of the dominant group, leaving the structural organization of racial oppression relatively unchallenged.

These frameworks have been introduced to aid in understanding racism as a complex system for creating and replicating social inequality within various domains and at multiple levels of social interaction. Racism is systemic, mediated at individual and institutional levels, and can be openly or subtly expressed. The recognition of racism in its various forms is only the first step in antiracism work. The social processes and practices sustaining inequality must be deconstructed with concise language that has the conceptual power to detect and clarify the racist underpinnings of white normalcy in everyday practices. The objective is to develop an awareness capable of grasping the mechanisms by which racial inequality is socially reproduced and disrupt the process.

BEYOND (AND WITHIN) RACISM: POWER AND PRIVILEGE IN CBPR

Similar to racism, the concepts of power and privilege are central to CBPR, particularly in feminist and Indigenous participatory research (Fine, 2004; Lonczak et al., 2013). In-depth work in the field has explored how participatory approaches challenge, reinforce, or change power relationships between trained researchers and community groups. However, this too is complicated. "Though practitioners of participatory research routinely draw on the concept that knowledge is power, they seldom publicly share how power dynamics between researchers and community partners have played out in particular partnerships . . ." (Garzón et al., 2013, p. 72). Discourse on power and privilege frequently is intertwined with explorations of race and racism, and appropriately so, given the interlocking systems of oppression in which race or ethnicity bear long and deep relationships to the power and privilege experienced. Yet power and privilege also are played out when, for example, an African American researcher with a PhD is heavily advantaged financially with status and perceived authority in a CBPR project, when compared to the lead community partner who is also an African American woman but lives in poverty and has a high school diploma.

Further, and particularly in CBPR and related partnerships, conventional conceptualizations of power and privilege may not capture the nuances involved. Privilege, for example, is frequently defined as "unearned access to resources" because of one's advantaged social location, whereas power is the ability to decide who will have access to resources as well as "the capacity to influence the behaviors of others or one's self, or the course of events" (Myers & Ogino, 2016, p. 8). These terms are all examples of linguistic racial accommodation, which don't convey historical and structural reasons for lack of resource access or how the capacity to influence people and events was acquired.

CBPR STRATEGIES TO COMBAT RACISM

CBPR partnerships should consider incorporating strategies that help clarify the multilevel mechanisms through which racism, power, and privilege can affect partnering processes and research outcomes. This would include the ways the partnerships themselves may inadvertently reinscribe positions of power through racially accommodative language based on white privilege within partnering processes (Yonas et al., 2006). Especially important for diverse partnerships is the need to create an atmosphere that fosters open communication about partners' lived experiences negotiating racial oppression and privilege. Periodic sessions (formal or informal) encouraging reflexivity about partners' experience with racism may generate useful insights that can inform research design, knowledge production, and identify areas where racism is unintentionally being reproduced within the partnership (see Chapter 8 on formal antiracism training). Team reflections about race and racism, however difficult, may yield a synergism contributing knowledge and research for combatting social, racial, and health inequities.

CBPR CASE STUDIES: PRACTICAL APPLICATIONS

In this section, we use examples from two case studies that examine how racism, power, and privilege can be reproduced *unintentionally* within a CBPR partnership and showcase new theoretical conceptions of identity that should be considered within diverse partnerships and research teams. We will draw on our conceptual and theoretical frames to provide recommendations to help CBPR researchers and partnerships be aware of subtle forms of racism, power, and privilege and how they can be addressed among partners. These case studies offer a chance to examine more deeply the ways American Indians, Blacks, Latinos, and other people of color may be subjected to systemic racism and marginalization through the interpersonal dynamics of communication. What is considered acceptable ways of communication are subject to many factors, such as type of discourse (formal-informal), positionality within the power hierarchy, identity, and communicative context or setting (Muhammad et al., 2015). Applying a microlevel lens examining how communication is marginalized within participatory research illustrates how racism can be reproduced within partnerships *unintentionally,* including when navigating pressures to conform to institutional research process and when reporting on scientific data, which privileges dominant group values and communication styles.

West Oakland Environmental Indicators Project

The largely African American and Latino community of West Oakland, California, has a long and proud history of activism, dating to its role as the birthplace of the Pullman Porters' Union and later of the Black Panthers Party (Rhomberg, 2004). Bounded on three sides by freeways, however, and home to the state's second busiest port and other trucking-related industries, West Oakland has also long suffered high rates of illnesses exacerbated by air pollution, including asthma hospitalization rates in children seven times the state average (Pacific Institute & West Oakland Environmental Indicators Project, 2002). To address these issues, a CBPR partnership was established in 1999 between a local environmental justice group, now known as the nonprofit West Oakland Environmental Indicators Project (WOEIP), and a local nonprofit research institute, the Pacific Institute (PI). Through its Community Strategies for Sustainability and

Justice (CSSJ) program, PI helped train residents who undertook air sampling, truck counts, and other methods that demonstrated highly disproportionate exposures borne by its mostly low-income African American and Latino residents. The fifteen-year WOEIP-PI partnership is best known for its use of its data collection and strong media and policy advocacy to help create systems-level changes (e.g., a truck route ordinance). In 2016, WOEIP was involved in citywide efforts to successfully ban the storage of coal at the Port of Oakland. But the partnership also has engaged in deep reflection and dialogue on its own processes as these relate to power and privilege (see Garzón et al., 2013; Gonzales et al., 2011), to which we now turn.

The intersections among race, ethnicity, gender, and class were among the areas explored by the partnership in relation to power and privilege. Within PI, a highly educated Latina who co-led CSSJ noted that she had experienced "racialized and gendered stereotypes" causing her to need to be "twice as good as my white male counterpart to get the same level of respect and recognition." She went on to note that "it throws people off when the researcher in the room is not a white male, because the expectation is that women of color should be the recipients, and not the providers of services" (Garzón et al., 2013, p. 74). By contrast, the white male who co-led WOEIP noted that although he was acutely aware of the unearned power his race and gender accorded him in other spheres (e.g., in being able to get a police response when his neighbors of color could not), within the partnership he clearly didn't "carry the weight" that his African American female colead did in their community work, and he routinely deferred to her for that reason (p. 74).

Microaggression occurred in the course of the partnership's work. The act of translation for community and decision-maker audiences was a common role that CSSJ and WOEIP staff members played for each other. In community meetings, WOEIP staff members often would elaborate on what CSSJ staff members said by using less formal and more emotive language. By contrast, when drafting technical documents, CSSJ staff members would often wordsmith what WOEIP staff members said to conform to a scientific writing style by editing statements that could be interpreted as anecdotal or emotional. Although this often worked well, a CSSJ leader noted that WOEIP staff members had sometimes "called me on being too academic," and WOEIP staff members also sometimes felt that their words had just been reiterated in a more "jargony" way.

WOEIP and CSSJ partners commented on such dynamics in further reflecting on their communication styles and related power differences. A WOEIP staffer thus remarked that "the ability to have technical skills to write . . . gives power to the research group" and sometimes results in power dynamics and perceived devaluating that takes the form of unconscious micro-insults. WOEIP staff members noted that they thus didn't have "the ability to put things into print, reports, or responding to email, but as a result had to deal with how [CSSJ] gets disappointed on not getting deliverables in a timely manner" (Garzón et al., 2013, p. 75). Conversely, CSSJ staff members often felt uncomfortable refraining from expressing themselves in front of WOEIP in order to show deference to the community partner. As one staff member reflected:

> One thing I noticed myself doing a lot of is giving WOEIP staff space to talk. By not taking up space I gave them space to talk, but I don't think I was actively listening . . . I felt like I was reproducing the dynamic of when residents speak to decision makers. There is no real engagement there . . .

Finally, and despite deep recognition of the mutual benefits of working in partnership, tensions also played out concerning power dynamics and were reflected in a partner's comment that "I had to learn the difference [among] being authentic in my testimony, telling the truth based on my experience, and being tactful."

Central tenets of CBPR recognize the value of local knowledge and the idea of community as a fundamental unit of identity (see Chapter 3). Does community cultural identity, knowledge, expertise, and communication style only have value as long as it remains within the confines of the *community* or bracketed with quotations as qualitative data (Reyes Cruz, 2008)? The practice tacitly suggests that during the process of dominant group *cultural translation,* the feelings, thoughts, and experiences of people of color must be expressed in a format that privileges the perspective of the oppressor and not the oppressed to have scientific validity. Revising communication styles to conform to "scientific writing" standards is a type of oppression that imposes dominant group standards depriving the speaker of his or her cultural communication (Sue et al., 2007). The potential to reproduce systemic racism through microaggression within this CBPR partnership was witnessed in two ways: (1) as micro-insults, when institutional norms devalued the ways people of color expressed themselves about their lived experience as anecdotal or emotional communication and therefore inferior styles (Sue, 2007); and (2) as micro-invalidations, by conceptualizing language expressed by community partners as somehow lacking scientific merit because it lacked conformity to dominant group technical communication standards.

UNM CBPR Team Reflections

CBPR academic practitioners have recognized the potential for reproduction of gender, racial, ethnic, and socioeconomic inequalities and power differentials within the research process and within the production of scientific knowledge itself. Researchers also may have power and privilege from their class, education, racial-ethnic backgrounds, or other identity positions. Both of these positionalities (power and privilege) have the potential for reproducing systemic health inequities and disadvantaging community partners. Reflection on issues of power, identity, and positionality has led the research team at the Center for Participatory Research at the University of New Mexico (UNM-CPR) to examine in greater detail the need for theoretical frameworks for understanding power and privilege and their effects on research partnering processes and outcomes (Muhammad et al., 2015). This team has sought to better understand research positionality through examining their ascribed and achieved identities that confer status on an individual researcher, such as race and ethnicity or level of education attained. They have grappled with how to better share power as a defining factor in building effective academic-community collaborations.

A panel, "Insider/Outsider: Our Ascribed and Achieved Identities as Researchers," conducted at the 2011 University of New Mexico "CBPR for Health" annual summer institute, uncovered these issues, reflecting on their own personal life experiences, motivations, and connections between themselves and communities they partner with (e.g., such as the differences for a Latina scholar working in her own community versus working in one very different in history or origin).

From the panel, a Chicana scholar spoke about the inextricable link between her personal and professional identities. For her, CBPR is not merely a research paradigm but "a way of life." She stated a researcher committed to the ideals of CBPR must be willing to undergo a process of deconstruction. In other words, researchers must be willing to have one's various identities and lived experiences confronted within the context of societal power inequity as a necessary process for building genuine CBPR teams and partnerships. A Native scholar shared this view but from a slightly different perspective. The CBPR team approach enabled her to more seamlessly bridge core identity beliefs with her research. "You know I've always said that CBPR allowed me to be who I am . . . I haven't had to be someone else in the research process." This comfort resonated as a way to handle the stress often felt by researchers of color working within dominant group institutions that perceive them as subordinated to others. Tensions may arise when researchers feel compelled to sublimate one's cultural identity, appearance, or style of communicating to conform to majority group norms about knowledge construction.

The importance of CBPR research reinforcing the life experiences of scholars of color does not necessarily extend to researchers from more outside identities. A white researcher from an academic middle class background discussed how she never claimed similar life experiences to the tribes she works with, though she has developed long-term relationships and friendships with tribal partners. She is well aware that she has power and privilege not just as an academic but also attributable to the characteristic of whiteness. "My question has always been, how can I do participatory research with integrity and use the resources and power that I have to work with communities in a positive way." A Black academic researcher also saw his racial identity as a resource to be used within the research environment. While conducting field work in southern rural Missouri, he talked about noticing the local cultural norm discouraged discussion of racial inequality and used that insight to enhance data collection through private conversations. In this community, whites often denied that racism still existed, yet Blacks acknowledged its existence but preferred not to dwell on the past, and they were able to talk with the Black researcher more directly about their experiences than if he had been white. The scholars of color on the panel expressed their strong attachment for racial, ethnic, or cultural identity as protective and a valuable research skill. One scholar concurred about the importance of having a clear understanding of her identity as a researcher of color, "I feel as an American Indian woman, with me strongly attached to my identity and my community, that I am able to address some of the most persistent health disparities among American Indian women."

DISRUPTING THE POTENTIAL FOR REINSCRIPTION OF RACISM IN CBPR

In this chapter, racism is conceptualized as a comprehensive interaction among systemic-institutional, interpersonal, covert, and internalized racism, often embodied in linguistic racial accommodations. These understandings manifest themselves in multiple positions of power and privilege that can permeate partnerships, often in unintentional ways, and affect the capacity of the partnership to challenge external inequities. The examples presented here show how CBPR practitioners working with communities of color can consider incorporating partnering processes that dislodge the centrality of white privilege throughout all phases of the research. People of color have well learned that open criticism of institutional policies and practices as being racist can result in retaliation and the denial of benefits (i.e., grants, community investment, employment promotions).

A genuine commitment to the ideals of CBPR and social justice is essential to avoid the co-optation of CBPR under the influence of instrumentalist variants of participatory research

(Trickett, 2011) that exploits communities of color for funding and professional advancement while replicating power hierarchies and white hegemony in knowledge production. Several aspects of the research process can unintentionally (or covertly) reinscribe systemic racism at critical junctures across the life span of the partnership and therefore need to be elevated to a conscious antiracism reflection and action (Yonas et al., 2006). For examples of deliberate work against covert and overt systemic racism, see Chapter 8 on a CBPR project within two cancer care institutions and Chapter 22 on participatory action research efforts to challenge the unjust criminal system. (See also anti-racism training in Yonas et al., 2013.)

In conclusion, recommendations are provided on how to add antiracism enhancements to traditional CBPR in three key research areas.

Community Capacity Building

A fundamental aim of CBPR is to enhance the skills, provide opportunities for training, and expand the knowledge base of community and university partners and stakeholders. The question facing the next generation of academically trained CBPR practitioners is, to what extent are academic institutions, funding bureaucracies, academic publishers and journal editors, and academic researchers willing to participate in a social and intellectual revolution that undermines the present system of inequality?

A popular strategy used to frame this often-difficult dialogue about racism and community capacity relies on Cazenave's (2016) *linguistic racial accommodation*. It is not uncommon for researchers, policy experts, community partners, and activists, for example, to reject the notion of a "deficit" assessment of community resources, choosing instead to emphasize community assets as a focal point for discussion. Although an important change of framework, this assets approach can unfortunately fail to address the structural factors that contributed to the destabilization of communities of color. This approach is tantamount to asking a person whose home has been burglarized to focus more on *what the thief left than what was stolen*. Community capacity building, especially for communities of color, is directly linked to the principle of restorative justice. More specifically, it comes with the recognition that white privilege is an unearned benefit and, therefore, creates a responsibility to act to counter historical oppression of people of color.

Equitable Distribution of Funding

Another major challenge for participatory research is the inherent bias favoring academic and research institutions over the control and distribution of resources. It is now a standard requirement for most federally funded CBPR and community-engaged research projects to have at least one of the partners be a community-based organization. Usually, grant applications are submitted on behalf of a CBPR partnership consisting of academic and community partners. Although community groups or partners may be increasingly receiving budget subcontracts, universities and research institutions as the centers for expert knowledge and as financial intermediaries enjoy the bulk of grant funding primarily through university indirect costs and academic salaries. Community partners may receive nominal stipends (individually or as an organization) as compensation for their participation. Community-based organizations who partner with universities on CBPR projects are often located in impoverished, racially segregated, environmentally hazardous, violent, and politically isolated communities of color. Why?

Because communities so affected by structural inequality and systemic racism also just happen to contain easily identifiable research populations (racial segregation) with high prevalence of negative health outcomes that politicians, funders, universities, research institutions, and academically trained researchers are concerned about. Systemic racism and the relative obscurity of its functioning within present funding effectively *reproduces* racial and ethnic inequality through academic research and helps to keep communities of color in a state of dependency and subordination to academic institutions. An alternative to the current research funding structure is to direct more money toward development of federally funded permanent community research institutions and paid community research staff within existing or new community-based organizations similar to a federally qualified health center or centers of excellence. Just as it was shown that certain protections for human subjects was morally correct, similar arguments and advocacy can be made against the economic injustices pertaining to current research funding practices.

Researcher Identity and Positionality

Researcher identity and positionality reflect statuses (in part) derived from dominant group social and academic institutions and may have an impact on the valuation of community knowledge and outcomes. Under CBPR research processes, external and internalized power dimensions are the underlying context for academic and community collaboration (Wallerstein & Duran, 2008). CBPR partnerships face additional forms of power hierarchy: that which is most described, the relationships between academics and community partners, and that which may exist within the academic team between the principal investigator (often still from a white and more privileged background) and other investigators or research staff (Lingard, Schryer, Spafford, & Campbell, 2007).

Scholars of color on the research team may experience their own knowledge being marginalized in the academy, because their communities have been led to believe that their cultural heritage and knowledge is devalued by mainstream society. Historically, they have seen their communities as often the objects of research, with the knowledge generated appropriated to reflect the theories and requirements of the academy. At the same time, they face the contradiction that they are the academics, too, and question which knowledge paradigms to embrace.

One important strategy is to include academic team members whose identities (i.e., gender, race, ethnicity, sexual orientation, and class) intersect or bridge with those of the community partners. If there is not a cultural match of research team members with the community population, it becomes essential to work diligently to diversify your institution's faculty members and students and seek a cultural broker from the community itself. Changing the face of the academy is an important structural way to make a difference in knowledge production, because diverse academies foster trust, effective communication, access to local knowledge, and the valuing of epistemological diversity.

CONCLUSION

One under-theorized outcome of CBPR is liberation from traditional forms of knowledge production for the community and the academics involved in the work. When the ideals of CBPR are faithfully adhered to, the community is better able to free itself from the social structural factors that have historically silenced its voices of concern and marginalized its aspirations for hope (i.e., from colonization, racism, sexism, and economic exploitation). The academic researcher may likewise find release from personal and cultural biases that can develop through the achieved status of rigorous academic training and through the ascribed status arising from individual power, privilege, and prestige accruing as an academic. It is essential to acknowledge the continued importance of cultural humility (see Appendix 4) even when there are shared communities of identity between researchers and community partners. Level of formal education, institutional affiliation, lived experience, and roles in the partnership can also create power differentials that need to be navigated carefully and can take on even more significance when other identity markers such as race and gender are shared. Deconstructing these issues from one's personal positionality, within the partnership and within societal structures, can be the beginning to the long journey of the struggle for racial justice.

QUESTIONS FOR DISCUSSION

1. Describe how systemic racism is able to function with little observation in today's society. Can you give examples of your personal experience with incidences of covert racism, privilege, or microaggression?
2. Why is researcher identity and positionality important to consider when forming a CBPR partnership?
3. Consider the different phases of CBPR research. In what ways can microaggression, micro-invalidation, and micro-insult become a usual part of a community-academic partnership?

REFERENCES

Cazenave, N. A. (2016). *Conceptualizing racism: Breaking the chains of racially accommodative language*. Lanham, MD: Rowman & Littlefield.

Chavez, V., Duran, B., Baker, Q., Avila, M., & Wallerstein, N. (2008). The dance of race and privilege in community-based participatory research. In M. Minkler & N. Wallerstein, (Eds.), *Community-based participatory research in health* (pp. 81–97). San Francisco, CA: Jossey-Bass.

Coates, R. D. (2011). Covert racism: An introduction. In R. D. Coates (Ed.), *Covert racism: Theories, institutions, and experiences* (Studies in Critical Social Sciences). Leiden, the Netherlands: Koninklijke Brill NV.

Feagin, J. R. (2006). *Systemic racism: A theory of oppression*. New York, NY: Taylor & Francis.

Fine M. (Ed.). (2004). *Off white: Readings on power, privilege, and resistance*. New York, NY: Routledge.

Garzón, C., Beveridge, B., Gordon, M., Martin, C., Matalon, E., & Moore, E. (2013). Power, privilege, and the process of community-based participatory research: Critical reflections on forging an empowered partnership for environmental justice in West Oakland, California. *Environmental Justice, 6*(2), 71–78.

Gee, G. C., & Ford, C. (2011). Structural racism and health inequities: Old issues, new directions. *Du Bois Review, 8*(1), 115–132.

Gonzales, P., Minkler, M., Garcia, A., Gordon, M., Garzón, C., Palaniappan, M., Prakash, S., & Beveridge, B. (2011). Community-based participatory research and policy advocacy to reduce diesel exposure in West Oakland, California. *American Journal of Public Health, 101*(Suppl 1), S166–S175.

Jones, C. P. (2000). Levels of racism: A theoretic framework and a gardener's tale. *American Journal of Public Health, 8*, 1212–1215.

King, M., Smith, A., & Gracey, M. (2009). Indigenous health part 2: The underlying causes of the health gap. *Lancet, 374,* 76–85.

Lingard, L., Schryer, C. F., Spafford, M. M., & Campbell, S. L. (2007). Negotiating the politics of identity in an interdisciplinary research team. *Qualitative Research, 7*(4), 501–519.

Lonczak, H. S., Thomas, L. R., Donovan, D., Austin, L., Sigo, R. L., Lawrence, N., & Suquamish Tribe. (2013). Navigating the tide together: Early collaboration between tribal and academic partners in a CBPR Study. *Pimatisiwin, 11*(3), 395–409

Muhammad, M., Wallerstein, N., Sussman, A. L., Avila, M., Belone, L., & Duran. B. (2015). Reflections on researcher identity and power: The impact of positionality on community-based participatory research (CBPR) processes and outcomes. *Critical Sociology, 41*(7–8), 1045–1063.

Myers, A., & Ogino, Y. (2016). *Power, privilege, & oppression.* Retrieved from www.scrippscollege.edu/xbk/wp-content/uploads/sites/35/files/Power-Privilege-and-Oppression.pdf

Pacific Institute & West Oakland Environmental Indicators Project. (2002). *Neighborhood knowledge for change: The West Oakland environmental indicators project.* Oakland, CA: Pacific Institute.

Reyes Cruz, M. (2008). What if I just cite Graciela? Working toward decolonizing knowledge through critical ethnography. *Qualitative Inquiry, 14*(4), 651–658.

Rhomberg, C. (2004). *No there there: Race, class, and political community in Oakland.* Berkeley: University of California Press.

Sherover-Marcuse, R. (1986). *Emancipation and consciousness: Dogmatic and dialectical perspectives in the early Marx.* Malden, MA: Blackwell.

Smedley, A., & Smedley, B. (2005). Race as biology is fiction, racism as a social problem is real: Anthropological and historical perspectives on the social construction of race. *American Psychologist, 60,* 16–26.

Smedley, B. (2012). The lived experience of race and its health consequences. *American Journal of Public Health, 102,* 933–935. doi:10.2105/AJPH.2011.300643

Sue, D. W., Capodilupo, C. M., Torino, G. C., Bucceri, J. M., Holder, A., Nadal, K. L., & Esquilin, M. (2007). Racial microaggressions in everyday life: Implications for clinical practice. *American Psychologist, 62*(4), 271–286.

Trickett, E. J. (2011). Community-based participatory research as worldview or instrumental strategy: Is it lost in translation(al) research? *American Journal of Public Health, 101*(8), 1353–1355.

Wallerstein, N. B., & Duran B. (2006). Using community-based participatory research to address health disparities. *Health Promotion Practice, 7,* 312–323.

Wallerstein, N., & Duran B. (2008). The theoretical, practical, and historical roots of CBPR. In M. Minkler & N. Wallerstein (Eds.), *Community-based participatory research for health: From process to outcomes* (2nd ed., pp. 25–46). San Francisco, CA: Jossey-Bass.

Williams, D. R. (2012). Miles to go before we sleep: Racial inequities in health. *Journal of Health and Social Behavior, 53*(3), 279–295.

Yonas, M. A., Jones, N., Eng, E., Vines, A. I., Aronson, R., Griffith, D. M., White, B., & DuBose, M. (2006). The art and science of integrating undoing racism with CBPR: Challenges of pursuing NIH funding to investigate cancer care and racial equity. *Journal of Urban Health: Bulletin of the New York Academy of Medicine, 83*(6), 1004–1012.

Yonas, M. A., Aronson, R., Coad, N., Eng, E., Petteway, R., Schaal, J., & Webb, L. (2013). Infrastructure for equitable decision making in research. In B. A. Israel, E. Eng, A. J. Schulz, & E. A. Parker (Eds.), *Methods for community-based participatory research* (2nd ed., pp. 97–126). San Francisco, CA: Jossey-Bass.

CHAPTER 5

TRUST DEVELOPMENT IN CBPR PARTNERSHIPS

JULIE E. LUCERO, KATHRINE E. WRIGHT, AND ABIGAIL REESE

TRUST IS FOUNDATIONAL to all human relationships and becomes exceedingly important in relationships in which risk and safety are concerned. Associations developed because of health research are one such type of relationship. Community-academic partnerships are examples of situations in which researchers are granted a position to help in the goal of improving health, yet they pose a real threat of opportunistic behavior. Research has often been concerning to underserved communities because of the historical practices that contribute to risk and destabilizing safety. These have included undermining of autonomy, coercion and power imbalances, research without community benefit, interpretation and reporting of data resulting in community stigma or cultural misunderstanding, and general lack of reconciling community concerns (Cochran et al., 2008; Cook & Jackson, 2012). Related to risk is conflict, and when trying to resolve or lessen risk, conflict can emerge because of inherent differences in perceptions, culture, goals, and values (Cochran et al., 2008; Lucero & Wallerstein, 2013; Pondy, 1992). Therefore, conscious reconciliation of these differences has the potential to mitigate conflict, decrease risk, improve safety, and build trust.

Community-based participatory research (CBPR), a research approach that falls under the umbrella of community-engaged research, seeks to democratize research and promote health equity. Through the democratization process, partners can reconcile conflict-causing differences and challenge the position of power, knowledge creation, and oppression within historic research endeavors (Chavez et al., 2008; Freeman et al., 2006). Despite the promise of equity, many underserved communities may still be wary of CBPR research because of the history of inappropriate research and opportunistic researchers (Cochran et al., 2008). It is impossible to ignore the importance of trust, yet the trust development process in research partnerships is often not a conscious process and is assumed to be present or absent.

The majority of trust and CBPR literature conceptualizes trust as an outcome and acknowledges that research on trust development is lacking. Although numerous CBPR scholars have discussed the importance of trust and offer anecdotal suggestions, very few systematically research it. CBPR scholars often report the presence of trust as personal attributes of the researcher, such as authenticity, action, listening, commitment, recognizing the expertise of community, voicing expectations, taking a facilitator role as opposed to a director role, and getting to know the community (Christopher, Watts, McCormick, & Young, 2008; Hora, Prochaska, Bolin, & Ory, 2007; Jones et al., 2008). However, time is the variable necessary for the community to decide whether the demonstrations of trust-building personal attributes are genuine.

CBPR and trust literature suggests that a process of trust development begins with demonstrating trust-building behaviors and ends with sustaining trust. However, this process of trust development lacks empirical support. Trust development in early CBPR literature was assumed and reported from perceptions of the academic partners, an age-old criticism (Molyneux, Peshu, & Marsh, 2005). However, in recent years community voices have begun to be represented more in efforts such as the journal *Progress in Community Health Partnerships*. To bridge the gap, the CBPR literature needs to represent all partner voices.

Another limitation of trust research is that trust is often investigated and measured as a binary variable despite the documentation of several observed trust types (Connell & Mannion, 2006; Lucero & Wallerstein, 2013). The conceptualization of trust as present or absent limits the understanding of trust as a complex, dynamic, and multidimensional construct. A binary conceptualization also keeps key components hidden, including individual and systematic factors, of trust maintenance as well as trust functioning in the phases of partnership and research processes. In one study of CBPR that looked across the research spectrum, trust was identified as a critical element within all phases of research, not just in partnership development (Belone et al., 2016). The field will benefit from the integration of trust types, a missing component of current models.

The extant CBPR literature has yet to document the process of trust development, leaving it under-theorized. Organizational communication and behavior literature is useful in theorizing the components involved in trust development, because CBPR partnerships are composed of two or more organizations working to achieve a common goal. This chapter presents a trust typology as an alternative to binary distinctions of trust in CBPR. The typology is discussed and qualitative and quantitative data are presented from data collected during two different but related projects to support the existence of these types in practice. Although the focus of this chapter is at the partnership level, the typology can also be used to inform partnerships about the level of trust between the partnership and the community.

STUDY BACKGROUND

From 2006–2008, supplemental funding was secured from the National Center for Minority Health and Health Disparities through the Native American Research Centers for Health mechanism to understand what constructs matter most to CBPR partnerships and outcomes (Wallerstein et al., 2008). The product of the pilot grant was a CBPR conceptual model. Through a

TABLE 5.1 Trust Typology Model with Characteristics

Trust Types	Characteristics
Critical-reflective trust	Trust is at the place where mistakes and other issues resulting from differences can be talked about and resolved.
Proxy trust	Partners are trusted because someone who is trusted invited them.
Functional trust	Partners are working together for a specific purpose and time frame, but mistrust may still be present.
Neutral trust	Partners are still getting to know each other; there is neither trust nor mistrust.
Role-based trust	Trust is based on a member's title or role with limited or no direct interaction.
Trust deficit (suspicion)	Partnership members do not trust each other.

literature review, web-based survey, and a series of community consultations, historical mistrust and trust-mistrust between a community and a specific research team was highly ranked by participants as important elements for the success of CBPR projects (Belone et al., 2016). During the community consultations, participants stated that trust resides throughout the process of CBPR and is not isolated from historical mistrust as a contextual factor (Belone et al., 2016). As a result, the development of a trust typology ensued (see Lucero, 2013, for more detail). In the development of this trust development framework, the need to support the product with evidence was imminent.

First, qualitative support was provided by data collected during the community consultation focus groups that preceded the Research for Improved Health (RIH) study to illustrate the trust types that exist in practice. A brief discussion of the community consultation process and data generation is described here because it is not presented elsewhere in the book. The quantitative measurement of the trust typology was done with data from the RIH study (see Chapters 6 and 17). Results from the RIH survey illustrate how to measure trust types.

This iteration of the typology includes six types that were validated by community experiences and supported within interorganizational literature (Table 5.1). It is important to understand that this typology should not be interpreted as being anchored at opposite poles. The authors do not assume that partnerships begin in trust deficit. Rather, a partnership can start and move between trust types. For each project, a required or ideal type of trust will need to be determined by partnership members (Wicks, Berman, & Jones, 1999).

TRUST TYPOLOGY: SUPPORT FOR A DEVELOPMENTAL FRAMEWORK

Several iterations of the trust typology were developed. The version presented here proved salient as evidenced by the following section.

Community Consultation

In 2009, six focus groups were conducted with American Indian, African American, Chinese origin, Puerto Rican, Mexican, and a few white community members to review and revise the CBPR conceptual model (full details are found in Belone et al., 2016). The focus group method was used to fulfill two aims: (1) seek face validity of the model and (2) determine if the model could be used for self-reflection and diagnosis. Partnerships were asked to "think about the major drivers and barriers to authentic participation in the CBPR project" and to reflect on "which issues [outlined in the model] matter the most to your partnership now?" Each discussion ended by asking partnerships to determine what they needed to strengthen their partnership or provide advice on best practices. In each focus group, trust was identified as a key issue. For this reason and with permission of the principal investigator, these focus group data were used for secondary analysis to answer the question of which trust types exist in practice. Secondary analysis of qualitative data is useful when investigating sensitive topics in elusive populations (Long-Sutehall, Sque, & Addington-Hall, 2010). A synthesized matrix and reports on validated, expanded, and new constructs from six community consultations were reviewed, analyzed, and reported next. Each type of trust is presented with exemplar quotes from the community consultations.

Partnerships in *critical reflective (CR) trust* are characterized as having open communication. Mistakes and other issues resulting from differences can be discussed and resolved. CR trust is similar to Rousseau, Sitkin, Burt, and Camerer's (1998) relational trust. Relational trust develops over time and through repeated interactions. Repeated interactions provide evidence of reliability and dependability of partners and give rise to positive expectations. Interdependence between partners increases over time as new opportunities and initiatives are pursued. As one community partner stated,

> If there wasn't the kind of trust and collaboration that was there before, I think this would have been an even more challenging process. I think because of the relationships it just helps to know that we're all doing our best to try and make this work part of trust is knowing that you're aware, that you're mindful of other people's capacity.

CR trust contains aspects of identification-based trust (Lewicki & Bunker, 1995) and cognitive-based trust (McAllister, 1995). Identification-based trust requires values and goals to be shared by partners, and cognitive-based trust is an individual's beliefs about another person's reliability, dependability, and competence. Further, the notion of citizenship behaviors in organizations, or going above and beyond to help team members and the team to be successful, is central to critical reflective trust. These relationships share ethical values and interpersonal relationships. The importance of this aspect of critical reflective trust was demonstrated in the course of the community consultations:

> So, you know, that's that trust factor, and that's also that bond, or being able to recognize that we at some point in time might mess up in an area, you know; that we can trust each other that you're not saying this to hurt me but to help me grow who I am, you know, things like that.

As with any trust type, the potential for growth or deterioration exists. In CR, trust partnership nurturing is ongoing and small mistakes do not critically affect the partnership. In sum, critical reflective trust is thought to develop over time, with ongoing interactions with reliable behavior and demonstrated care and concern for partners, community, and health issues. The centrality of respect and safety to group dynamics was referenced repeatedly by community partners: "our relationship, it's created a safety net where we feel free as individuals to be able to do the work that needs to be done in order to meet our goals. But if for some reason we mess up, there's a net there."

Proxy trust occurs in partnerships when members are trusted because someone who is trusted invited them. This is similar to giving an unfamiliar person the "benefit of the doubt" for a period of time. This can occur in a negative space as well and is called *proxy mistrust*. Early knowledge about partners or knowledge about a partner's reputation is thought to affect trust in small group teams (McKnight, Cummings, & Chervany, 1998). Knowledge about team members can arise from prior personal experience working together or from others' prior experience with team members. Race, ethnicity, and cultural background of team members can influence proxy trust by influencing the trust that community members have in the research team. For example, having partners who mirror community characteristics can increase the community's trust in the research team.

> One time when we were doing surveys in the East Side Detroit and wanted to hire some kind of temp agency in Ann Arbor with these young students to come down to the East Side of Detroit to knock on folks doors and do surveys. And none of the young people look like the people on the East Side of Detroit and I was trying to explain that folks aren't even gonna open the door. They are going to look out the window and say, "I'm not opening the door." So, in fact, what they did was hire and train residents from the East Side to actually implement the surveys which really turned out great. To add to that, it really should be a reflection on . . . a mirror of the community that's involved.

Webber (2008) found prior experiences to be positively associated with early development of trust in a team environment, but this association did not predict trust at later stages of team functioning, suggesting that proxy or familiarity with team members offers a probationary period that must be maintained through positive interactions and resolution of key issues. Proxy trust also has added benefits for the partnership, such as decreasing the time factor (assuming the relationships continue to establish trust). For example:

> I would certainly say that the fact that [research partner], you had this long-standing relationship with an organization that you actually helped found and the fact that you previously had worked with [research partner] and there were all these relationships between various partners that were very strong. There was a lot of trust going and I think we saved a lot of time.

Functional trust occurs when members of a partnership are working together for a specific function and time frame. Panteli and Sockalingam (2005) call this type co-alliance trust, which results when organizations make equal contributions of resources, competencies, and knowledge for specific projects and time frames. Additionally, Shapiro (1987) and Sitkin and Roth (1993) conceptualize a type of trust based on formal legal agreements, formal rules, and memoranda of agreement. Formal agreements can diminish mistrust by explicating roles and responsibilities, expectations, and decision-making processes. Ground rules and agreements were identified as a priority by a community partner, "When we were writing renewal, we educated our brand-new community advisory committee; we went over principles of CBPR and laid a foundation right there, and I had pushed very hard for that."

Aspects of knowledge-based trust (KBT) (Lewicki & Bunker, 1995) also fit within functional trust. In KBT, partners possess enough knowledge to understand and predict behavior partly because of the "fit" of partners. Functional trust depends on the function of the partnership. Therefore, functional trust is task and time dependent; based on equitable contributions of resources, competencies, and knowledge; may include formal arrangements; and partners possess enough knowledge of each other to predict behavior and commitment.

Neutral trust means partners are still getting to know each other; neither trust nor mistrust exists at this point. In this stage, individuals rely on the purpose or task of the relationship to buttress interpersonal trust. Neutral trust resembles swift trust, a type of trust that needs to form very quickly to make progress (Meyerson, Weick, & Kramer, 1996). Swift trust is time, task, and goal dependent and is driven more by contextual cues, such as economics, than by interpersonal relations. Neutral trust, similar to swift trust, is fragile because situations requiring quick decisions about trust without the ability to weigh the risks might be more prone to conflict than relationships that grow together and develop shared goals and values along the way. The establishment of a successful partnership depends on the ability to sustain trust between partners past the initial development of trust. One community member explained the importance of contextual factors and the continual development of trust:

> I think one of the things that actually [member] said at one point was the difference of working with someone [at university] and here; that cultural factor piece was that you really need to spend the time to get to know people before you can start doing the work, doing the tasks, and I think that is an important contextual factor, that culture. How things operate in your experience versus someone else needs to be thought about because you might never feel the move from point A to point B because what someone needs from their experience is to get to know you first, or vice versa, and I think that affects those group dynamics, and we don't talk about that much, but I think it's important.

Once tasks are complete, individuals or organizations will evaluate the relationships and determine whether they dissolve or continue their relationships based on needs of their organization or community. The following quote illustrates the decision making that community members undertake to determine whether it makes sense to continue with a partnership:

> We demand a certain level not only of respect but time and resources that sometimes people aren't prepared to give. You know they come in thinking well we could do this thing and you end up putting more time into it and you find that it's like a job. So in some ways we demand a lot. So that's another aspect of partnerships is that we will tend to work towards groups or organizations that are willing to invest the time that we're willing to invest into a project. If we see that a group is laissez-faire with our relationship then we'll evaluate that partnership and see if it's useful to have that.

Role-based trust is based on the titles or roles of members with limited or no direct interaction prior to the relationship. Presumptive trust (Webb, 1996), or role-based trust, suggested that people who function in certain roles—a physician for example—are trained to have patients' best interest in mind thereby reducing uncertainty even if other trust-building characteristics are missing. Role-based trust can be quite fragile and produce failures in cooperation and coordination because trust based on roles is short term and requires reinforcement through meeting established expectations. One community partner lamented the lack of follow-through from a group of researchers granted role-based trust:

> Like the last group that came from the university to collect data, I was making sure they were going to do what they said they were going to do. I invited them to sit with the community and the community leaders, let everyone know that they were collecting data. They even came back and spoke after collecting their data and made all these promises [they didn't keep]; and that was it. I think following through is very important, is very key for staying in the trust of the community.

Because of the historical experience of research in marginalized communities, it has been assumed that trust based on the position a person holds is equivalent to no trust during relationship development. In fact, our community consultations indicate that suspicion toward the researchers is more likely to be present: "Often, they [researchers] just assume that we don't have an agenda, that we do not have the plan, that we do not lead our own lives, that we do not have a plan for our future, and so they just push their own agenda."

Trust deficit (suspicion) means partnership members do not trust each other because of historical relationships or conduct. It is likely that trust will not develop between partners. One community member reflected on the community's historical mistrust with research partners: "Someone is always testing us for something. Let's not let the community feel like they are just guinea pigs again and when it's over with its smoke and mirrors again." Deutsch (1958) introduced suspicion as an *expectation* of a malevolent event; this personality trait is a result of personal and observed experience. The trust deficit type is the most sensitive to the disposition of the actors and the trust situation. Trust disposition is based on early trust-related experiences and eventually becomes a stable personality characteristic (Hardin, 1996; Rotter, 1971, 1980). The implication of suspicion as a personality trait is that individuals with a pessimistic disposition toward trust will demonstrate lower levels of trust on initial contact. The historical context contributes to past experiences and colors trust deficit. Focus group members identified the actions of outsiders and the omission of results to the community as a reason for historical mistrust (Belone et al., 2016).

> I believe that in the past we have seen so many other org[anizations] and different people coming here to do different things, and it didn't happen. It didn't happen, or they would use the information they got from this area and do whatever they were gonna do with it, and we never got back the results from whatever they were doing. So some of it may have been mistrust . . . I believe some of it, not a lot of it, but some of it may be mistrust.
>
> That's where I thought that the trust and the mistrust had to be addressed because a lot of times when you walk into a community if you're from the outside there is no openness until they can trust you and so take the time on group dynamics and get to know people and that equates to developing trust.

Data from the community consultation focus groups provided ample support for the six trust types. More data was found for critical reflective, proxy trust, and trust deficit. Less support was available for functional, role-based, and neutral trust, but data still supported praxis, the interactive understanding of the theory and practice of trust as a dynamic concept, that can change over time. The next step was the quantitative measurement of the trust typology in the RIH study.

Research for Improved Health (RIH)

RIH was a mixed methods study that included a key informant and community engagement (CE) web-based surveys (Lucero et al., 2016; see Chapters 6 and 17 for details). As the trust typology provides a new view on trust, the social trust scale was used to establish construct validity. This scale is four-item forced-choice measure designed to assess the general confidence that one has in the integrity, ability, and character of others (Figueroa, Kincaid, Rani, & Lewis, 2002). Higher scores on a five-point Likert scale indicate higher levels of trust. The means plot in Figure 5.1 reveals higher scores for the social trust scale and corresponds with critical reflective trust. Similarly low scores on the social trust scale correspond with suspicion. This provides some validity for the trust typology measure.

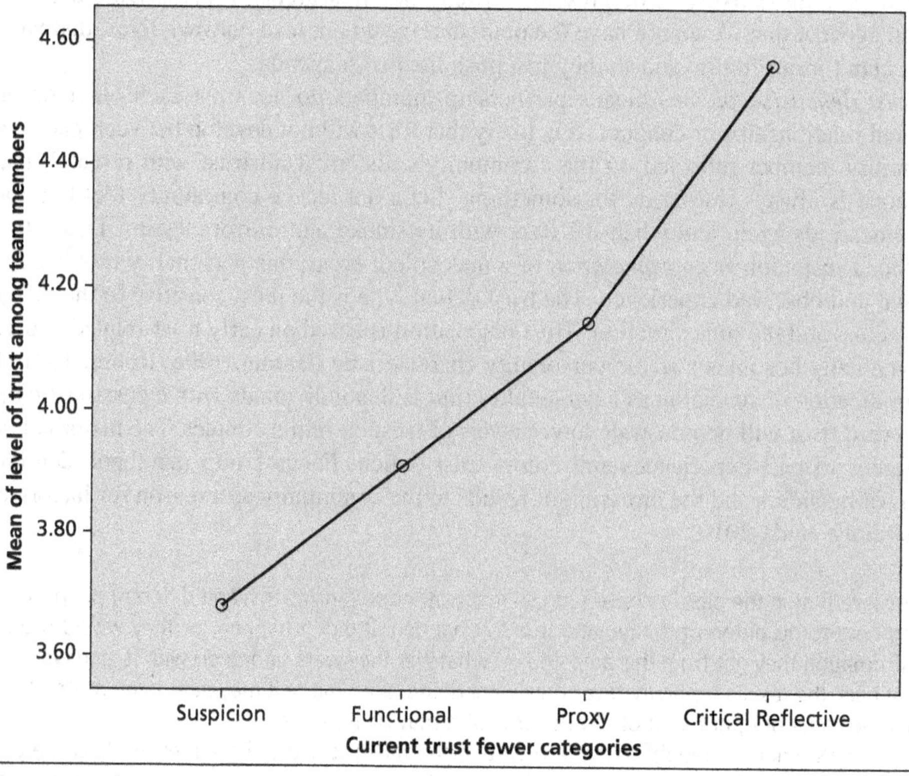

FIGURE 5.1 *Means Plot of Social Trust and Trust Types*

As agreement between the two scales existed, a measure was created to operationalize the trust typology. The trust typology resulted in a three-item forced-choice measure designed to assess the change of trust types over time. The measure asked about level of trust at the beginning of the partnership, level currently, and level desired for the future, using a category scale with responses ranging from critical reflexive trust to no trust (see Table 5.1). The majority of survey participants reported critical reflective trust in partnerships at the time they responded to the RIH questionnaire. To have enough data in each cell for analysis, the types suggestive of less trust were combined to create a four-level typology: critical reflective trust ($n=296$), proxy trust ($n=56$), functional trust ($n=64$), and suspicion ($n=16$). Conceptually this categorization makes sense because the types of no trust, proxy mistrust, unearned trust, and neutral trust all suggest suspicion. These results were reported elsewhere; see Lucero et al. (2016) for more information.

CONCLUSION

Investigating and measuring trust as a binary variable is a limitation of trust research, because scholars have documented several types of observed trust (Connell & Mannion, 2006; McKnight & Chervany, 2006). The conceptualization of trust as present or absent limits the understanding of trust as a complex and multidimensional construct. This chapter presents a trust typology as an alternative measure. As it stands, the use of the typology at the different time periods enables partners to reflect on trust over time rather than assuming it has been present or absent. In the quantitative data, participants reported movement in trust levels over time. This reinforces the assertion of trust being a process and not just an outcome. The typology can assist partners in determining the different types of trust present within the partnership (e.g., community at proxy and researchers at critical reflective). It can be used as a reflection tool, and can help partnership members address divergent perspectives and attempt to resolve differences.

Although innovative, typologies are problematic in research because significant variation and overlap exist within each category, making it extremely difficult to use a typology as a dependent variable. However, the typology is useful in organizing theory as part of exploratory research. The next step in trust development theory is to develop a new measure using trust types as latent variables. A new measure should include the totality of the trust environment using a systems perspective. The vision for the new instrument is for partnerships to implement it at multiple time points to determine the type they are functioning within and determine if that is where the members want to be. If not, members need to decide what kind of trust they want to achieve and what they need to get there. Evidence from the community consultations that led to the development of this trust typology indicates that the goal of partners regarding trust is an environment in which partners share similar goals, feel that safety outweighs risks, and members are responsible for the partnership. Once the partnership achieves an appropriate level or type of trust, energy reserved for conflict mediation can be redirected into the research project and health outcomes.

QUESTIONS FOR DISCUSSION

1. Reflect on partnerships you know or have participated in. How has trust in these partnerships changed over time? In what ways did they trust, and where are they now?
2. If you are seeking to strengthen trust in a partnership, what strategies could you imagine would be helpful?

REFERENCES

Belone, L., Lucero, J. E., Duran, B., Tafoya, G., Baker, E. A., Chan, D., Chang, C., Greene-Moton, E., Kelley, M. A., & Wallerstein, N. (2016). Community-based participatory research conceptual model: Community partner consultation and face validity. *Qualitative Health Research, 26*(1), 117–135. doi:10.1177/1049732314557084

Chavez, V., Duran, B., Baker, Q. E., Avila, M. M., & Wallerstein, N. (2008). The dance of race and privilege in community-based participatory research. In M. Minkler & N. Wallerstein (Eds.), *Community-based participatory research for health: From process to outcomes* (2nd ed., pp. 91–106). San Francisco, CA: Jossey-Bass.

Christopher, S., Watts, V., McCormick, A., & Young, S. (2008). Building and maintaining trust in a community-based participatory research partnership. *American Journal of Public Health, 98*(8), 1398–1406.

Cochran, P.A.L., Marshall, C. A., Garcia-Downing, C., Kendall, E., Cook, D., McCubbin, L., & Gover, R.M.S. (2008). Indigenous ways of knowing: Implications for participatory research and community. *American Journal of Public Health, 98*(1), 22–27.

Connell, N. A. D., & Mannion, R. (2006). Conceptualisations of trust in the organisational literature: Some indicators from a complementary perspective. *Journal of Health Organization and Management, 20*(5), 417–433.

Cook, B. D., & Jackson, T. R. (2012). Eighty years of bad blood: The evolution of human research after the Tuskegee Study. *Journal of Healthcare, Science, and Humanities, 2*(2), 31–58.

Deutsch, M. (1958). Trust and suspicion. *Journal of Conflict Resolution, 2*(4), 265–279.

Freeman, E. R., Brugge, D., Bennett-Bradley, W. M., Levy, J. I., & Carrasco, E. (2006). Challenges of conducting community-based participatory research in Boston's neighborhoods to reduce disparities in asthma. *Journal of Urban Health, 4*(6), 1013–1021.

Figueroa, M. E., Kincaid, D. L., Rani, M., & Lewis, G. (2002). Communication for social change: An integrated model for measuring the process and its outcomes. (*The Communication for Social Change Working Paper Series*, No.1). New York: The Rockefeller Foundation.

Hardin, R. (1996). Trustworthiness. *Ethics, 107*(1), 26–42.

Hora, K. L., Prochaska, J. D., Bolin, J. N., & Ory, M. G. (2007). Lessons learned utilizing the CBPR model to address disease management guidelines in rural communities. *Texas Public Health Journal, 59*(2), 17–21.

Jones, K. M., Gray, A. H., Paleo, J., Branden, C. J., & Lesser, J. (2008). Community and scholars unifying for recovery. *Issues in Mental Health Nursing, 29*(5), 495–503.

Lewicki, R. J., & Bunker, B. B. (1995). Developing and maintaining trust in work relationships. In R. M. Kramer & T. R. Tyler (Eds.), *Trust in organizations: Frontiers of theory and research* (pp. 114–139). Thousand Oaks, CA: Sage.

Long-Sutehall, T., Sque, M., & Addington-Hall, J. (2010). Secondary analysis of qualitative data: A valuable method for exploring sensitive issues with an elusive population? *Journal of Research in Nursing, 16*(4), 335–344. Retrieved February 10, 2017, from www.wlv.ac.uk/pdf/Secondary%20analysis%20JRN3815531.pdf

Lucero, J., Wallerstein, N., Duran, B., Alegria, M., Greene-Moton, E., Israel, B., Kastelic, S., Magarati, M., Oetzel, J., Pearson, C., Schulz, A., Villegas, M., & White Hat, E. (2016). Development of a mixed methods investigation of process and outcomes of community-based participatory research. *Journal of Mixed Methods*. doi:10.1177/1558689816633309

Lucero, J. E. (2013). *Trust as an ethical construct in community-based participatory research partnerships (published doctoral dissertation)*. Albuquerque, NM: University of New Mexico.

Lucero, J. E., & Wallerstein, N. (2013). Trust in community-academic research partnerships: Increasing the consciousness of conflict and trust development. In J. Oetzel & S. Ting-Toomey (Eds.), *Sage handbook of conflict communication: Integrating theory, research, and practice* (2nd ed.). Thousand Oaks, CA: Sage.

McAllister, D. J. (1995). Affect- and cognitive-based trust as foundations for interpersonal cooperation in organizations. *Academy of Management Journal, 38*(1), 24–59.

McKnight, D. H., & Chervany, N. L. (2006). Reflections on an initial trust-building model. In R. Bachmann & A. Zaheer (Eds.), *Handbook of trust research* (pp. 29–51). Cheltenham, UK: Edward Elgar Publishing.

McKnight, D. H., Cummings, L. L., & Chervany, N. L. (1998). Initial trust formation in new organizational relationships. *Academy of Management Review, 23*(3), 473–490. doi:10.5465/AMR.1998.926622

Meyerson, D., Weick, K., & Kramer, R. M. (1996). Swift trust and temporary groups. In R. M. Kramer & T. R. Tyler (Eds.), *Trust in organizations: Frontiers of theory and research* (pp. 166–195). Thousand Oaks, CA: Sage.

Molyneux, C., Peshu, N., & Marsh, K. (2005). Trust and informed consent: Insights from community members on the Kenyan coast. *Social Science and Medicine, 67*(7), 1463–1473.

Panteli, N., & Sockalingam, S. (2005). Trust and conflict within virtual interorganizational alliances: A framework for facilitating knowledge sharing. *Decision Support Systems, 39*(4), 599–617.

Pondy, L. R. (1992). Conflict and negotiation in organizations: Historical and contemporary perspectives. *Journal of Organizational Behavior, 13*(3), 257–261.

Rotter, J. B. (1971). Generalized expectancies for interpersonal trust. *American Psychologist, 26*(5), 443–452.

Rotter, J. B. (1980). Interpersonal trust, trustworthiness, and gullibility. *American Psychologist, 35*(1), 1–7.

Rousseau, D. M., Sitkin, S. B., Burt, R. S., & Camerer, C. (1998). Not so different after all. A cross discipline view of trust. *Academy of Management Review, 23*(3), 393–404.

Shapiro, S. P. (1987). The social control of impersonal trust. *American Journal of Sociology, 93*(3), 623–658.

Sitkin, S. B., & Roth, N. L. (1993). Explaining the limited effectiveness of legalistic "remedies" for trust/distrust. *Organization Science, 4*(3), 367–392.

Wallerstein, N., Oetzel, J., Duran, B., Tafoya, G., Belone, L., & Rae, R. (2008). CBPR: What predicts outcomes? In M. Minkler & N. Wallerstein (Eds.), *Community-based participatory research for health: From process to outcomes* (2nd ed.). San Francisco, CA: Jossey-Bass.

Webb, G. (1996). Trust and crises. In R. M. Kramer & T. R. Tyler (Eds.), *Trust in organizations* (pp. 288–302). Thousand Oaks, CA: Sage.

Webber, S. S. (2008). Development of cognitive and affective trust in teams: A longitudinal study. *Small Group Research, 39*(6), 746–769. doi:10.1177/1046496408323569

Wicks, A. C., Berman, S. J., & Jones, T. M. (1999). The structure of optimal trust: Moral and strategic implications. *Academy of Management Review, 24*(1), 99–116.

PART 3

CBPR CONCEPTUAL MODEL: CONTEXT AND PROMISING RELATIONSHIP PRACTICES

One of the most studied features of CBPR is partnership processes or dynamics. Numerous studies have examined the key elements of what makes a high-functioning partnership. The argument (with growing evidence to this effect) is that if partnering practices are effective, then intervention and research design will reflect mutual learning and partner synergy, or ability to work together effectively. These dynamics and the research or intervention then also have a positive impact on system, capacity, and health outcomes (see Chapters 6 and 17 along with Appendix 6).

Partnership processes are the means of structuring the work and interacting among partners and include three elements. First, individual characteristics (e.g., displaying cultural humility and being bridges among different groups) shape the interactions. Second, structures of the partnership include formal agreements, sharing of resources, and alignment with CBPR principles. Third, relationships, or how partners interact with one another, including features such as participatory decision making, trust, dialogue, and influence.

However, partnership processes do not operate in a vacuum and thus CBPR models, theories, and practice need to account for context. The emphasis on context is one of the hallmarks of CBPR. Context includes local and larger politics and policy trends, socio-economic-cultural characteristics, historical collaborations of trust-mistrust, university and community capacities and readiness, and the importance of health issues being researched. Contextual factors provide a backdrop for influence on partnership processes, that is, on partnership structures and members and on relationships, including how they are managed and strengthened.

The chapters in this section all consider the role of context for shaping partnership processes and the importance of seeking equitable group dynamics practices for sustainability of a successful partnership. In Chapter 6, Sarah L. Kastelic, Nina Wallerstein, Bonnie Duran, and John G. Oetzel introduce the history of the Research for Improved Health (RIH) study and the development of the CBPR conceptual model that is used to organize this book. Further, this chapter provides an overview of the RIH research design of mixed qualitative and quantitative methods, the data collection of a multilevel survey and in-depth case studies, and integration of quantitative and qualitative data analyses. Although the CBPR model has been further developed and refined, the authors argue that the model is a dynamic tool that should be adapted by local partnerships and used creatively.

In Chapter 7, Emily J. Ozer and Amber Akemi Piatt provide an overview of youth-led participatory action research (YPAR), discussing key contexts for youth research processes, identifying relevant curricular resources, and highlighting potential dilemmas and choice points in engaging in YPAR. They provide illustrative examples from the United States and other country contexts such as Guatemala, Brazil, Portugal, and Australia. The authors consider the value of YPAR for promoting equity and positive development, particularly for the majority of young people in the world who must negotiate racism, economic inequalities, violence, and other threats to healthy development. YPAR engages young people's expertise in scientific inquiry about youth development and health. Finally, they consider the challenge of "scaling" YPAR and related participatory approaches into broader systems change efforts and initiatives, capitalizing on social media and web-based platforms while maintaining the integrity and spirit of the approach.

In Chapter 8, Eugenia Eng and colleagues present a case study grounded in the history and context of racism, particularly institutional racism. Today's effects from institutional racism are subtle and require careful and authentic identification and recognition. This chapter describes how the Greensboro Health Disparities Collaborative applied antiracism principles to an NIH-funded CBPR project designed to test a system change intervention to enhance race-specific equity in quality and completion of cancer care at two cancer centers in Greensboro, North Carolina, and Pittsburgh, Pennsylvania. The authors present four intervention components to address the context of transparency and accountability for racial equity, including staff equity trainings, an analysis of patient interviews of their experiences with the power and authority in the system, nurse navigators, and real-time physician champions. Initial findings from integrating a CBPR approach with antiracism principles indicate benefits of this collaborative approach.

In Chapter 9, Magdalena Ávila, Shannon Sanchez-Youngman, Michael Muhammad, Lauro Silva, and Paula Domingo de Garcia introduce a CBPR case on environmental justice in the South Valley of Albuquerque, New Mexico. This chapter examines context and the promises and pitfalls of their policy partnership through a lay health worker (promotora) intervention to address policy targets. The South Valley Partners for Environmental Justice were able to achieve some of their key goals over their ten-year partnership, including the training and empowering of a cadre of community researchers. However, the case also illustrates the impacts of context and partnering processes when there is misalignment among community members and academic researchers. More specifically, the case reveals how conflicting ways of knowing and divergent social justice tactics contributed tensions that eroded trust among the partners. Additional challenges included the historical context and inhospitable policy environment that further contributed to misalignment in dynamics.

CHAPTER 6

SOCIO-ECOLOGIC FRAMEWORK FOR CBPR

DEVELOPMENT AND TESTING OF A MODEL

SARAH L. KASTELIC, NINA WALLERSTEIN, BONNIE DURAN, AND JOHN G. OETZEL

THE SIGNIFICANCE OF stakeholder knowledge and participation in research addressing complex health problems has grown exponentially (Barkin, Schlundt, & Smith, 2013) and is reflected in multiple national NIH and CDC initiatives (Ahmed & Palermo, 2010; Greenlund & Giles, 2012; Selby, Beal, & Frank, 2012) in the United States. Additionally, the Patient Protection and Affordable Care Act's focus on eliminating disparities relies on community-engaged research (CEnR), including engagement of patient stakeholders, to align academic health centers with community priorities. Multidirectional learning is especially important for research projects among disenfranchised and hard-to-reach populations and academic institutions with insidious traditions of knowledge asymmetry (Michener et al., 2012). Internationally, there has been a concurrent growing interest in public participation in government-funded health research through engagement of service users and nonprofessionals as a strategy for democratization of knowledge and to address health inequities. (For more historical and theoretical background on CBPR and CEnR, see Chapter 2.)

The move toward wider use of CBPR and CEnR approaches is also motivated by protests from, and lack of research participation by, groups historically ignored or subject to unethical and biased research questions and methods (Duran & Duran, 1995; Tuhiwai Smith, 1999). CBPR efforts with historically marginalized groups are commonly aimed at "decolonizing" essentialist narratives (racial, cultural, gender, etc.) created by "scientific" discourse that serves, in part, as the philosophical and moral grounds for the colonization and stratification of the global enterprise to this day. CBPR prevents ongoing abuses by prioritizing community-defined research questions, ensuring community-level benefit, and promoting knowledge democracy that privileges well-established community-derived theories of etiology and change (Hicks et al., 2012; Trickett, 2011).

An important contribution to illustrating the legitimacy and value of CBPR was the development of a conceptual model to serve as a guide for elucidating potential pathways of partnering practices to outcome and capture barriers and promoters of effective CBPR partnerships. Model development was the starting point of a three-stage federally funded research process to support the study of the art and science of community-academic research partnerships: (1) creation of the model (2006–2009), (2) first national testing of measures of the model (2009–2013), and (3) refinement of measures (including translation into Spanish) and intervention study (2015–2020). This chapter summarizes this iterative development and expanded use of the model in the United States and internationally. Based on the first national testing of the model, we also offer analyses of potential pathways of promising practices contributing to outcomes. Chapter 17 provides complementary information on using the CBPR conceptual model for evaluation, on measures and metrics to assess constructs within the model (see also Appendix 10), and on empirical data assessing relationships among partnership practices and outcomes.

STAGE ONE: CREATING THE MODEL

In 2006, believing in CBPR as a methodology to promote community wisdom in health research, Nina Wallerstein from the University of New Mexico Center for Participatory Research (UNM CPR) and Bonnie Duran from the University of Washington Indigenous Wellness Research Institute (UW IWRI) started, with pilot funding from the National Institute of Minority Health and Health Disparities (NIMHD), to create an overarching research design to study CBPR. Throughout this pilot and into the next stages, we convened and were guided by a "think tank" of community and academic CBPR practitioners providing expert consultation throughout the project. Face-to-face meetings, when possible, were supplemented by conference calls and guidance by subcommittees.

Using multiple data collection methodologies, we first conducted an interdisciplinary review of academic literature, building on search terms from the first Agency for Health Care Research and Quality review of CBPR (Viswanathan et al., 2004) about community participation, engagement, and collaborative forms of inquiry and partnership. Literature was reviewed from disciplines as varied as ethnic and Indigenous studies, business administration, communication, education, as well as the social sciences, law, public health, and other biomedical and nursing sciences. Results identified evaluations primarily of CBPR principles and processes, and coalition, organizational, and group dynamic measures. An earlier model provided important concepts and constructs (Schulz, Israel, & Lantz, 2003), but there was little research on associations of practices with outcomes (summarized in Wallerstein et al., 2008). From 2002 to 2008, 258 articles were identified in a review of the CBPR (and related) literature. Forty-six instruments, including 224 individual measures of characteristics in the CBPR conceptual model, were reviewed, and reliability and validity were assessed if possible (Sandoval et al., 2012).

The research team then conducted an Internet survey of more than one hundred CBPR projects, collecting data about the resonance of the partnering and outcome constructs identified through the literature review and think tank guidance. This preliminary investigation resulted in the first iteration of the CBPR conceptual model, which was further validated through qualitative community consultation with six partnerships (Belone et al., 2016).

In creating the conceptual model, we wanted to explicate the specific domains, such as contexts, partnership characteristics and processes, that contribute to research and intervention designs and that ultimately influence outcomes of CBPR. By definition and through guiding principles (Israel, Eng, Schulz, & Parker, 2013; Minkler & Wallerstein, 2008), effective, authentic CBPR requires local identification of health problems and builds on community contexts, including local strengths and resources, to participate in the project and address health inequities. The CBPR model adopted this transformational framework to showcase how partnering practices could have a broad range of outcomes, from increased synergy as a short-term output; to intermediate-level policy, system, and capacity changes; to more long-term opportunities for social justice, equity, and health outcomes.

We also saw the model as embedding a theory of change from Paulo Freire's educational pedagogy of conscientization and praxis: an ongoing cycle of partners listening and engaging in dialogue with each other, making decisions and choosing actions as a result of their dialogues, reflecting on those actions, and then continuing with another cycle of listening, dialogue, action, and reflection (Freire, 1970, 1982; Wallerstein & Auerbach, 2004). Thus, the conceptual model was created to facilitate CBPR partnerships' ability to put their partnership in a framework that supports ongoing collective reflection and evaluation for strengthening the quality and effectiveness of their partnership to reach desired outcomes.

The model was intentionally created as a dynamic tool that has changed over time as research identifies other factors that promote or inhibit effective, authentic CBPR; and understanding of how domains and variables may interact deepens and becomes more nuanced. Even with the first iteration of the model, we saw the model as a framework to be adapted by partnerships in ways that most closely reflect each project's and partnership's goals. The intention was never to offer the singular, authoritative view on community-academic partnership characteristics, processes, and outcomes, that is, to become the "CBPR police," determining who is "doing CBPR right." Rather, we sought to offer through literature, data from the field, and ongoing expert consultation the best available thinking about contexts, partnering processes, interventions and research, and outcomes. Undoubtedly the hundreds of community-academic research partnerships in the United States (let alone throughout the world) have varying contexts, dynamics, health interventions or programs, research designs and outcomes, and priorities. In fact, the most salient question continues to be, under what conditions or contexts are which engagement and partnering practices the most effective to contribute to research and intervention design and to best affect a wide range of research, systems, capacity, and health and equity outcomes?

What follows is a conceptual model that seeks to be of use to community-academic partnerships and can be adjusted or customized in ways that emphasize any partnership's realities and goals (see Figure 6.1). Some model adaptations are presented here as well as in Chapter 17. Through multiple iterations and applications, the model continues to grow and be refined over time. The domains and constructs of the 2017 version of the conceptual model are described in the next sections (http://cpr.unm.edu/research-projects/cbpr-project/cbpr-model.html).

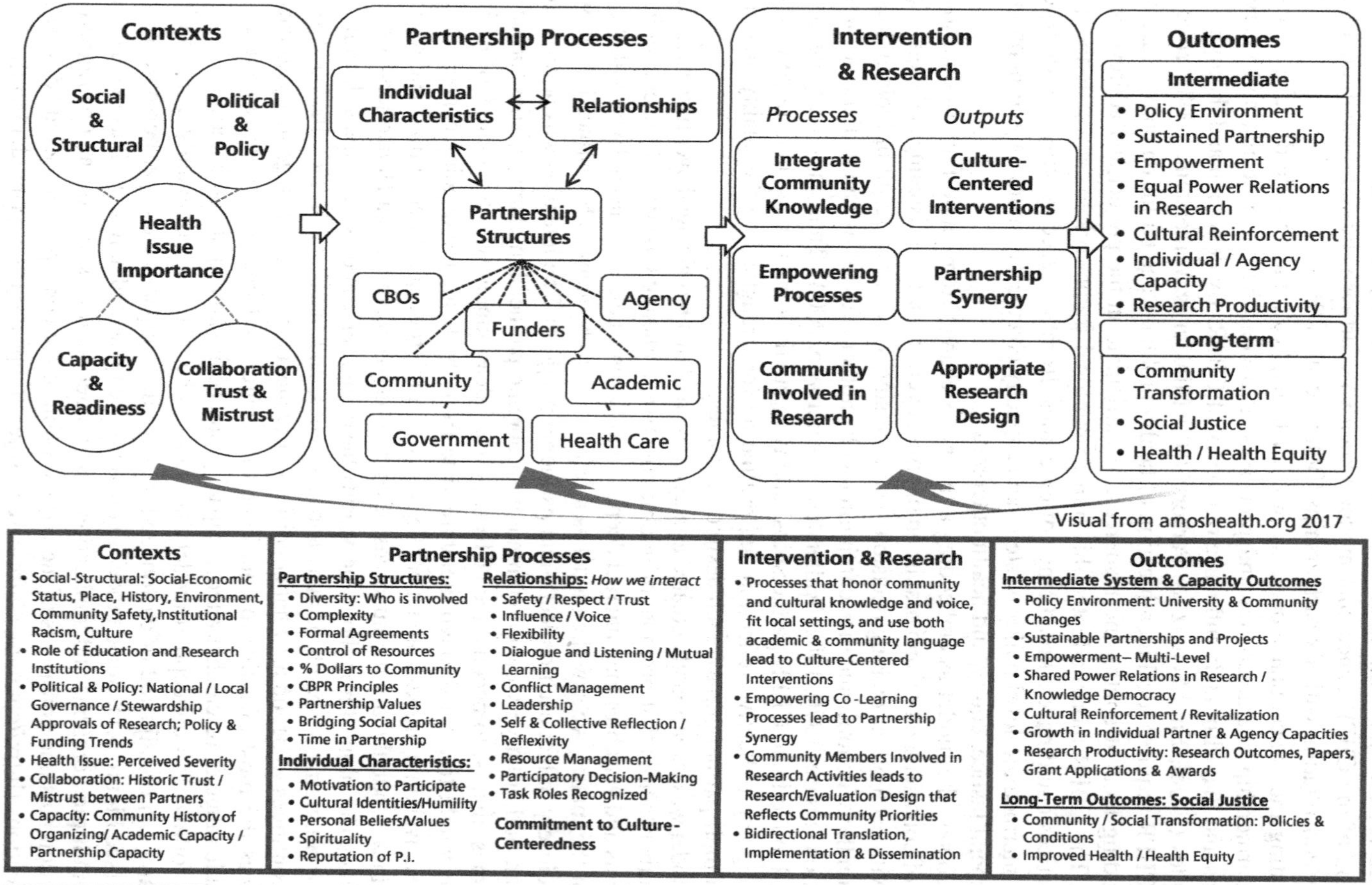

FIGURE 6.1 *CBPR Conceptual Model*

Source: Adapted from Wallerstein et al. (2008) and Wallerstein and Duran (2010, p. S1). Visual from amoshealth.org (2016).

The conceptual model is organized into four overarching domains: contexts, partnership processes, intervention and research, and outcomes. Although it may initially appear complex, the basic domains of the model are straightforward. The model hypothesizes that the context of any given community-academic partnership grounds the partnership processes, which include individual characteristics, relationships, and partnership structures. In turn, the context and partnership processes, with community involvement in all research stages, can affect and alter the "science" or the design of the research and health interventions. The implementation of research methods and interventions then can affect intermediate system and capacity outcomes within communities and academia as well as long-term changes in community health conditions and health equity.

Within each domain, several predominant constructs have been identified. The relative importance of the constructs may vary by partnership. In the context domain, five constructs (see Box 6.1) follow a socio-ecologic framework commonly used in public health. Social-structural and political factors are the highest level of social determinants, followed by organizational capacities of academic and community institutions, which are followed by interpersonal collaboration and levels of trust and mistrust, and perceptions of importance of health issues.

To highlight just a few factors, the perceived importance of the health issue describes the partners' perceived severity of the health problem(s) and, relatedly, the urgency of the health issue(s) being addressed by the partnership. The collaboration context accounts for the historic trust or mistrust between the partners. The capacity and readiness context addresses multiple capacities: the community's history of organizing or prior research experience; the academic institution's capacity to engage with communities; and their mutual capacity to partner.

The partnership processes domain (see Box 6.2) links the individual, interpersonal, and organization levels of the socio-ecologic framework and consists specifically of individual characteristics, structural features, and relationships among the academic, community, agency, health systems, and community-based organizations.

Among other things, the individual characteristics account for the core values, participation motivation, cultural identities and cultural humility (see Appendix 4), and personal belief systems and spirituality of the individuals involved in the partnership. The structural features account for the diversity of who is participating, as organizations or individuals; complexity of kinds of stakeholders participating; formal agreements or lack thereof; as well as team members'

Box 6.1 **Contexts**

- Social-structural: social-economic status, place, history, environment, community safety, institutional racism, culture, role of education and research institutions
- Political policy: national, local governance, stewardship, approvals of research, policy and funding trends
- Health issue: perceived severity by partners
- Collaboration: historic trust-mistrust between partners
- Capacity: community history of organizing, academic capacity, partnership capacity

Box 6.2 Partnership Processes

Partnership Structures

- Diversity: who is involved
- Complexity
- Formal agreements
- Control of resources
- Percentage of dollars to community
- CBPR principles
- Partnership values
- Bridging social capital
- Time in partnership

Individual Characteristics

- Motivation to participate
- Cultural identities, humility
- Personal belief, values
- Spirituality
- Reputation of PI

Relationships: How We Interact

- Safety/respect/trust
- Community voice/influence
- Flexibility
- Dialogue and listening, mutual learning
- Conflict management
- Leadership
- Self- and collective reflection, reflexivity
- Resource management
- Participatory decision making
- Task roles recognized

Commitment to Culture-Centeredness

capacity to bridge across cultures and positions of power. The relationships between stakeholders in partnership, or how the partnership interacts, include constructs such as safety, community voice and influence or lack thereof, dialogue and listening, self- and collective reflexivity practices, use of participatory decision making, and task roles recognized.

In the science or intervention and research domain, processes lead to outputs (see Box 6.3). The ability to integrate community and cultural knowledge and voice leads to a culture-centered nature of the intervention and a fit with local settings. Empowering processes lead to partnership synergy. The third construct, community members involved in research activities, leads to appropriate research design. Taken together, the processes lead to the bidirectional translation, implementation, and dissemination of research.

In the outcomes domain (see Box 6.4), partnering processes and their impact on research and interventions may produce multilevel impacts, from system and capacity outcomes for the community and academic partners as well as the potential for improved health and health equity. Intermediate system and capacity outcomes may include policy environment changes, whether the intervention is sustainable and culturally centered for broader reach, changes in power relations and knowledge democracy, and changes in cultural reinforcement—whether the intervention supports cultural revitalization or cultural continuity in the community. The

Box 6.3 Intervention and Research

Processes and Outputs

- Processes that honor community and cultural knowledge and voice, fit local settings, and use academic and community language leading to culture-centered interventions
- Empowering co-learning processes lead to partnership synergy
- Community members involved in research activities lead to research and evaluation designs that reflect community priorities
- Bidirectional translation, implementation, and dissemination

Box 6.4 Outcomes

Intermediate System and Capacity Outcomes

- Policy environment changes in universities and communities
- Sustainable partnerships and projects
- Empowerment: multilevel
- Shared power relations in research, knowledge democracy
- Cultural reinforcement, revitalization
- Growth in partner and agencies capacities
- Research productivity: research outcomes, papers, grant applications, and awards

Long-Term Outcomes: Social Justice

- Community/social transformation: policies, programs, conditions
- Improved health, health equity

long-term improved health outcomes include potentially transformed social and economic conditions, reduced health disparities, and increased social justice.

The CBPR conceptual model hypothesizes multiple pathways that context affects: partnership dynamics, research and intervention design, and outcomes. With feedback loops, outcomes can circle back to affect other domains, which then influence each other. A policy outcome, for example, which the partnership advocated for, could open up the policy environment to more input by the partnership, which could then bring in other stakeholders to identify additional data for action, thus creating more community capacities to use research to effect policy and community changes. These interactions, which may proceed partially along linear pathways, may also therefore be thought of as dynamic complex systems of reciprocal or mutual influence.

Once the initial model was created, we sought further community consultations, starting in 2009, to establish community face validity and make revisions as necessary. Qualitative data were gathered from six focus groups drawn from a purposive sample of the think tank members' community partners. The aims of the focus groups were to gain community partner perspectives on the conceptual model (i.e., the meanings, strengths, and weaknesses of the four domains and various constructs) and to adapt the model based on community wisdom about the constructs and deepen understandings about new constructs added to the model (Belone et al., 2016).

The six CBPR projects that participated in the focus group research included four geographically and ethnically diverse partnerships: two in the Midwest (one rural and one urban), one in the West, and one in the Southwest, as well as two national CBPR nonprofit organizations. Findings from the community consultations included (1) the model had strong face validity across geographically, racially, and ethnically diverse partnerships, with support for existing constructs and suggestions for new constructs; (2) the dimensions and constructs were useful prompts for discussion of partnership practices within specific communities; and (3) four cross-cutting constructs were seen in all domains of the model—trust development (also see Chapter 5), capacity, mutual learning, and power dynamics. The conversations underscored the usefulness of the conceptual model in promoting self- and collective reflection and a continual process evaluation for partnerships.

In summary, this first-stage exploratory pilot yielded an initial model and an interdisciplinary literature review of measurement instruments for constructs in the model (Pearson et al., 2011; Sandoval et al., 2012) to contribute to theory about effective, authentic CBPR. Testing the model was the next step.

STAGE TWO: RESEARCH FOR IMPROVED HEALTH: TESTING AND STRENGTHENING THE MODEL

As UNM CPR and UW IWRI came to the end of their three-year NIMHD-funded pilot, they sought additional support and a new partner to continue the process of refining and testing the conceptual model, all with an eye toward creating tools and information that support the continual strengthening of CBPR science. In 2008, co-PIs Wallerstein and Duran invited the National Congress of American Indians Policy Research Center (NCAI PRC) to join their think tank of CBPR practitioners and to partner as a new PI on their next funding application.

A grant from the Native American Research Centers for Health (NARCH), a funding partnership between the Indian Health Service and the National Institutes of Health, supported the next phase of work to test the model.[1] Wallerstein and Duran intentionally selected a junior investigator to mentor in the PI role. NCAI PRC director Sarah (Hicks) Kastelic brought a focus on CBPR in American Indian/Alaska Native (AI/AN) tribal communities and thereby strengthened the Indigenous lens of the role of governance, stewardship, and Indigenous knowledge within the model. Founded in 2003, the NCAI PRC's mission was to provide tribal leaders with the best available knowledge to make strategic policy decisions in a framework of Native wisdom that positively affects the future of Native peoples.[2] This mission positioned NCAI PRC to credibly lead a project to engage with community-academic partnerships including communities of color and tribal communities to further test the conceptual model.

This new partnership of three organizations and their teams represented several principles of CBPR: the coming together of different knowledge bases, recognition that each knowledge base brought complementary strengths, the shared goals of research for the purpose of community benefit and equity, and research capacity building of a more junior investigator from the community partner. This last principle, although not specifically within the CBPR literature, has been threaded throughout the years in this initiative, as well as in others around the country, to welcome new scholars, students, and community partners into a community of practice and mutual learning. For CBPR as a field, mentorship, in particular of scholars of color, has been a common practice with the goal of changing the face of the academy to bring in colleagues who can best serve and understand the communities they come from (see Chapter 19 for particular pipeline programs).

The NARCH V grant (2009–2013) funded a mixed-methods, cross-site research study entitled "Research for Improved Health: A Study of Community-Academic Partnerships" (RIH) to test the CBPR conceptual model and its four domains across a wide variety of federally funded community engaged and CBPR projects. Two Internet surveys of about two hundred partnerships and seven in-depth case studies were used to explore the following study aims: (1) describe the variability of CBPR characteristics across dimensions in the CBPR conceptual model to identify differences and commonalities across partnerships; (2) describe and assess the impact of governance on CBPR processes and outcomes across AI/AN and other communities of color; (3) examine the associations among group dynamic processes and three major CBPR outcomes: culturally responsive and centered interventions, strengthened research infrastructure and other community capacities, and new health-enhancing policies and practices, under varying conditions and contexts; and (4) identify promising practices, assessment tools, and future research needs for the field of CBPR. The intention was for NCAI, in particular, to bring those practices and tools to tribal leaders and researchers (Hicks et al., 2012). Again, the think tank of CBPR community and academic practitioners advised the research team in an ongoing fashion, including quantitative and qualitative instrument development and data analysis (see http://cpr.unm.edu/research-projects/cbpr-project/research-for-improved-health.html).

As described in significant detail by Lucero et al. (2016) (and with some information in Chapter 17), the RIH research design integrated mixed methods at each stage of the research process. Further, by revisiting stages to integrate new knowledge gleaned from practice, the research team had significant innovation in what they termed an "expanded iterative integration . . . grounded in an *Indigenous-transformative* [emphasis added] paradigm that recognized different ways of knowing at each stage and at critical decision points" (Lucero et al., 2016, p. 3).

The study design began with shared sample finalization and inclusion criteria for the quantitative web-based survey and qualitative case studies. The qualitative research began first, as the quantitative instruments were still being designed. The quantitative and qualitative instruments drew on the literature review during the pilot. The first case study was conducted, and results of the analysis were integrated into the survey design; further, qualitative materials were revised. This integration of practice, reflection, and new knowledge strengthened the qualitative materials and informed quantitative instrument development, recruitment, and instrument revision. The case studies continued on parallel track with the implementation of the web-based survey. Quantitative and qualitative analyses were conducted, and data validation occurred.

The sampling frame was constructed using a 2009 download of all federally funded CBPR and community-engaged research projects from the NIH RePORTER database. (For sampling details, see Pearson et al., 2015.) Of the participating community-academic partnerships, 45 percent were funded by three federal agencies: National Institute on Minority Health and Health Disparities (19.1 percent), National Cancer Institute (13.3 percent), and the Centers for Disease Control (12.6 percent). The majority of participating projects were intervention research (66 percent) as opposed to descriptive research (20.7 percent) or other research, such as dissemination and implementation or policy projects (13.3 percent). Nearly 59 percent of projects were funded by NIH R mechanisms. The average length of the project was 4.6 years. Twenty-one percent of projects served AI/AN populations ($n = 63$); 23 percent served other minority populations (Hispanic/Latino [$n = 24$], African American [$n = 20$], and Asian American [$n = 7$]); and 55 percent served no specified population ($n = 85$) or multiple populations ($n = 17$).

With oversampling of AI/AN projects because of targeted outreach to NARCH projects, we were able to identify specific issues related to governance differences between AI/AN projects and those of other populations. Projects serving AI/AN populations were more likely to share resources and power, including making key decisions together; more likely to have formal written research agreements, including publication guidelines and review, intellectual property agreements, and data sharing and use guidelines; and, generally, less well-funded (i.e., received less total funds than projects serving multiple race–unspecified racial groups). (For additional findings related to the relationship of CEnR research approval type to governance processes, productivity, and perceived outcomes, see Oetzel et al., 2015.) There were no significant differences between AI/AN-serving projects and those serving multiple races or unspecified racial groups in partners' engagement throughout the research process. Across all projects, community partners were engaged in an average of 6.5 research activities.

In addition to the survey, seven diverse case studies were identified from distinct regions, subpopulations, and health and social issues (see Table 6.1). The goal of the case studies was to complement and triangulate with the survey data and to focus more specifically on the mechanisms and pathways of how partnering practices may contribute to short-term, intermediate, and long-term outcomes. (For case study descriptions, see Chapters 9 and 11; Devia et al. [2017]; Lucero et al. [under review]; Wallerstein et al. [under review].)

Achievement of synergy as a proximal outcome, for example, as the capacity of partners to get the tasks of research done collaboratively, can promote a series of intermediate outcomes, such as greater equality between academics and community members in their decision-making and respect for each other's knowledge and, therefore, the co-development of interventions that would be centered within local cultural values and contexts. This cultural fit would then lead to a higher likelihood of sustainability of these interventions and increased chance of health improvement over the long run.

TABLE 6.1 Projects and Health and Social Issues

	Region	Population	Partners
Healing of the Canoe: Substance abuse prevention, youth life skills	Pacific Northwest	Native youth	University of Washington and two tribes
Men on the Move: Cardiovascular disease prevention, men's employment	Boothill, Missouri	African American men	St. Louis University; community members
Bronx HealthREACH: Faith-based diabetes management and prevention, unequal access to care	Bronx, New York	African American and Latino congregations	Institute for Family Health, New York University, churches, and community organizations
Lay health workers to increase colorectal cancer screening and nutrition education	San Francisco	Residents of Chinatown (55–64)	University of California, San Francisco; San Francisco State; NICOS (Community partner), Chinatown Health Department
Tribal Nation: Barriers to Cancer Prevention	South Dakota	Native adults	Black Hills Center for American Indian Health and tribe
South Valley Partners for Environmental Justice: Policies to reduce unequal exposure to toxins	Albuquerque, New Mexico	Hispanic population	University of New Mexico, Bernalillo County, Rio Grande Community Development Corporation, community partners
Assessment of health issues for Deaf and hearing impaired	Rochester, New York	Deaf or hearing impaired	Center for Deaf Health, University of Rochester, partners from Deaf community

With the case study and the survey data together, we conducted a mixed-method analysis of the RIH data to examine how all domains relate to each other. This analysis involved a structural equation model (SEM) to test the complex relationships as well integration of case study data to add depth and better understanding of the mechanisms of change to the statistical analysis.

We could not include every variable from the original conceptual model and so focused on specific variables within each domain. The tested model was a good fit with the data and included two context variables (partnership capacity and final approval), with paths to the partnership processes domain to two larger constructs: (1) partnership structures, including, for example, shared control over resources and percentage of resources to community, and (2) relationships, including, for example, leadership, trust, and participatory decision making), which led to the intervention and research domain (e.g., community involvement in research and synergy). Although interrelated, two pathways emerged. The material structural pathway, starting with final approval of the project on behalf of the community by a tribal government or health board compared to other approvals, is associated with a greater percentage of resources to the community. The percentage of resources, along with shared control of the resources, is associated with higher levels of community involvement in the research. The second relationship pathway starts with partnership capacity shaping partnership values, which is associated with stronger relationships and then synergy. Both of these pathways were positively associated with intermediate outcomes, and then intermediate outcomes are positively associated with long-term outcomes of community transformation and health outcomes.

Case study examples added the time element and directionality of how pathways worked. For example, in the San Francisco Chinatown case study on effectiveness of lay health workers, partners included a well-esteemed community organization. By receiving a subcontract and research training, the community organization (NICOS Chinese Health Coalition) controlled resources to hire staff members for each research step. Interviewees discussed how their collaborative structures led to greater involvement of community members in the research and collective decision making, which led to enhanced synergy, contributing to outcomes of intervention effectiveness, enhanced research capacity for NICOS, and increased recognition by academics of NICOS's goals for workforce development, a community benefit far beyond specific grant aims. Together, the qualitative data, coupled with the SEM analysis, demonstrated support for the robustness of the CBPR model (Oetzel et al., in press).

Through analysis of the model, we learned that effective partnering may not be a generic "promising practice," but dependent on holistic contextual factors (including those supported by survey data such as partner capacity to be advocates). When viewed organically, effective partnerships apply symbiotic strategies in response to their environments (e.g., history or political policy context) and their ability to transform internal group-level relationship dynamics (e.g., power sharing, trust, co-learning, and community voice) into greater partnership synergy and broad capacity and system changes. Another RIH case study, Bronx Health REACH, for example, worked with church pastors steeped in the civil rights movement as their historical context to demand their voice be heard. The power of the community partners supported strong equitable relationships with their academic partners, such as power sharing, which created a formidable synergy that was able to advocate for improved food environments and school nutrition policies to reduce excess rates of diabetes (Devia et al., 2017; Kaplan et al., 2009). The qualitative data therefore recommends adoption of promising practices with consideration of contexts and implications for actions within specific political-cultural conditions.

As RIH funding ended in 2013, the research partners shared instruments and materials widely to openly invite stakeholders to explore and use the model.[3] One example has been NCAI's subsequent NARCH grant to create a dissemination and implementation tool kit for several of the constructs, including trust and culture, and to highlight the role of governance and sovereignty in partnership evaluation.[4]

STAGE THREE: CONTINUING TO ADAPT AND EXPAND THE MODEL: DISCOVERING NEW USES

On the heels of RIH, UNM CPR and UW IWRI sought additional partners to continue to adapt, expand, and test the CBPR conceptual model. With support from the National Institute of Nursing Research (2015–2020), UNM CPR and UW IWRI recruited other University of Washington colleagues, Community-Campus Partnerships for Health, the National Indian Child Welfare Association, University of Waikato, New Zealand, and Rand Corporation to join "Engage for Equity (E^2)," a national study of community and academic partnerships, to continue development of measures and metrics of CBPR practices and outcomes. The specific aims are to (1) reconvene the national think tank of academic and community CBPR experts for their oversight and guidance; (2) refine, translate into Spanish, and test finalized metrics and measures with up to two hundred federally funded partnerships; and (3) conduct a randomized control trial comparing a workshop intervention that integrates partnership evaluation and self-reflection tools for forty partnerships versus access to materials and resources on the web. The Engage for Equity team has begun to deepen our understanding of theories of change that may matter in partnerships, such as the role of empowering processes or the role of culture-centeredness approaches in creating successful outcomes.

It is clear that the CBPR conceptual model has strong resonance and meaning in the field of community-engaged research and CBPR science. The model continues to evolve as a dynamic tool to explore, support, evaluate, and strengthen CBPR science. The research partners believe that rather than serving as a static model of the one "true" perspective on CBPR, the model serves a field-building and unifying purpose. The CBPR conceptual model has been continually promoted as a dynamic tool to be adapted by local partnerships and used creatively.

In the last five years, the research partners have learned much about how community and academic partnerships are organically making the model their own, adapting its content and format in ways that support their perspectives and experiences. For example, Lisa Gibbs, principal investigator of Teeth Tales, a CBPR study addressing children's oral health for Australian families in Melbourne from migrant backgrounds, adapted the conceptual model in 2014 (see Figure 6.2). With multiple community partners, including immigrant Pakistani and Arabic organizations, the University of Melbourne adapted the model in the final research stages to represent their study experience. They reflected on the model dimensions, kept relevant constructs, and added their own. Partners found it a useful summary exercise to identify and assess their most important partnering practices and outcomes.[5]

More recently, the Minnesota Rochester Healthy Community Partnership,[6] a ten-year established CBPR partnership working with the Somali, Hispanic, and Cambodian communities to promote community health and well-being, approached UNM CPR about support and tools for evaluating their partnership. (See Chapter 17 for a description of how they adapted the model, surveys, and interview instruments to evaluate their history and current partnering practices to envision future directions.)

The model has also been translated into Spanish and Portuguese.[7] A nonprofit health system, AMOS Health and Hope (Amoshealth.org), for example, has used the model to strengthen their training of community health workers (promotores) as coresearchers of maternal and child health inequities in remote rural underserved areas of Nicaragua. The promotores collect data

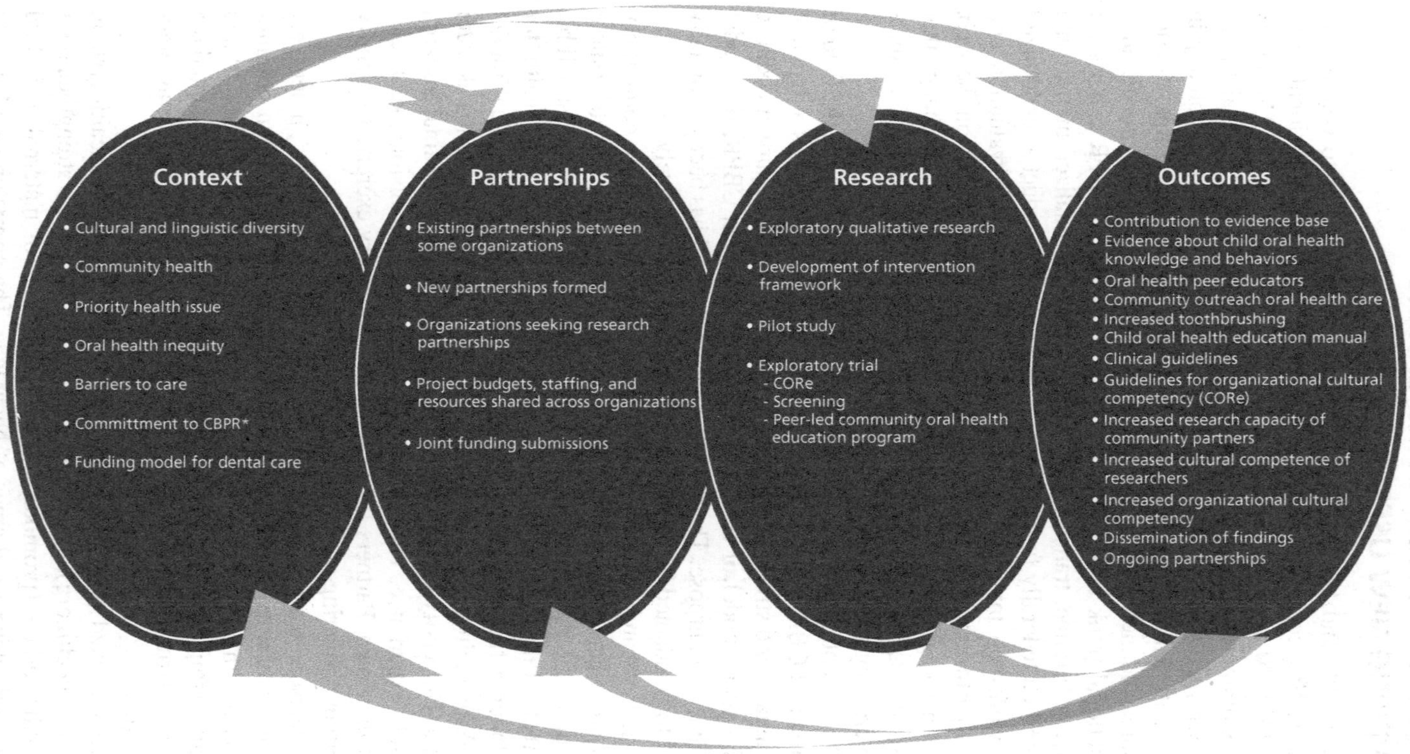

Context
• Cultural and linguistic diversity
• Community health
• Priority health issue
• Oral health inequity
• Barriers to care
• Committment to CBPR*
• Funding model for dental care
Partnerships
• Existing partnerships between some organizations
• New partnerships formed
• Organizations seeking research partnerships
• Project budgets, staffing, and resources shared across organizations
• Joint funding submissions
Research
• Exploratory qualitative research
• Development of intervention framework
• Pilot study
• Exploratory trial
- CORe
- Screening
- Peer-led community oral health education program
Outcomes
• Contribution to evidence base
• Evidence about child oral health knowledge and behaviors
• Oral health peer educators
• Community outreach oral health care
• Increased toothbrushing
• Child oral health education manual
• Clinical guidelines
• Guidelines for organizational cultural competency (CORe)
• Increased research capacity of community partners
• Increased cultural competence of researchers
• Increased organizational cultural competency
• Dissemination of findings
• Ongoing partnerships

FIGURE 6.2 *Teeth Tales Model*

Note: CBPR = community-based participatory research.

Source: Adapted from http://mspgh.unimelb.edu.au/centres-institutes/centre-for-health-equity/research-group/jack-brockhoff-child-health-wellbeing-program/research/physical-health-and-wellbeing/teeth-tales

on households to monitor family health and to identify community empowerment strategies, such as women's and youth groups, to address root causes of ill health (see Chapter 18). AMOS is also using the model to train medical students and faculty members on how to integrate community participation into research projects. The Spanish, Portuguese, and English versions have each been integrated into the empowerment, social participation, and participatory research curriculum (in three languages) on the UNM Center for Participatory Research website.[8]

Finally, the conceptual model is being used as a visioning and planning tool for new partnerships to brainstorm their desired outcomes and the partnering processes they would like to have. New teams often start with brainstorming in the fourth domain, the outcomes they would like to see. They then return to the first two domains of the model: identifying core contextual issues important to their communities and discussing partnership dynamics, that is, how they plan to integrate CBPR principles and strategies into their partnering practices or whether they need or want to develop formal agreements. They can then think ahead as to how their decision-making practices will affect their interventions and research design and methods, and ultimately, return to desired outcomes.

This newer use of the model as a reflection tool for setting a planning or evaluation agenda provides partnerships an opportunity to adapt the model for their own use. For CBPR visioning facilitation guides for planning and evaluation purposes, see http://cpr.unm.edu/research-projects/cbpr-project/facilitation_tools.html.

These self-created plans can then be revisited on an annual basis and form part of an ongoing cycle of evaluation and reflection opportunities for recognition of achievements and recommendations for the future. As a living, breathing document, we hope that the CBPR conceptual model can be useful for your own reflections and actions in current and future collaborative research endeavors.

CONCLUSION

Future stages of work on the conceptual model include evolution of how best to apply the model for planning, collective evaluation, and ongoing reflection on partnering practices and outcomes. Cross-partnership dialogue about model use may lead to further evolution or potential reinterpretation of the model. Future research will focus on better understanding the pathways among variables in the domains or better identifying theories of change that lead to system, capacity, and social justice outcomes. We hope that partnerships can be better positioned to make deliberate choices about which context, relationship, or structural processes or other partnering factors are important to them and their research, in order for them to achieve their own desired outcomes.

QUESTIONS FOR DISCUSSION

1. What is the value of the CBPR conceptual model? How can it be used?
2. How has the evolution of this model supported a larger CBPR research agenda, including improving CBPR science?
3. What are the potential dangers of putting forth a model of CBPR (even if you acknowledge variability and no one "right" way)?

ACKNOWLEDGMENTS

The research described in this chapter was supported by NARCH (U261HS300293; U261IHS0036-04-00), with Indian Health Service in partnership with the National Institute of General Medical Sciences, National Institute of Minority Health and Health Disparities, National Institute on Drug Abuse, National Center for Research Resources, Office of Behavioral Social Sciences Research, National Cancer Institute, and Health Resources Services Administration. We thank the research team and members of the think tank and community scientific advisory board for their collaboration. We also appreciate Dr. Malia Villegas who stepped in as PI for Dr. Sarah Kastelic, when Sarah left the directorship of NCAI's Policy Research Center. Most important, we thank the academic and community partners who participated in the surveys and case studies.

NOTES

1. See www.nigms.nih.gov/Research/CRCB/NARCH/Pages/default.aspx.
2. See www.ncai.org/policy-research-center/about-prc/mission.
3. See quantitative and qualitative instruments at http://cpr.unm.edu/research-projects/cbpr-project/research-for-improved-health.html.
4. See www.ncai.org/policy-research-center/initiatives/projects/narch.
5. http://cpr.unm.edu/research-projects/cbpr-project/background-to-teeth-tales.html.
6. See http://rochesterhealthy.org/website/.
7. http://cpr.unm.edu/research-projects/cbpr-project/cbpr-model.html.
8. See http://cpr.unm.edu/curricula--classes/empowerment-curriculum.html.

REFERENCES

Ahmed, S. M., & Palermo, A. G. (2010). Community engagement in research: Frameworks for education and peer review. *American Journal of Public Health, 100*(8), 1380–1387. doi:10.2105/AJPH.2009.178137

Barkin, S., Schlundt, D., & Smith, P. (2013). Community-engaged research perspectives: Then and now. *Academic Pediatrics, 13*(2), 93–97.

Belone, L., Lucero, J. E., Duran, B., Tafoya, G., Baker, E. A., Chan, D., . . . Wallerstein, N. (2016). Community-based participatory research conceptual model: Community partner consultation and face validity. *Qualitative Health Research, 26,* 117–135.

Devia, C., Baker, E., Sanchez-Youngman, S., Barnidge, E., Golub, M., Motton, F., Muhammad, M., Ruddock, C., Vicuña, B., & Wallerstein, N. (2017). CBPR to advance social and racial equity: Urban and rural partnerships in black and Latino communities. *International Journal for Equity in Health, 16,* 17. doi:10.1186/s12939-016-0509-3

Duran, E., & Duran, B. (1995). *Native American postcolonial psychology.* Albany State University of New York Press.

Freire, P. (1970). *Pedagogy of the oppressed.* New York, NY: Seabury Press.

Freire, P. (Ed.). (1982). *Creating alternative research methods: Learning to do it by doing it.* Toronto, Canada: Participatory Research Network.

Greenlund, K. J., & Giles, W. H. (2012). The Prevention Research Centers program: Translating research into public health practice and impact. *American Journal of Preventive Medicine, 43*(3 Suppl 2), S91–S92. doi:10.1016/j.amepre.2012.06.002

Hicks, S., Duran, B., Wallerstein, N., Avila, M., Belone, L., Lucero, J., . . . White Hat, E. W. (2012). Evaluating community-based participatory research to improve community-partnered science and community health. *Progress in Community Health Partnership: Research, Education, and Action, 6,* 289–299.

Israel, B. A., Eng, E., Schulz, A. J., & Parker, E. A. (Eds.). (2013). *Methods in community-based participatory research for health* (2nd ed.). San Francisco, CA: Jossey-Bass.

Kaplan, S. A., Ruddock, C., Golub, M., Davis, J. D., Foley, R.C.D., . . . Calman, N. (2009). Stirring up the mud: Using a community-based participatory approach to address health disparities through a faith-based initiative. *Journal of Health Care for the Poor and Underserved, 20,* 1111–1123.

Lucero, J., Wallerstein, N., Duran, B., Alegria, M., Greene-Moton, E., Israel, B., . . . White Hat, E. (2016). Development of a mixed-methods investigation of process and outcomes of community-based participatory research. *Journal of Mixed Methods Research.* Advance online publication. doi:10.1177/1558689816633309

Lucero, J., et al. (under review). CBPR as negotiation: A cancer screening case study from Chinatown, San Francisco. *Journal of Health Psychology.*

Michener, L., Cook, J., Ahmed, S. M., Yonas, M. A., Coyne-Beasley, T., & Aguilar-Gaxiola, S. (2012). Aligning the goals of community-engaged research: Why and how academic health centers can successfully engage with communities to improve health. *Academic Medicine, 87*(3), 285–291. doi:10.1097/ACM.0b013e3182441680

Minkler, M., & Wallerstein, N. (Eds.). (2008). *Community-based participatory research for health: From process to outcomes* (2nd ed.). San Francisco, CA: Jossey-Bass.

Oetzel, J. G., Villegas, M., White Hat, E., Duran, B., & Wallerstein, N. (2015). Governance of community-engaged research: Exploring the associations of final approval with processes and outcomes. *American Journal of Public Health, 105,* 1161–1167.

Oetzel, J. G., Wallerstein, N., Duran, B., Villegas, M., Sanchez-Youngman, S., et al. (in press). Community-engaged research for health: A test of the CBPR conceptual model. *BioMed Research International.*

Pearson, C., Duran, B., Martin, D., Lucero, J., Sandoval, J., Oetzel, J., Tafoya, G., Belone, L., Avila, M., Wallerstein, N., & Hicks, S. (2011). *CBPR variable matrix: Research for improved health in academic-community partnerships* [Interactive model]. Retrieved from http://ces4health.info/index.aspx

Pearson, C. R., Duran, B., Oetzel, J., Margarati, M., Villegas, M., Lucero, J., & Wallerstein, N. (2015). Research for improved health: Variability and impact of structural characteristics in federally funded community engaged research projects. *Progress in Community Health Partnerships: Research, Education, and Action, 9,* 17–29.

Sandoval, J. A., Lucero, J., Oetzel, J., Avila, M., Belone, L., Mau, M., & Wallerstein, N. W. (2012). Process and outcome constructs for evaluating community-based participatory research projects: A matrix of existing measures. *Health Education Research, 27,* 680–690.

Schulz, A. J., Israel, B. A., & Lantz, P. (2003). Instrument for evaluating dimensions of group dynamics within community-based participatory research partnerships. *Evaluation and Program Planning, 26,* 249–262.

Selby, J. V., Beal, A. C., & Frank, L. (2012). The Patient-Centered Outcomes Research Institute (PCORI) national priorities for research and initial research agenda. *JAMA, 307*(15), 1583–1584. doi:10.1001/jama.2012.500

Trickett, E. J. (2011). Community-based participatory research as worldview or instrumental strategy: Is it lost in translation(al) research? *American Journal of Public Health, 101*(8), 1353–1355. doi:10.2105/AJPH.2011.300124

Tuhiwai Smith, L. (1999). *Decolonizing methodologies: Research and Indigenous peoples.* New York, NY: Zed Books.

Viswanathan, M., Ammerman, A., Eng, E., Garlehner, G., Lohr, K. N., Griffith, D., . . . Whitener, L. (2004, August). *Community-based participatory research: Assessing the evidence summary* (AHRQ Pub. No. 04-E022-1). Rockville, MD: Agency for Healthcare Research and Quality. Retrieved from https://archive.ahrq.gov/clinic/epcsums/cbprsum.pdf

Wallerstein, N., & Auerbach, E. (2004). *Problem-posing at work: Popular educators guide.* Edmonton, Canada: Grass Roots Press.

Wallerstein, N., & Duran, B. (2010). Community-based participatory research contributions to intervention research: The intersection of science and practice to improve health equity. *American Journal Public Health, 100*(Suppl 1), S40–S46.

Wallerstein, N., Oetzel, J., Duran, B., Magarati, M., Pearson, C., Belone, L., Davis, J., Dewindt, L., Lucero, J., Ruddock, C., Sutter, E., Villegas, M., Dutta, M. (under review). Conceptualizing and measuring the culture-centered approach in community based participatory research. *Social Science and Medicine.*

Wallerstein, N. B., Oetzel, J., Duran, B., Tafoya, G., Belone, L., & Rae, R. (2008). What predicts outcomes in CBPR? In M. Minkler & N. Wallerstein (Eds.), *Community-based participatory research for health: From process to outcomes* (pp. 371–394). San Francisco, CA: Jossey-Bass.

CHAPTER 7

YOUTH-LED PARTICIPATORY ACTION RESEARCH (YPAR)

PRINCIPLES APPLIED TO THE US AND DIVERSE GLOBAL SETTINGS

EMILY J. OZER AND AMBER AKEMI PIATT

YOUTH-LED PARTICIPATORY ACTION research (YPAR) is an approach to inquiry and social change that engages young people in identifying problems relevant to their own lives, conducting research to understand the problems, and advocating for changes based on research evidence (Brown & Rodríguez, 2009; London, Zimmerman, & Erbstein, 2003; Ozer & Douglas, 2015). YPAR, similar to other forms of community-based participatory research (CBPR), is focused on increasing the power of marginalized groups in improving real-world problems via iterative cycles of inquiry and action (Minkler & Wallerstein, 2003). YPAR research and practice has grown in recent years: a 2016 Psychinfo database search, for example, shows more than three hundred citations using the term *youth-led participatory action research.* YPAR spans fields including public health, education, and community psychology, with youth researchers addressing diverse topics, such as neighborhood food access (Breckwich Vásquez et al., 2007), invasive pest management in the Ecuadorian Andes (Dangles et al., 2010), educational inequalities (Ozer & Wright, 2012), water quality in a rural Colombian watershed (Roa García & Brown, 2009), and community education about the judicial system (Stovall & Delgado, 2009).

CBPR focuses on equity and empowerment, as well as generating knowledge that is informed by insider experts on the nature of the problems studied. YPAR deserves specific consideration for how it can contribute positively to the development of children and adolescents who participate (Ozer, 2016; Ozer & Russo, 2016). YPAR is a particularly promising approach for disadvantaged youth in early to mid-adolescence because these are developmental periods characterized by fluidity and transition for individual and collective senses of identity and purpose (Damon, Menon, & Cotton Bronk, 2003; Ozer, Ritterman, & Wanis, 2010). YPAR that involves youth in analyzing and changing the conditions that influence their schools and communities provides opportunities for youth to identify as leaders with purpose (Damon et al., 2003; Spencer, Fegley, & Harpalani, 2003), rather than seeing themselves in terms of negative stereotypes held by others (Cahill, Rios-Moore, & Threatts, 2008). Further, YPAR seeks to enhance critical consciousness—critical reflection, motivation, and action—that pushes youth to investigate broader structural conditions that shape behavior rather than just individual-level explanations (Watts, Diemer, & Voight, 2011).

A small but growing research literature indicates that YPAR is well suited to create and strengthen opportunities for youth to enhance their own knowledge, skills, and motivation; address inequities in health, education, and other systems; and expand the opportunities for meaningful influence in the settings in which young people grow and develop (Berg, Coman, & Schensul, 2009; Cargo et al., 2003; Holden, Evans, Hinnant, & Messeri, 2005; Mitra, 2004; Ozer & Douglas, 2013). Individual-level gains found in qualitative YPAR research include increases in adolescents' sense of purpose, perceived support from caring adults, and positive attitudes toward school (Mitra, 2004; Wilson et al., 2007).

In this chapter, we provide an overview of key YPAR practices, examples of YPAR projects from around the world, and important choice points and challenges that are likely to be faced in practice. Similar to other researchers, we view YPAR as multidimensional: an intervention to promote positive youth development and improve inequitable conditions that undermine it, a re-visioning of young people not as problems to be "fixed" but rather as expert cocreators of knowledge, and an approach toward engaging youth and their expertise in research conducted about them. In practice, YPAR projects can vary with respect to focusing more explicitly on political empowerment versus enhancing youth's inquiry and action skills and their participation in improving and designing settings and programs intended to serve them.

KEY YPAR PRINCIPLES

As in any research, there are many paths and choice points in YPAR. YPAR needs to be responsive to the context of youth, particularly to the resources and limitations of the institutions and communities engaged in efforts related to youth participation, and thus by definition will not look exactly the same across settings. That said, there are core principles and practices in this approach that are important to articulate, including (1) bringing youth participants into the training and practice of research, critical thinking, and change strategy; (2) carefully attending to intentional power sharing between youth and adults, especially considering that youth do not exert the same power in school or out-of-school contexts; and (3) integrating iterative research and action phases into the project (Ozer et al., 2010).

Context: Youth as Experts and Knowledge Creators

Regardless of specific emphases, all YPAR projects assert that youth are capable of generating expert knowledge of value in addressing problems that affect their development and well-being. Youth can be valued partners in the scientific enterprise and agents for changes in systems and communities beyond the traditional role of serving as passive participants in research that seek to affect them. Positive views of youth—particularly youth of color—as providing expertise and leadership potential run counter to dominant stereotypical views of adolescents as sources of worry or threat (Camino & Zeldin, 2002) and as a group lacking in agency, wholly governed by hormones and peer pressure.

Researchers who study youth development with YPAR have identified how research validity is strengthened via partnership with youth researchers, including in defining research questions, developing instruments, and interpreting findings (Fine, 2008; Langhout & Thomas, 2010). The role of YPAR in providing an insider phenomenological perspective on youth development, especially for the investigation of sensitive, hidden, or hard-to-report phenomena, is discussed in greater detail in Ozer (2016).

Relationships: Adult-Youth Power Sharing

Sharing of power between adult facilitators and youth researchers requires intentionality and care given the inequality of adult-youth relationships, especially within the inherent hierarchy of K–12 school settings (Kohfeldt, Chhun, Grace, & Langhout, 2011; Ozer, Newlan, Douglas, & Hubbard, 2013; Zeldin, Christens, & Powers, 2013). We note that power sharing regarding key decisions and processes in YPAR does not mean that all ideas made by the youth should be followed uncritically. Rather, it means that the perspectives and interpretations of the youth researchers must be considered by the group for their strengths and limitations rather than outright overruled by an adult. The plan and process for decision making should be discussed openly and followed so that there are no surprises.

Engaging in YPAR requires preparing the ground early through activities that develop trusting relationships and communication skills among the youth participants and between the adult and youth participants (see Mirra, Garcia, & Morrell [2015] for in-depth analysis of building trust and negotiating power within a long-term educational partnership for YPAR). Conducting YPAR calls for effective adult facilitators who can train and guide teams of youth researchers on the journey without fully taking over steering the ship. Our research, and that of others concerned with the balance of power in youth development programs (Larson, Walker, & Pearce, 2005), analyzes how effective adult facilitators use strategies to maintain youth control over key aspects of the YPAR projects, such as defining the problem, choosing the design, interpreting data, and deciding on action steps, while at the same time providing helpful structure, such as breaking down tasks and keeping timelines. Importantly, in addition to guiding the organizational and learning processes of research and action, effective adult facilitators help students resolve conflicts—substantive and personal—and navigate the political complexities of seeking to make changes in institutions such as schools in which they have little power.

In addition to these "non-negotiables," other youth development activities that generally occur as part of high-quality YPAR projects include skill-building exercises related to working in groups to achieve goals and the expansion of youth's social network with peers and adult leaders (Ozer & Douglas, 2015).

Balancing Research and Action

Although this chapter focuses on YPAR, there are other approaches, such as youth organizing, action civics, and city planning, that often similarly emphasize equity and social change (Center for Cities and Schools, 2016; Generation Citizen, 2016; Kirshner, 2015; Kirshner & Ginwright, 2012). Of these related approaches, YPAR tends to be the most focused on generating and engaging with data—coupled with taking action based on those data. Because YPAR projects differ in context, group dynamics, issues, methods, and opportunity for social change, there is no easy formula for how to best integrate iterative cycles of research and action in a YPAR project. Research and action are not mutually exclusive: actions driven by well-designed and well-implemented research can deliver more targeted, meaningful impacts, and research that is driven by an action-oriented agenda can often be more relevant and useful.

YPAR PHASES AND SUPPORT RESOURCES

There are multiple curricula that can help scaffold groups interested in conducting YPAR projects; these curricula provide interactive activities that can be adapted to various development and educational levels. For our initial UC Berkeley–SF Peer Resources Project (2003–2011) that supported and studied YPAR in public high schools (Ozer & Douglas, 2013; Ozer et al., 2008), we drew from existing curricula (Anyon et al., 2007; London, 2001; Schensul, Berg, & Sydlo, 2004) to create a hybrid that fit the goals and pedagogical approaches of SF Peer Resources' middle and high school elective classes. In our recent efforts to develop an interactive web platform—the YPAR Hub—to help diffuse YPAR, we synthesized the contributions of multiple curricula; the result is a website with downloadable lesson plans and practical tips for adult facilitators, as well as examples of YPAR in the United States and internationally. Some of these resources are discussed in the following sections as we walk through phases of YPAR.

Issue Selection

It is critical that the issues tackled by the YPAR groups reflect the authentic concerns of the youth researchers—in other words, that the problems or questions are ones that they genuinely care about and want to influence. Before deciding on a topic, however, it is also important for the adult facilitators and youth researchers to be strategic in considering the potential allies, resources, and time they would have for any given issue. Who else will care about this issue? What are the existing governance structures and opportunities for the group to report back their findings? Even in the early stages of YPAR projects, thinking ahead to possible action steps and to the timing for getting on the calendar of key stakeholders for reporting back is highly recommended to make sure that there will be an audience for the results.

Multiple strategies can help support young people to identify an issue that they are motivated to work on and that is addressable within the time frame of the project. Although some YPAR groups target big community-level issues, such as reducing the number of liquor stores or air pollution in their neighborhoods, others take on more discrete issues, such as having clean bathrooms, drinking fountains, or adequate athletic equipment at their schools. Many examples of successful YPAR projects start with an open-ended issue selection process, guided by (1) defining their community and then (2) assessing the strengths and problems of that community. Once the group has agreed on a more narrow area of interest, they can then define their research questions, hypotheses, and methods.

For example, when *Voces y Manos* conducted a YPAR project with Indigenous youth in rural Guatemala, they used a layered issue selection process. First, a small group of the older adolescents in the organization developed and facilitated internal focus groups with the younger adolescents who were guided by open-ended questions to learn what topics mattered to the group. The older adolescents recorded and transcribed the sessions, then identified the themes that emerged. They brought back the main emergent themes to the full group of adolescents—burdensome cost of school-related resources, lack of trust with teachers, fear of free expression in schools, gender inequities, and subjectivity of classroom grading—to dig into creating indicators for each of the issue areas. The full group then developed a survey that was later administered to a random sample of high school students in the municipality.

Although YPAR projects often start with an open-ended issue selection process, it is also common that the choice of topics is more constrained. This can occur for many reasons, such as when the YPAR project is developed in the context of an existing initiative to study a particular issue or evaluate services, or when the organization has a specific mandate to justify its existence or funding. For example, in the UC Berkeley–SF Peer Resources study, student cohorts sometimes began the school year knowing they were charged with addressing a particular topic, such as supporting youth of color with the transition to high school. The fact that these YPAR projects were conducted in elective high school classes meant that new students entered into the project every year or even every semester. When the prior year's YPAR cohort had made progress, such as increasing the ethnic diversity of the school or working to improve the cultural responsiveness of the teaching, there was a clear benefit to sticking with the same issue across cohorts to better sustain traction on influencing policies and practices. At the same time, there was recognition that it was important for new cohorts to work on issues that they genuinely wanted to change rather than solely carrying the torch of the prior cohort. In examining constrained cases of "bounded empowerment," we identified processes that facilitated youth ownership and sustained work, such as teachers' framing and buy-in strategies (e.g., asking students to further refine an existing research question or shape unfinished phases of a project); micro-power compensation (e.g., providing opportunities for autonomous decision making on specific tasks within the predetermined project); and alignment of student interests across cohorts (i.e., natural agreement across cohorts on what an important issue focus would be in their community) (Ozer et al., 2013). Thus, even when the topic is constrained, it is important that each youth cohort selects or adapts an issue that matters to it and is feasible to advance within the time frame.

Once an issue has been identified, it must be framed strategically. YPAR seeks to engage young people in social-ecological analyses to address issues that matter to them while identifying the root causes that create and perpetuate those problems. By identifying root causes as best as they can, youth researchers and adult facilitators seek to enact solutions that address the upstream sources of problems in order to foster meaningful, sustainable change. The framing of the issue shapes the research design, methodology, analysis, and action agendas; it also communicates the parameters of possible solutions to researchers, stakeholders, allies, and affiliates. For example, the framing of issues can inadvertently reinforce negative attitudes toward youth by placing blame on the individual (e.g., "local students steal from neighborhood convenience stores at high rates") rather than acknowledging the influence of the conditions in which youth live (e.g., "local students experience high poverty because of the elimination of city rent control policies and subpar minimum wages").

Research Design and Methods

After landing on a topic with the guidance of adult facilitators, youth researchers engage in decision-making processes about the research design, methods, and interpretation of the data collected. Any issue can be studied with many designs and methods, so it is important to be strategic and inclusive in this core phase of YPAR. YPAR projects often focus on complex areas of inquiry and thus can be sliced many ways. Further, given that the researchers likely have personal experience with a limited range of methods—surveys, for example, are most common—it is important to use curricula that expose them to the rationales for prioritizing different types of research methods and data. Understanding the relative advantages and disadvantages of different forms of data is important not only for gaining insight into the issue that youth researchers are working on but also for promoting important intellectual competencies related to critical thinking and arguing from evidence, areas that are central to current educational standards and priorities in the United States and other countries (Kornbluh, Ozer, Kirshner, & Allen, 2015).

After deciding on an issue and defining a research question, one of the first steps that the research team must take is to search for existing data available to answer their question. Youth researchers may decide that they will be informed by existing data sets while also generating some new data on a particular aspect of the issue that needs to be understood through data from their own school or community. For example, youth interested in violence prevention might start with understanding published data on county crime levels and then decide to conduct surveys or observations in their own school or neighborhood to inform local action steps. Fortunately, there are new online resources that provide guidance in identifying and understanding existing data sets regarding health, education, housing, civic life, and other areas of interest (Center for Regional Change, 2014; YPAR Hub, 2015).

If new data are needed, selecting research methods that best shine a light on the issue at hand can necessitate balancing many competing needs and constraints, such as funding, equipment, time, and expertise. To support this process, the YPAR Hub has a decision tree to help guide groups through some of the choice points inherent to YPAR. Some research methods commonly used within the YPAR approach include focus groups, interviews, mapping, observations, photovoice, and surveys. Mapping, for example, is best suited for investigating issues that are tied to geographic locations whereas photovoice works well with issues that can be represented visually, either literally or symbolically (see Langhout, Fernandez, Wyldbore, & Savala [2015] for a detailed case example). Surveys generally enable researchers to gather data from a larger number of people cost-effectively whereas interviews provide for more in-depth investigation into individuals' experiences and opinions. Many projects opt to employ multiple methods to capitalize on the benefits of each.

As an example of choosing research methods, we consider *Viramundo,* a nongovernmental organization in Brazil that conducted YPAR to document disparities between wealthy neighborhoods in Rio de Janeiro and the neighboring slums, or *favelas,* in Rocinha (F. Wittlin, personal communication, October 10, 2015). The research team opted to use community communication technologies, such as participatory photography and videography, in their data collection. They videotaped interviews with community members on the streets and in homes in the city and in the slums responding to questions about bias and discrimination against the *favelas*. The research team then compiled and edited the content into a publicly available video. The viewer is thus able to not only gather the text content of what the respondents say but also their nonverbal communication (e.g., raised eyebrows, shrugged shoulders) and their settings (e.g., busy commercial street, dilapidated home). This visually oriented method facilitated *Viramundo*'s ability to best answer their specific research question and also gave them powerful material to engage with the media as part of their action plan for change. (See also Chapter 23 on international youth mapping.)

Data Analysis and Interpretation

A key point to consider in working with and interpreting data is how to do high-quality generation and analysis of evidence that is appropriate to the developmental and educational level of the research team and viable within time and financial constraints. It is important to make this as fun and interactive as possible, especially given that some youth may come to the project with negative experiences with learning with numbers in math and science. Even the term *research* may have negative connotations; it is better to focus on questions they want to answer rather than framing the process as a "big research project." Fortunately, data analysis does not need to be complicated to be systematic. For groups that want to keep it simple and do not have access to the Internet, much can be learned by looking at patterns using basic statistics such as means, medians, and ranges for different groups. Qualitative analysis of data can also be conducted through activities such as having youth sort hard copies of quotes in envelopes or tables around a room as part of a thematic coding process. For groups with access to the Internet, there are good free versions of computer programs, such as SurveyMonkey, that enable respondents to enter numeric or text survey data directly into the computer program; this saves time on data entry and can be used for easy generation of tables and graphs.

One way to reduce the pressure of data interpretation is to invite students to reflect on surprises between what they expected versus what they found as well as patterns among their sample. Guided questions can help youth researchers to highlight the key points of their findings and to note any meaningful differences among subjects (e.g., "Would you have expected English language learners to report more bullying than native English speakers? Do male and female students feel equally safe at school?"). Arguing from evidence is an important critical thinking and educational competency; thus, strategies in data interpretation in which youth researchers state a claim and provide supporting evidence help prepare the research team to provide a compelling report back to stakeholders and develop skills for weighing evidence. See the YPAR Hub home page (http://yparhub.berkeley.edu) for a video of how youth researchers gathered supporting evidence to improve teaching practices.

Voces y Manos, the organization in Guatemala previously discussed, provides an excellent example of the use of survey methods in an international context. The youth researchers surveyed high school students in their municipality to learn more about their issue from a maximum number of people at a minimal financial cost. After data collection, adult facilitators provided youth researchers with hands-on training in analyzing data, and the youth learned skills such as generating graphs from survey data. In the data interpretation and analysis phase, the youth researchers realized that the results pointed to multiple manifestations of systemic issues related to poverty and disempowerment in their communities. Though many students chronically struggled with similar issues (e.g., lack of trust with teachers), they did not have a centralized place where they could safely seek support or request a review of their schools' practices. They concluded that the themes they studied were symptoms of a lack of infrastructure expressly designed to support local youth, and the youth researchers decided to focus their action phase on pressuring elected officials to commit to fund a preexisting but unfunded Office of Childhood and Adolescence. This office could then be reasonably charged with sustainably addressing and alleviating issues for youth in their community.

Outcomes: Reporting Back and Taking Action

After data collection and interpretation are complete, youth researchers and adult facilitators identify specific actions that they can take to address the problem, work to report their findings and proposals to relevant stakeholders, and negotiate the political and logistical complexities of working for change. For example, YPAR groups in the UC Berkeley Peer Resources project used report back activities such as peer education presentations to students, student-led professional development sessions for teachers, and slideshow presentations of key findings to teachers, school administrators, district decision makers, university partners, and funders.

Voces y Manos also employed a creative report back strategy that advanced their specific action plan. After deciding that the group wanted to use their data to make policy and budget recommendations for their municipality, they knew they needed to engage the target that could implement their requested change: their local mayoral candidates. As such, the youth researchers held a public forum to present their findings and policy proposal. They worked with a coalition of local organizations and youth organizers and involved local radio, television outlets, and social media to ensure that the forum reached a large number of residents and raised the profile of the event. Furthermore, students received trainings in digital literacy, print literacy, and numeracy (demonstrated in their PowerPoint presentations) that enabled them to engage in scientific discourse. Furthermore, the public forum was livestreamed for those who could not attend in person (e.g., *Voces y Manos* alumni, international donors). In all, 250 people in their small community participated in person—including all seven mayoral candidates—and an additional six hundred people watched remotely. By the end of the public forum, all mayoral candidates signed an agreement that they would implement the youth researchers' policy proposal to fund their Office of Childhood and Adolescence.

Another innovative report back was implemented by the Dream Teens, a national project in Portugal seeking to integrate youth voice into public policies that affect their lives and communities (Aventura Social, 2015). After working online in small groups with support from university teams to conduct the research, all youth researchers convened in person to reflect on and deliver recommendations to the National Secretary of Health. Following this event, the government ministry posted the Dream Teens' recommendations on their website, and key officials reported that the recommendations were "crucial" for tailoring national policies related to youth.

Finally, YPAR projects can find inspiration for report back strategies in the larger CBPR field. For example, a campaign against discriminatory police practices in New York with the CUNY Public Science Project projected findings onto the sides of buildings at night, and the

Morris Justice Project in New York City created portraits of community members that challenged negative stereotypes about their neighborhood and distributed postcards with statistics comparing disproportionate unwarranted police stops in their neighborhood to those in a high-income neighborhood.

Scaling, Embedding, and Institutionalizing Change

Beyond promoting the skills and empowerment of the youth who participate in YPAR, a key goal of most YPAR projects is to make a meaningful difference in the problem that the youth set out to address. As noted in the academic literature (Sarason, 1996) and known all too well by those in practice, changing policies and institutions that affect the lives of youth is difficult—for well-connected adults let alone youth who do not enjoy the same rights and privileges as adults. Despite the challenges, there are important examples of YPAR projects that made a difference in influencing settings, policies, and systems that we consider here and on the YPAR Hub. In the United States, there are published examples of youth research and evaluation being integrated into the work of youth-serving entities such as San Francisco's Department of Children, Youth, and Their Families (Youth IMPACT, 2001) and organizations such as Girls, Inc. (Chen, Weiss, & Nicholson, 2010). Educational systems have been a major site of YPAR in the United States (Cammarota & Fine, 2008; Kirshner, 2007; Ozer & Douglas, 2013). In other work (Ozer, 2016; Ozer et al., 2010), we used social-ecological and developmental theoretical frames to consider how YPAR can help address the "developmental mismatch" of secondary schools (Eccles & Roeser, 2011) by promoting greater opportunities for youth agency and influence through meaningful roles in school governance (Ozer & Douglas, 2013; Ozer & Wright, 2012).

An important challenge for YPAR is embedding YPAR and related participatory youth approaches into systems-change efforts to expand the impact on policies and practices that affect youth development while simultaneously maintaining the integrity of YPAR's key principles and rigor. In addition to the web platforms already discussed in this chapter, there are noteworthy efforts under way to bring YPAR and other youth voice efforts to scale—some of which rely on social media to connect youth across schools, communities, and even countries (Aventura Social, 2015; Kornbluh, Neal, & Ozer, 2016). For example, UNICEF recently launched U Report, a text message–based platform focused on engaging young people in developing countries to provide data on important issues.

In Australia, the Improving Children's Lives Initiative at the University of Melbourne formed a partnership with *Behind the News,* a children's news program that is broadcast into K–12 schools by the Australian Broadcast Commission (L. Gibbs, personal communication, March 10, 2016; The University of Melbourne, 2016). *Behind the News* has developed an interactive approach to news journalism with students. Working with University of Melbourne as a research partner, the program will invite children to identify and respond to issues of concern to them, and the university team will then analyze the responses and report back to students in order to support further action.

Finally, another step that should aid the scaling of YPAR is the recent launch of the Kids in Action network by the International Collaboration for Participatory Health Research (ICPHR) to invite registration of participatory health research projects with children up to age fourteen years to use a peer support process that will promote best practices and facilitate positive local and collective outcomes (www.icphr.org/kids-in-action.html).

CONCLUSION

This chapter provided an overview of YPAR's key processes and phases, with a focus on illustrative examples from the United States and other countries, such as Guatemala, Brazil, Portugal, and Australia, while identifying relevant curricular activities for each phase. We proposed that YPAR has value in promoting positive youth development, particularly for the majority of young people in the world who must negotiate racism, economic inequity, violence, and other threats to their well-being. We suggested that the potential benefits of YPAR are multidimensional; it is not just an approach for strengthening young people's learning and development while improving community conditions but also for engaging young people's expertise in scientific inquiry about youth development and health. Finally, we considered current steps to scale YPAR that aim to deepen its broad impact, capitalizing on social and web-based platforms while seeking to maintain the integrity and spirit of the approach.

QUESTIONS FOR DISCUSSION

1. Considering the principles and complexities of YPAR, what might be some challenges to conducting YPAR at scale with large numbers of students across communities, and what current strategies and platforms are being used to help address these challenges?
2. Think about a school that you currently attend or did in the past. If you were to pick an area to improve, what would be on your short list? Pick one to reflect on in a YPAR thought experiment. Drawing on the examples in the chapter, including web resources, consider the stakeholders you would want to engage in this research and what kinds of research designs and methods might generate actionable evidence to help support improvements.

ACKNOWLEDGMENTS

The first author's research on YPAR described here was supported by a William T. Grant Scholars' Award and the Centers for Disease Control and Prevention. The authors thank Michael Bakal, Flavio Wittlin, and Lisa Gibbs for details about their work; Julia Levinson for research assistance; the high school students who participated in YPAR projects; SF Peer Resources (especially Elizabeth Hubbard, Gary Cruz, Adee Horn, Morgan Wallace, and Pui Ling Tam); SFUSD for research collaboration; and the UC Berkeley student teams.

REFERENCES

Anyon, Y., Brink, K., Crawford, M., Fernández, M., Hofstedt, M., Osberg, J., & Strobel, K. (2007). *Youth Engaged in Leadership and Learning (YELL): A handbook for program staff, teachers, and community leaders*. Stanford, CA: John W. Gardner Center for Youth and Their Communities.

Aventura Social. (2015). Dream Teens. Retrieved from www.dreamteens-en.aventurasocial.com/

Berg, M., Coman, E., & Schensul, J. J. (2009). Youth action research for prevention: A multi-level intervention designed to increase efficacy and empowerment among urban youth. *American Journal of Community Psychology, 43*, 345–359.

Breckwich Vásquez, V., Lanza, D., Hennessey-Lavery, S., Facente, S., Halpin, H. A., & Minkler, M. (2007). Addressing food security through public policy action in a community-based participatory research partnership. *Health Promotion Practice, 8*(4), 342–349.

Brown, T. M., & Rodríguez, L. F. (2009). *Youth in participatory action research*. San Francisco, CA: Jossey-Bass.

Cahill, C., Rios-Moore, I., & Threatts, T. (2008). Open eyes-different eyes: PAR as a process of personal and social transformation. In J. Cammarota & M. Fine (Eds.), *Revolutionizing education: Youth participatory action research in motion*. New York, NY: Routledge.

Camino, L., & Zeldin, S. (2002). From periphery to center: Pathways for youth civic engagement in the day-to-day life of communities. *Applied Developmental Science, 6*(4), 213–220.

Cammarota, J., & Fine, M. (Eds.). (2008). *Revolutionizing education: Youth participatory action research*. New York, NY: Routledge.

Cargo, M., Grams, G., Ottoson, J., Ward, P., & Green, L. (2003). Empowerment as fostering positive youth development and citizenship. *American Journal of Health Behavior, 27*(Supplement 1), S66–S79.

Center for Cities and Schools. (2016). *Y-PLAN*. Retrieved from http://y-plan.berkeley.edu/

Center for Regional Change. (2014). Welcome to the UC Davis Center for Regional Change. Retrieved from http://regionalchange.ucdavis.edu/

Chen, P., Weiss, F. L., & Nicholson, H. J. (2010). Girls Study Girls Inc.: Engaging girls in evaluation through participatory action research. *American Journal of Community Psychology, 46*(1–2), 228–237.

Damon, W., Menon, J., & Cotton Bronk, K. (2003). The development of purpose during adolescence. *Applied Developmental Science, 7*(3), 119–128.

Dangles, O., Carpio, F. C., Villares, M., Yumisaca, F., Liger, B., Rebaudo, F., & Silvain, J. F. (2010). Community-based participatory research helps farmers and scientists to manage invasive pests in the Ecuadorian Andes. *Ambio, 39*(4), 325–335.

Eccles, J. S., & Roeser, R. (2011). Schools as developmental contexts during adolescence. *Journal of Research on Adolescence, 21*, 225–241.

Fine, M. (2008). An epilogue of sorts. In J. Cammarota & M. Fine (Eds.), *Revolutionizing education: Youth participatory action research in motion* (pp. 213–234). New York, NY: Routledge.

Generation Citizen. (2016). *Generation Citizen*. Retrieved from www.generationcitizen.org/

Holden, D., Evans, W. D., Hinnant, L., & Messeri, P. (2005). Modeling psychological empowerment among youth involved in local tobacco control efforts. *Health Education and Behavior, 32*(2), 264–278.

Kirshner, B. (2007). Supporting youth participation in school reform: Preliminary notes from a university-community partnership. *Children, Youth and Environments, 17*(2), 354–363.

Kirshner, B. (2015). *Youth activism in an era of education inequality*. New York: New York University Press.

Kirshner, B., & Ginwright, S. (2012). Youth organizing as a developmental context for African American and Latino adolescents. *Child Development Perspectives, 6*(3), 288–294.

Kohfeldt, D., Chhun, L., Grace, S., & Langhout, R. D. (2011). Youth empowerment in context: Exploring tensions in school-basedyPAR. *American Journal of Community Psychology, 47*(1–2), 28–45.

Kornbluh, M., Neal, J. W., & Ozer, E. J. (2016). Scaling-up youth-led social justice efforts through an online school-based social network. *American Journal of Community Psychology, 57*(3–4), 266–279.

Kornbluh, M., Ozer, E. J., Kirshner, B., & Allen, C. D. (2015). Youth participatory action research as an approach to sociopolitical development and the new academic standards: Considerations for educators. *Urban Review, 47*(5), 868–892.

Langhout, R. D., Fernandez, J. S., Wyldbore, D., & Savala, J. (2015). Photovoice and house meetings as tools within participatory action research. In L. A. Jason & D. S. Glenwick (Eds.), *Handbook of methodological approaches to community-based research: Qualitative, quantitative, and mixed methods* (pp. 82–92). New York, NY: Oxford University Press.

Langhout, R. D., & Thomas, E. (2010). Imagining participatory action research in collaboration with children: An introduction. *American Journal of Community Psychology, 26*(1–2), 60–66.

Larson, R., Walker, K., & Pearce, N. (2005). A comparison of youth-driven and adult-driven youth programs: Balancing inputs from youth and adults. *Journal of Community Psychology, 33*(1), 57–74.

London, J. (2001). *Youth REP: Step by step: An introduction to youth-led evaluation and research*. Oakland, CA: Youth in Focus.

London, J., Zimmerman, K., & Erbstein, N. (2003). Youth-led research and evaluation: Tools for youth, organizational, and community development. *New Directions for Evaluation, 2003*(98), 33–45.

Minkler, M., & Wallerstein, N. (2003). Introduction to community-based participatory research. In M. Minkler & N. Wallerstein (Eds.), *Community-based participatory research for health* (pp. 3–26). San Francisco, CA: Jossey-Bass.

Mirra, N., Garcia, A., & Morrell, E. (2015). *Doing youth participatory action research: Transforming inquiry with researchers, educators, and students*. New York, NY: Routledge.

Mitra, D. L. (2004). The significance of students: Can increasing student voice in schools lead to gains in youth development? *Teachers College Record, 106*(4), 651–688.

Ozer, E. J. (2016). Youth-led participatory action research: Developmental and equity perspectives. In S. S. Horn, M. D. Ruck, & L. S. Liben (Eds.), *Advances in child development and behavior* (pp. 189–207). Burlington, MA: Academic Press.

Ozer, E. J., Cantor, J. P., Cruz, G. W., Fox, B., Hubbard, E., & Moret, L. (2008). The diffusion of youth-led participatory research in urban schools: The role of the prevention support system in implementation and sustainability. *American Journal of Community Psychology, 41*(3–4), 278–289.

Ozer, E. J., & Douglas, L. (2013). The impact of participatory research on urban teens: An experimental evaluation. *American Journal of Community Psychology, 51*, 66–75.

Ozer, E. J., & Douglas, L. (2015). Assessing the key processes of youth-led participatory research: Psychometric analysis and application of an observational rating scale. *Youth & Society, 47*(1), 29–50.

Ozer, E. J., Newlan, S., Douglas, L., & Hubbard, E. (2013). "Bounded" empowerment: Analyzing tensions in the practice of youth-led participatory research in urban public schools. *American Journal of Community Psychology, 52*(1–2), 13–26.

Ozer, E. J., Ritterman, M., & Wanis, M. (2010). Participatory action research (PAR) in middle school: Opportunities, constraints, and key processes. *American Journal of Community Psychology, 46*, 152–166.

Ozer, E. J., & Russo, I. (2016). Development and context across the lifespan: A community psychology synthesis. In M. A. Bond, C. B. Keys, & I. Serrano-Garcia (Eds.), *Handbook of community psychology* (pp. 421–436). Washington, DC: American Psychological Association.

Ozer, E. J., & Wright, D. (2012). Beyond school spirit: The effects of youth-led participatory action research in two urban high schools. *Journal of Research on Adolescence, 22*(2), 267–283.

Roa García, C. E., & Brown, S. (2009). Assessing water use and quality through youth participatory research in a rural Andean watershed. *Journal of Environmental Management, 90*(10), 3040–3047.

Sarason, S. B. (1996). *Revisiting "The culture of the school and the problem of change."* New York, NY: Teachers College Press.

Schensul, J. L., Berg, M. J., & Sydlo, S. (2004). Core elements of participatory action research for educational empowerment and risk prevention with urban youth. *Practicing Anthropology, 26*(2), 5–9.

Spencer, M. B., Fegley, S. G., & Harpalani, V. (2003). A theoretical and empirical examination of identity as coping: Linking coping resources to the self processes of African American youth. *Applied Developmental Science, 7*(3), 181–188.

Stovall, D., & Delgado, N. (2009). "Knowing the ledge": Participatory action research as legal studies for urban high school youth. *New Directions for Youth Development, 2009*(123), 67–81.

The University of Melbourne. (2016). *Children's Lives Research Initiative*. Retrieved from http://research.unimelb.edu.au/hallmark-initiatives/childrens-lives-research-initiative—welcome

Watts, R. J., Diemer, M. A., & Voight, A. M. (2011). Critical consciousness: Current status and future directions. *New Directions for Child and Adolescent Development, 2011*(134), 43–57.

Wilson, N., Dasho, S., Martin, A., Wallerstein, N., Wang, C., & Minkler, M. (2007). Engaging young adolescents in social action through photovoice: The Youth Empowerment Strategies (YES!) project. *The Journal of Early Adolescence, 27*(2), 241–261.

Youth IMPACT. (2001). *Youth voices inspiring creative change*. Retrieved from www.whatkidscando.org/archives/images/studentwork/YouthImpactReport.pdf

YPAR Hub. (2015). Investigate. Retrieved from http://yparhub.berkeley.edu/investigate-curriculum/

Zeldin, S., Christens, B. D., & Powers, J. L. (2013). The psychology and practice of youth-adult partnership: Bridging generations for youth development and community change. *American Journal of Community Psychology, 51*(3–4), 385–397.

CHAPTER 8

PARTNERSHIP, TRANSPARENCY, AND ACCOUNTABILITY

CHANGING SYSTEMS TO ENHANCE RACIAL EQUITY IN CANCER CARE AND OUTCOMES

EUGENIA ENG, JENNIFER SCHAAL, STEPHANIE BAKER, KRISTIN BLACK, SAMUEL CYKERT, NORA JONES, ALEXANDRA LIGHTFOOT, LINDA ROBERTSON, CLEO SAMUEL, BETH SMITH, AND KARI THATCHER

AS NOTED BY the Sullivan Commission (Sullivan, 2004), many visible racial barriers of the US health care system were eradicated by the civil rights era, but today's effects from institutional racism are subtle and require careful recognition. Institutional racism is a process of advantage and oppression, conscious or not, functioning as "a system of structuring opportunity and assigning value based on race phenotype, that unfairly disadvantages some. . ., unfairly advantages others. . ., and undermines the. . .potential of the whole society. . ." (Jones, 2003, p. 10). Race, a biologically specious construct, does little to describe the specific origins and causal pathways of race-specific inequities in quality and completion of health care (Williams & Rucker, 2000).

Despite decades of documenting racial disparities in cancer survival in the United States, variations in treatment persist. African American breast cancer patients continue to initiate treatment later (Gorin, Heck, Cheng, & Smith, 2006) and receive less treatment than their white counterparts (Bickell et al., 2006; Hershman et al., 2005; Voti et al., 2006). Non–small cell lung cancer represents more than 80 percent of all cases (Jemal et al., 2007), and the only reliable curative treatment for it is surgical resection, with five-year survival rates at about 50 percent for localized disease and 21 percent for regional (Ries et al., 2007). Alone or in consultation with their physicians, 24 percent of white patients and 36 percent of African American patients with Stage 1 or 2 disease decide not to pursue surgical resection (Bach, Cramer, Warren, & Begg, 1999; Cykert et al., 2010; Farjah et al., 2009) treatment. Patients who do not undergo appropriate lung resection surgery are limited to a median survival rate of less than one year (Bach et al., 1999). This racial variation in surgery has been directly linked to excess lung cancer mortality (Bach et al., 1999).

Although used for decades by community organizers working for civil rights and social change, the relevance of the antiracism framework to health care inequity has rarely been examined or applied to health systems change. This chapter is a case study of building a community-academic-health agency research partnership on antiracism training and collaborative processes within two cancer centers located in Greensboro, North Carolina, and Pittsburgh, Pennsylvania. Emphasis is given to how our partnership identified system-level barriers to transparency and accountability for racial equity in quality and completion of cancer care, which informed our design and testing of a system change intervention at both cancer centers. Finally, we offer insights on the potential of integrating CBPR principles and an antiracism framework as a part of the growing system change movement within US medical care and the National Institutes of Health (NIH).

HISTORY OF THE INTERSECTION OF CBPR AND ANTIRACISM TRAINING IN GREENSBORO

Citizens of Guilford County, North Carolina, have played a pivotal role in this nation's history of civil rights. On February 1, 1960, four students from NC A&T University conducted the first lunch counter sit-in. Also in Guilford County, Dr. George Simkins Jr. led African American doctors, dentists, and patients to prosecute the largest white-owned and white-serving-only hospital in the county, Moses Cone Memorial Hospital, for discrimination by maintaining racially separate medical facilities with taxpayers' money. The 1963 *Simkins v. Cone Health* decision marked the first time that federal courts applied the Equal Protection clause of the Fourteenth Amendment to prohibit racial discrimination by a private entity (Powell, 2006). The following year, Congress passed the Civil Rights Act of 1964, officially prohibiting private discrimination in public places.

The county seat is Greensboro, with a population of 282,586 (2014 estimate): 48.4 percent of residents are white and 40.6 percent are African American; 87.7 percent of residents have at least a high school diploma, and 35.7 percent have a bachelor's or higher degree. About one in five Greensboro residents (20.3 percent) live below poverty (US Census Bureau, 2015).

In 1997, The Partnership Project (TPP) was formed by three local organizations: Project Greensboro, Guilford College, and the City of Greensboro. TPP's mission was to deepen the capacity of fragile neighborhoods to take responsibility for community improvement. TPP's first director encouraged board members and staff members to attend the People's Institute for Survival and Beyond (PISAB) antiracism training in New Orleans to better understand the history of racism in the United States and address its current institutional manifestations.

The PISAB's two-day training focuses on a racial analysis of how and why institutions from all sectors in our society interact in maintaining a race-based hierarchy. The rationale is that gatekeepers from institutions work for equity with different understandings of racism, relying on discipline-specific frameworks, personal feelings, and popular opinion. A gatekeeper is anyone who works in an institution and has the power to give and deny access to their institution's resources or equity—ranging from information and services to use of the bathroom key. Regardless of the size of the gate, it is not owned by the gatekeepers but by the institution. Gatekeepers, however, are in control of who has access and when, by virtue of their work or personal relationship with patients and clients. Using this racial analysis, participating organizations establish a common lens and vocabulary to (1) critically analyze structural issues of race and class, rather than characteristics of individuals and groups, and (2) address the explicit and subtle ways that racialized patterns in American history, culture, and policies permeate structures and practices within and across systems, such as education, criminal justice, and health care, which create and sustain inequities (www.pisab.org).

TPP organized to bring the PISAB training to Greensboro. The first training was sponsored in 1997. The PISAB analysis took root and local community members built on it forming the Racial Equity Institute (REI), which now conducts quarterly trainings in Greensboro. Although TPP began as a community-building organization, introduction to PISAB's racial analysis transformed TPP to an antiracism training organization with the mission to educate community members and organizational leaders in understanding institutional racism and development of strategic actions to benefit communities. In 2007, TPP was reorganized as a 501(c)3 corporation.

TPP's mission was validated with empirical findings published in the Institute of Medicine (IOM) report, *Unequal Treatment* (Smedley, Stith, & Nelson, 2003). Reviewing ten years of studies on patient and provider attitudes, expectations, and behaviors, the IOM panel concluded that race and ethnicity of patients remained significant predictors of the quality of health care received, even after accounting for access to care and issues that arise from differing socioeconomic conditions. The panel offered recommendations for system-change improvements in medical care financing, allocation of care, availability of language translation, community-based care, and others.

Bolstered by these findings, TPP leaders sought funding from the Moses Cone-Wesley Long Community Health Foundation to build a coalition grounded in antiracism training and driven by community voices to address health inequities in Greensboro. The foundation encouraged TPP to approach the UNC's School of Public Health to recruit academic researchers for future collaboration. TPP invited faculty members Geni Eng and Anissa Vines and postdoctoral fellow Derek Griffith, given their record of CBPR health inequities research. Together, they applied successfully for an eighteen-month planning grant, awarded by the foundation in 2004 to TPP with a subcontract to UNC (Yonas et al., 2006). After eighteen months, thirty-four persons (50 percent community-based, 50 percent representing health agencies and academic institutions) had completed antiracism training, signed a "full-value contract" formalizing a commitment to shared goals, expectations, and values for working together and an agreement that all products generated, research or otherwise, belong to the group.

After completing training on how to apply for NIH funding, and on CBPR, the newly formed collaborative agreed to focus on documenting race-specific inequities in the local cancer care system, applying for an R21 for formative research to the National Cancer Institute (NCI).

We established ourselves as the Greensboro Health Disparities Collaborative (GHDC) with the mission to create structures and processes that respond to, empower, and facilitate communities in defining and resolving issues related to disparities in health. Working in subcommittees, we designed the Cancer Care and Racial Equity Study (CCARES), which NCI funded in 2006 to answer the following research questions:

> Did African American and White women with breast cancer in Guilford County, North Carolina, receive treatment at Cone Cancer Center that was the same?
> If the breast cancer care was not the same, how was it different and what could have been the reasons?

It is noteworthy that although the executive vice president of the Cone Health System had reviewed our CCARES application and submitted a letter of support for providing access to the facility's breast cancer patients and cancer registry database, the Cone Health Cancer Center (CHCC) was not yet a health agency partner with GHDC and UNC, although GHDC members included physicians and nonclinical staff members employed by Cone Health. Hence, GHDC orchestrated a community press conference to announce NCI funding of CCARES and invited Cone Health's vice president for oncology services and the CHCC medical director. Both attended the press conference, recognized the potential implications of CCARES findings for their cancer center, requested to join GHDC, and completed the two-day antiracism training.

ENGAGING CANCER CENTERS AS EQUAL PARTNERS IN SYSTEM CHANGE RESEARCH FOR HEALTH EQUITY

CCARES' formative research findings revealed a six-month delay in reporting cancer registry data to CHCC staff. Registry data revealed racial differences in histological tumor grade, surgical outcomes, insurance status, and physician recommendation of hormone therapy, chemotherapy, and radiation therapy (Yonas, Aronson, Schaal, et al., 2013). Associations with racial differences in treatment outcomes could not be examined because cancer registry data did not include hormone receptor status, patient refusal of treatment, dates for initiating and discontinuing or completing treatment, or discontinuing follow-up care. Cone Health's cancer care system lacked transparency on equity in quality and completion of care. Additionally, critical incident interviews with white ($n=27$) and African American ($n=23$) breast cancer patients treated at CHCC during the same period revealed 861 specific encounters described as having an impact, positive and negative, on their cancer care experience (Yonas, Aronson, Schaal, et al., 2013). Subtle but important racial differences on the impact from patient encounters within the cancer care system indicated lack of accountability for equity in quality of care. Implications from CCARES findings suggested the need for a prospective study to monitor each patient encounter during treatment, by race, to identify systemic causes for less than optimal care for African American patients.

Following the CBPR approach, GHDC presented and discussed the implications of CCARES findings to the fifty breast cancer survivors interviewed and CHCC administrators and clinicians *before* disseminating to the public. With a small grant from a local foundation, GHDC and UNC sponsored a private dinner for interviewees, a private meeting with CHCC staff members, and a public forum at the public library in Greensboro. Among the benefits of a separate meeting with CHCC staff members was the opportunity for the medical director and vice president for oncology services to commit to serving as an equal partner with GHDC and UNC in designing a follow-up system-change intervention study, informed by CCARES findings, and applying for NCI funding through the RO1 mechanism. During this period between funding, GHDC continued to meet monthly, planning and conducting activities toward achieving its mission, including academic and community presentations, developing community outreach, support of academic partners and their students, and establishing Sisters Network Greensboro (SNG), a local chapter of a national survivorship organization for African American breast cancer survivors.

THE SYSTEM CHANGE STUDY: ACCOUNTABILITY FOR CANCER CARE THROUGH UNDOING RACISM AND EQUITY (ACCURE)

In 2009, Dr. Yonas, the postdoctoral fellow integrally involved with CCARES, accepted a faculty position with the University of Pittsburgh Medical Center (UPMC) and recruited that cancer center as a CBPR partner to serve as the second site for the study. Our partnership submitted two RO1 applications to NCI. The second was revised, resubmitted, and funded in 2012.

Applying CBPR Principles to Prepare for Resubmitting Application

To organize for the resubmission to NCI, we divided into writing groups to revise specific sections, including specific aims, significance, preliminary studies, intervention, and research strategy. Following CBPR principles, each group included a representative from each of our academic, community, and cancer center partners. We held weekly conference calls to appraise one another on progress in thinking, and co–principal investigator (co-PI) Eng served as the coordinator for synthesizing written texts.

ACCURE System Change Study Design

ACCURE's research question was, "What are the structures built into cancer care systems that trigger vulnerabilities to implicit bias, and how can they be changed to reduce race-specific inequities in quality and completion of breast and lung cancer care?" Our ACCURE intervention study directed public health and translational clinical research attention to the concepts of transparency and accountability as mechanisms of systems change to achieve racial equity in cancer care.

We conducted a five-year study using interrupted time-series design, with an embedded randomized control trial (RCT) to test the effectiveness of the ACCURE intervention on optimizing therapy and narrowing treatment disparities between white and African American patients with a first diagnosis of Stage 1–2 breast and lung cancer receiving treatment at Greensboro's CHCC and the UPMC Cancer Center that contribute to excess mortality. For the RCT, a cohort of 150 Stage 1–2 breast and Stage 1–2 lung cancer patients from the two centers were randomized to the ACCURE navigator or usual care navigator.

The ACCURE intervention had two transparency (1 and 2) and two accountability (3 and 4) components: (1) an analysis of power and authority with cancer patients, (2) health care equity education and training (HEET) quarterly sessions with oncology providers and staff members, (3) a full-time ACCURE navigator at each center to act as a two-way communication bridge between patients and their encounters with the cancer care system, and (4) race-specific clinician feedback to physician champions (one for breast and one for lung cancer) at each cancer center. Components (3) and (4) used a real-time warning system derived from electronic health records that immediately indicated if a patient either missed an appointment or did not reach expected milestones in care.

As a first step in launching ACCURE, GHDC members were offered alternate human subjects research ethics training, developed and approved by UNC's institutional review board (IRB) for nontraditional investigators (Yonas, Aronson, Coad, et al., 2013). This training provided a community-friendly set of slides that covered the human subjects protections content of the web-based collaborative institutional training initiative and was delivered by an ACCURE co-PI with examples specific to ACCURE. Twenty-six GHDC members completed the training, indicating strong community interest in contributing to ACCURE's implementation. Their names and contact information were entered into the UNC IRB database. Being trained and certified enabled community members of GHDC to actively engage in all data collection and analysis throughout the ACCURE study. By ensuring community input alongside academic and cancer center input, the authenticity of data and the relationships among ACCURE partners were enhanced and strengthened. The ACCURE grant was administered by a steering committee with representatives from all academic, community, and cancer center partners who met weekly via conference calls and reported monthly to the GHDC.

Transparency Intervention Components

The antiracism training that is foundational to the GHDC posits that lack of transparency and accountability are the mechanisms that prevent systems from adequately addressing racial disparities. We began ACCURE by exploring the functioning of the system to make it transparent to the investigators.

Analysis of Power and Authority To understand similarities and differences in the delivery of cancer care between the two centers, our intervention began with ACCURE staff members shadowing usual-care nurse navigators for breast and lung cancer patients at each cancer center. From these observations and personal experiences, members of GHDC and SNG developed a visual representation of the cancer care system for ACCURE's "power analysis," an antiracism diagnostic tool that examines the origins and pathways within "systems of power and authority" that produce inequity. Figure 8.1 is the resulting diagram of the cancer care system, used during small-group discussions with white and African American cancer patients on encounters with gates and gatekeepers that encouraged or discouraged them from continuing their care.

For ACCURE's focus groups, we recruited forty-two white and African American patients who initiated treatment in January–December 2011 for their first diagnosis of Stage 1–2 breast or lung cancer at both cancer centers. Eligible participants, grouped by race, gender, and type of cancer, received a $15 incentive for a ninety-minute session to discuss these questions: "During your treatment these past [three or six] months, what were the things that were done—or not done—that made you think you *were* getting treated well? That made you think you *were not* getting treated well?" Two racially concordant TPP consultants, experienced in conducting a power analysis, served as the moderator and note taker at both sites. Discussions were digitally recorded and transcribed verbatim.

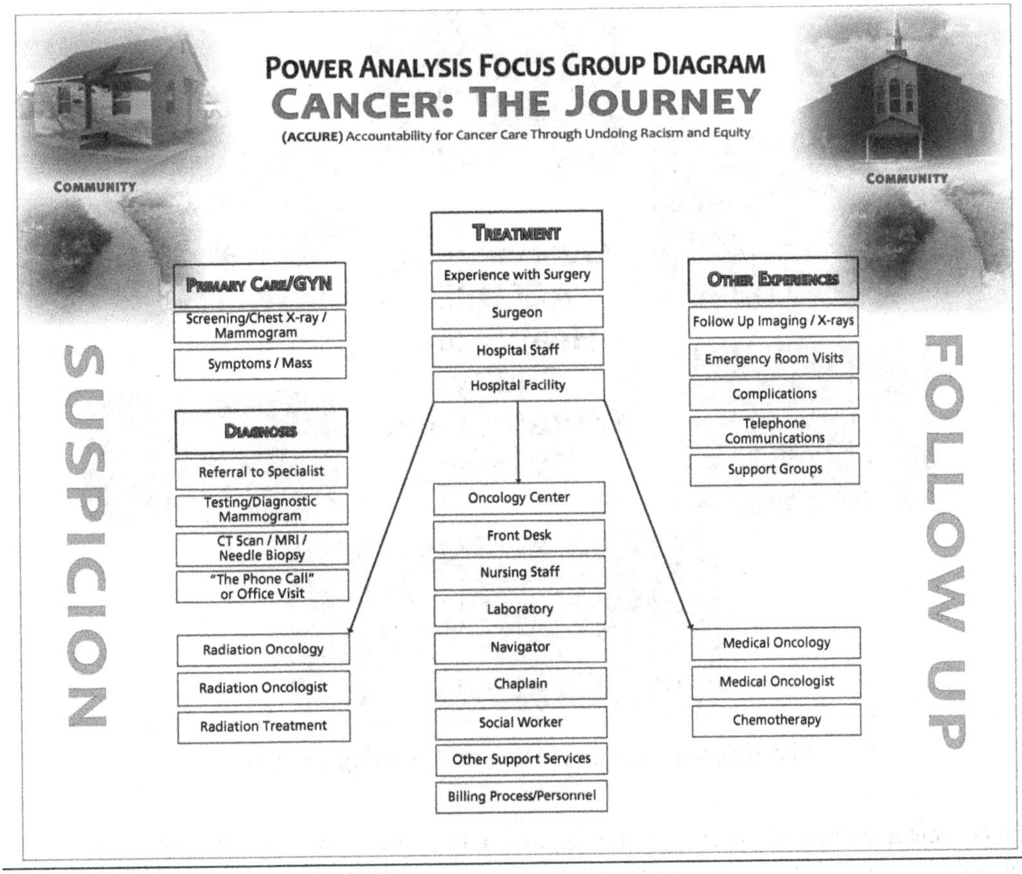

FIGURE 8.1 *Cancer Journey Diagram*

Note: The cancer journey diagram, developed by GHDC and Sisters Network Greensboro, a local affiliate of a national African American breast cancer survivorship organization, was a focal point for power analysis discussions and data analysis. It depicts a patient's journey through cancer care, beginning in the community, from diagnosis through therapy and return to the community following treatment.

For the analysis, eight pairs of academic and community partners were trained to code all transcripts. A small group of community and academic partners then used Atlas.ti, a text analysis software, to enter and retrieve coded text from verbatim transcripts and compare power analysis findings, by race and site, to identify "pressure point encounters." The greater the overlap in pressure point encounters reported by patients, the stronger the association by race on timely initiation of recommended care, adherence to, and completion of care (see Schaal et al., 2016, for more details). The findings from this power analysis were used to inform the remaining three components of ACCURE's intervention.

Healthcare Equity Education and Training (HEET) Sessions For system-wide application of findings from the power analysis on origins and pathways that undermine racial equity in cancer care, we offered quarterly one-hour HEET sessions for certified continuing education credit to

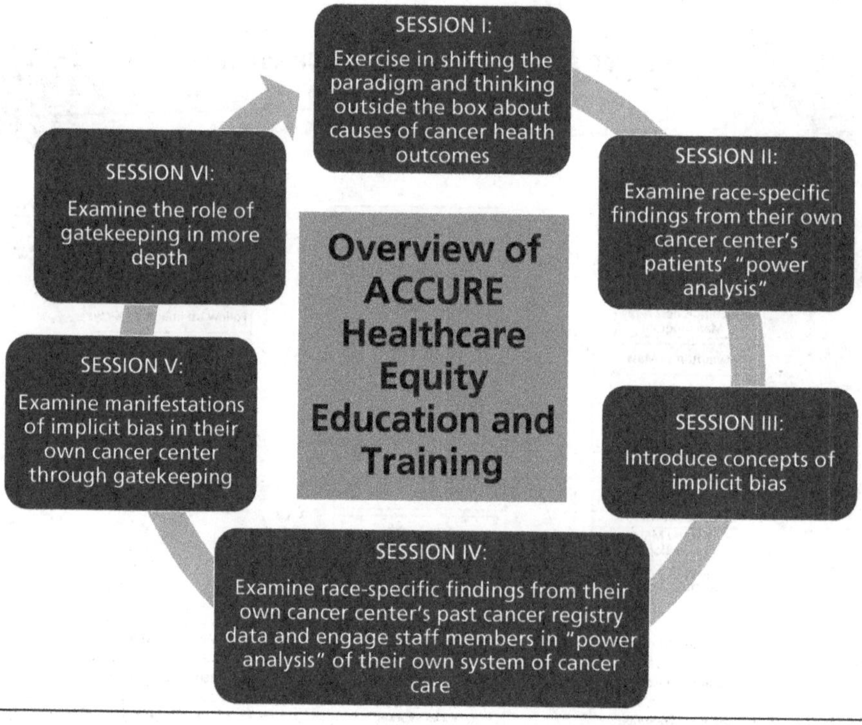

FIGURE 8.2 *Healthcare Equity Education and Training Sessions*

cancer center staff members at each site, beginning in year 2. These sessions presented and discussed principles gleaned from antiracism trainings and shared intermediate ACCURE findings by race on missed appointments, delays on treatment initiation, and premature discontinuation of recommended therapies. In addition, HEET sessions educated staff members regarding their roles as gatekeepers within their institutions.

A HEET planning committee, including representatives from TPP, REI, and ACCURE staff members from each cancer center, was responsible for publicizing, evaluating, designing the content, and selecting REI, community, and academic presenters. Figure 8.2 displays the content. We had projected that 50 percent of staff members at each cancer center would have attended HEET sessions by the end of the intervention. However, differences in the dissemination of information within an academic hospital versus a community hospital required modifications in the delivery format.

Accountability Intervention Components

In addition to transparency, systems must be accountable to their constituents to achieve equity. By establishing mechanisms for accountability, the health care system can begin to address racial disparities.

ACCURE Navigator Review of job descriptions for cancer patient nurse navigators at both cancer centers revealed variation in educational backgrounds (e.g., high school diploma, RN) and scope of responsibilities. The range of duties included direct patient contact, initial greeting and comfort care, social work tasks, follow-up to missed appointments, administrative responsibilities, and tasks related to protection of the institution.

Our grant complemented the usual care offered by a navigator by hiring and training an ACCURE navigator to serve as a two-way communication bridge to optimize accountability for (1) hearing how patients understand (health literacy) and how patients feel (medical mistrust) about the plan of care outlined for them and the policies and procedures they had recently and were currently encountering, (2) eliciting patient suggestions for reducing the impact of negative experiences, and (3) communicating solutions back to the cancer center. The ACCURE navigator was an experienced cancer care provider and educator with a bachelor's degree in nursing. We provided training designed to address specific issues interfering with completion of care that were uncovered by our previous studies and patient focus groups. Whereas the job descriptions for usual care navigators involved a reactive posture to respond to expressed patient concerns, the ACCURE navigator proactively reviewed the care plan with the patient face-to-face at the initiation of care and by telephone every two months thereafter. The purpose was to solicit patient understanding and specifically address questions and concerns raised by patients before a break in care occurs (i.e., before an appointment is missed). In addition to antiracism training, the ACCURE navigator was trained in the "ask-advise-assist" counseling technique to confirm patients' understanding of prognosis, treatment, and the follow-up care process.

To work system-wide, the ACCURE navigator was trained to use our specially developed automated real-time registry (RTR). RTR is a digital uploading process through which the ACCURE navigator obtained visit and procedure appointments for all consented patients. Automated warnings were transmitted to the navigator if a patient missed an appointment or an anticipated treatment milestone did not occur. With the warning trigger, the ACCURE navigator would contact the patient to address concerns or barriers related to missed appointments. For missed milestones, the care team, often using the ACCURE physician champion, would be informed and discussions would ensue on fulfilling the milestone.

Available as a resource to the ACCURE navigator at each cancer center were two oncologists (one for lung and one for breast cancer) designated as physician champions not only for their clinical expertise but also to assist in following up with providers when patients miss milestones in care. Because the ACCURE navigator and physician champions at each cancer center attended weekly clinical breast and thoracic oncology conferences, they brought RTR warnings, alerts, and patient insights directly to the clinical team regarding the lack of expected care progress for resolution in real time. The combination of accrued RTR data and findings from the analysis of power and authority were used to inform HEET sessions and the clinical performance reports, described in the following section.

Race-Specific Clinical Performance Reports (CPRs) In recent years, ACCURE's two cancer centers installed electronic medical record (EMR) software, designed specifically for medical oncology, providing a clear, fast, and flexible means of documenting patient information throughout the medical assessment and chemotherapy administration process. With the ability to include diagnostic images, lab results, full-featured scheduling, and external documentation, the software could provide (1) a complete picture of patient care and (2) generate a clinician worksheet to help medical oncologists efficiently plan, accurately order, and carefully monitor the chemotherapy process.

EMR data through successive definitions of meaningful use enabled real-time identification by ACCURE of patients who, through non-adherence, misperception, or nonstandard recommendation, fell out of accepted parameters of care. Table 8.1 displays the parameters defined for ACCURE with structured data that were pulled by automated reports. We used date of pathologic diagnosis or abnormal chest computerized tomography as the initiating trigger, determined reasonable parameters for therapeutic starting points, and incorporated accepted standards of care for effective therapy to define milestones and outcomes.

From these data, each cancer center generated CPRs that were specific to the institution as a whole. Each CPR presented race-specific data as shown in Table 8.1 on patients treated that time period, aggregated for all providers. Data from CPRs were disseminated quarterly through ACCURE's HEET sessions.

RESULTS AND LESSONS LEARNED

At the time of this writing, ACCURE is in its fifth and final year, and we are still completing our analyses of process and outcome evaluation data. Presented here are the outcome results from our embedded RCT of the ACCURE navigator intervention component with early-stage lung cancer patients.

ACCURE achieved parity that narrowed historical racial gaps in treatment and, at the same time, raised treatment completion rates for both races. We compared race-specific rates of completing potentially curative treatment (e.g., stereotactic body radiation or surgical resection) within four months of diagnosis of (1) 2,044 baseline patients at both cancer centers, who had received treatment, 2007–2011, before ACCURE began; (2) 393 patients randomly assigned to "usual care navigators," and (3) one hundred patients randomly assigned to the ACCURE navigators. Table 8.2 displays the results. Among baseline patients, we found a significant racial gap of 76 percent white versus 64 percent African American ($p < .05$) who received potentially curative lung cancer treatment. Among patients assigned to ACCURE navigators, this eleven percentage point racial gap disappeared; 96 percent of white ($n=75$) and African American ($n=25$) patients completed potentially curative treatment. Among the "usual care navigator" patients, we also saw a significant improvement ($p < .05$) in completion of potentially curative care, when compared to baseline. This finding may be the result of a spillover effect at the two cancer centers, whereby ACCURE navigator sensibilities and training may have influenced staff members outside of the project.

At a monthly GHDC meeting, one of ACCURE's physician champions, Dr. Matthew Manning, proposed submitting an abstract on these findings to be presented at the 2016 annual meeting of the American Society for Thoracic Radiation Oncology (ASTRO). He obtained approval from the GHDC Publications and Dissemination Committee, and several GHDC members served as coauthors. ASTRO accepted the abstract and designated it to be one of three presentations to receive a press conference. At a subsequent GHDC monthly meeting, Dr. Manning presented the PowerPoint slides, rehearsed the presentation, and received substantive constructive feedback from community and academic members on terminology used to describe the science and practice of ACCURE's intervention and the logical progression of the "story" to be told about ACCURE's CBPR approach. (For further information on

TABLE 8.1 Breast and Lung Cancer Treatment Outcome Measures

Outcome Measure	Cancer Diagnosis	Definition
Adequate completion of chemotherapy treatment	*Breast*	*Yes, if 80 percent of chemotherapy visits were completed* *No, otherwise*
	Stage 1b or 2 lung	*Yes, if three out of four chemotherapy visits were completed* *No, otherwise*
Surgery completed	*Lung*	*Yes, if surgery completed within four months of diagnosis* *No, otherwise*
Adherence to medical oncology follow-up appointments	*Stage 1 and 2 breast and lung*	*No, if three consecutive missed appointments* *Yes, otherwise*
Days to treatment initiation	Breast	Number of days from diagnosis to chemotherapy treatment initiation
Treatment started on time	Breast or lung	Yes, if chemotherapy started within 120 days of diagnosis (date of path report) No, otherwise
Surgery completed	Breast	Number of days from diagnosis to surgery
Start radiation therapy	Breast with lumpectomy (not mastectomy)—younger than age seventy	Yes, if patients start treatment No, otherwise
Completed radiation therapy	Breast with lumpectomy (not mastectomy)—younger than age seventy	Yes, if 80 percent of sessions completed No, otherwise
Adequate completion of chemotherapy treatment	Stage 3 colon	Yes, if six treatments completed within six months diagnosis No, otherwise

Note: Primary outcomes in italics text.

TABLE 8.2 Early Stage Lung Cancer Treatment Rates (Stereotactic Body Radiation Therapy and Surgical Resection) by Race and ACCURE Intervention Arm, by Percent

Race	Baseline: R + SBRT	Baseline: R	ACCURE: R + SBRT	ACCURE: R	Usual Care: R + SBRT	Usual Care: R
Black	64	55	96[a]	80[a]	85[a]	57
White	76	61	96[a]	79[a]	87[a]	55

R = surgical resection.
[a] $p < .05$ compared with baseline.

Dr. Manning's presentation see www.medscape.com/viewarticle/869840?nlid=109754_2981&src=wnl_dne_161006_mscpedit&uac=241217HR&impID=1210188&faf=1.) As a result of this preliminary success, additional system changes are being considered at Cone Health, for example, identifying potential transparency and accountability factors to racial differences in receiving low-dose CT scan screening for lung cancer.

Who benefited? By joining the principles of antiracism with CBPR in a clinical trial of a system change intervention, quality and completion of treatment was improved for early-stage cancer patients of all races. To achieve equity for African American patients, our intervention was intentionally focused on enhancing the cancer care system's transparency and accountability for the quality and completion of treatment received by African American patients. At both cancer centers we introduced innovations in (1) health care informatics that analyzed their own data by race (i.e., RTR, CPRs) and (2) patient-centered communication structures that were informed by antiracism training (i.e., specially trained nurse navigators and physician champions and HEET sessions for all staff members). Our preliminary outcome data indicate that, through systems change, all early-stage lung cancer patients benefited, achieving parity with 96 percent completing potentially curative treatment within four months of diagnosis.

Although findings from our process evaluation are promising, we note differences in the type of staff members who attended HEET sessions. At the cancer center affiliated with an academic teaching hospital, HEET sessions were offered during grand rounds, and HEET participants were primarily physicians. The other cancer center was a regional hospital that did not offer grand rounds, and HEET sessions were presented at the end of a workday and were attended by nurses, social workers, and other auxiliary staff members. We had intended to reach at least 50 percent of staff members at each cancer center with HEET sessions, but we had not anticipated how the preexisting culture and different structures for continuing education would shape participation.

What were the challenges and lessons learned? Our GHDC partnership and ACCURE research team were fully aware that securing NIH funding for a longitudinal clinical trial of a systems-change intervention to eliminate persistent racial inequities in cancer outcomes within medical care settings was a lofty goal. Nonetheless, we were certain that we could offer, at the very least, lessons learned on the dynamics of attempting to integrate the CBPR approach into a broader antiracism movement that would be relevant for achieving health equity.

One lesson is to find a balance between following the details of CBPR while not losing sight of the long-term vision of challenging the overarching context of antiracism. It was essential for us to recognize that GHDC's antiracism mission is broader than ACCURE's specific aims. Any study conducted by GHDC is a means toward an end. Although ACCURE established a steering committee who met weekly to guide administration and management of study activities and the budget, the final decision-making power rested with GHDC members on deviations from the initial proposal, personnel changes, interpretation of findings, publications and presentations, and proposed supplements. At the same time, GHDC leaders observed that the agendas for monthly GHDC meetings were so focused on the CBPR details of ACCURE that GHDC's antiracism mission was becoming eclipsed. As a solution, each GHDC meeting begins with a cochair raising a current societal event that is relevant to antiracism, ranging from voter registration to House Bill 2 in NC. In addition, bimonthly, short interactive exercises are designed and presented by GHDC's outreach committee on antiracism issues, such as microaggressions or a time line of our family's cultural roots.

A second lesson is to negotiate the balance of community and academic members in a long-term CBPR partnership. Over time, because of the innovative nature of this work, GHDC has drawn more and more membership from academic institutions. Additionally, community members have developed research experience and have been hired into institutional roles during ACCURE, subtly shifting the balance of voices around the table. As a result, GHDC is engaged in an ongoing conversations about who among us is, and is not, currently in a position to authentically speak from a community perspective. This question defies a categorical answer and charges us to use the analysis of power and authority as a mirror to reflect on our partnership and our gatekeeping.

A third lesson is to anticipate the gatekeeping role of academic CBPR partners during the post-award period. After receiving funding for ACCURE, it was essential for us to recognize that ACCURE's subcontracts between UNC and the two cancer centers were "business as usual," whereas, the subcontract with TPP, ACCURE's community-based organization partner, was not. With minimal cash flow and one part-time accountant, TPP has limited resources to adjust to changes in policies and procedures from NIH (e.g., new conditions for reconciling cash advances versus invoicing for reimbursing receipts), UNC's Office of Sponsored Research (e.g., newly required criminal background checks for paying community consultants), and UNC's IRB (e.g., no longer allowing cash incentives for participants and mandating gift cards for which merchants can demand a photo ID with no legal basis). Such adjustments placed extra burdens on ACCURE's project manager and co-PIs, who served as gatekeepers faced with the dilemma of how to serve as advocates for TPP, UNC, or both. Details on ACCURE's solutions can be found in *Academic Researcher's Guide for Pre- and Post-Award Grants Management When Conducting Community Engaged Research* (https://tracs.unc.edu/docs/cares/CAGAT_Academic_Researchers_Guide_v20150929.pdf). This guide was designed for academic researchers at UNC interested in gaining a greater understanding of, and information about, the grant submission and management process when conducting federally funded community-engaged research.

In conclusion, this case study of ACCURE is built on an understanding of the importance of structural racism and the integration of antiracism training and collaborative processes of CBPR within the two cancer centers. We have described and reflected on how involving cancer center providers and staff members to join a thirteen-year-old CBPR partnership, grounded in anti-racism training and CBPR, enabled us, in general, to investigate race-specific patient experiences with quality and completion of cancer care and, in particular, to uncover and address major barriers for African American patients.

QUESTIONS FOR DISCUSSION

1. The ACCURE case study is focused on the health care system. Which concepts, methods, and lessons learned from ACCURE would be relevant for addressing inequities within other systems, such as education, criminal justice, social welfare, and for-profit business?
2. The authors refer to gatekeeping roles among health care staff within a cancer center and partners within a CBPR partnership. Thinking back to your own experiences, how have you served as a gatekeeper? Moving forward, how do you foresee yourself, as an enlightened gatekeeper, to use your power and accountability for breaking down health inequities?

REFERENCES

Bach, P. B., Cramer, L. D., Warren, J. L., & Begg, C. B. (1999). Racial differences in the treatment of early-stage lung cancer. *New England Journal of Medicine, 341,* 1198–1205.

Bickell, N. A., Wang, J. J., Oluwole, S., Schrag, D., Godfrey, H., Hiotis, K., Mendez, J., & Guth, A. A. (2006). Missed opportunities: Racial disparities in adjuvant breast cancer treatment. *Journal of Clinical Oncology, 24,* 1357–1362.

Cykert, C., Dilworth-Anderson, P., Monroe, M. H., Walker, P., McGuire, F. R., Corbie-Smith, G., Edwards, L. J., & Bunton, A. J. (2010). Modifiable factors associated with decisions to undergo surgery among newly diagnosed patients with early stage lung cancer. *Journal of the American Medical Association, 303,* 2368–2376.

Farjah, F., Wood, D. E., Yanez, N. D., III, Vaughan, T. L., Symons, R. G., Krishnadasan, B., & Flum, D. R. (2009). Racial disparities among patients with lung cancer who were recommended operative therapy. *Archives of Surgery, 144,* 14–18.

Gorin, S. S., Heck, J. E., Cheng, B., & Smith, S. J. (2006). Delays in breast cancer diagnosis and treatment by racial/ethnic group. *Archives of Internal Medicine, 166,* 2244–2252.

Hershman, D., McBride, R., Jacobson, J. S., Lamerato, L., Roberts, K., Grann, V. R., & Neugut, A. I. (2005). Racial disparities in treatment and survival among women with early-stage breast cancer. *Journal of Clinical Oncology, 23,* 6639–6646.

Jemal, A., Siegel, R., Ward, E., Murray, T., Xu, J., & Thun, M. J. (2007). Cancer statistics, 2007. *CA: A Cancer Journal for Clinicians, 57,* 43–66.

Jones, C. P. (2003). Confronting institutionalized racism. *Phylon, 50*(1–2), 7–22.

Powell, W. (2006). *Encyclopedia of North Carolina.* Chapel Hill, NC: University of North Carolina Press.

Ries, L.A.G., Melbert, D., Krapcho, M., Mariotto, A., Miller, B. A., Feuer, E. J., & Reichman, M. (2007). *SEER cancer statistics review, 1975–2004.* Bethesda, MD: National Cancer Institute. Retrieved from seer.cancer.gov/csr/1975–2001

Schaal, J. C., Lightfoot, A. F., Black, K. Z., Stein, K., White, S. B., Cothern, C., Gilbert, K., Hardy, C. Y., Jeon, J. Y., Mann, L., Mouw, M. S., Robertson, L., Waters, E. M., Yonas, M. A., & Eng, E. (2016). Community-guided focus group analysis on cancer disparities. *Progress in Community Health Partnerships: Research Education Action, 10*(1), 159–166.

Smedley, B. D., Stith, A. Y., & Nelson, A. R. (Eds.). (2003). *Unequal treatment: Confronting racial and ethnic disparities in health care.* Washington, DC: National Academies Press.

Sullivan, L. W. (2004). *Missing persons: Minorities in the health professions; A report of the Sullivan Commission on Diversity in the Healthcare Workforce.* Alexandria, VA: The Sullivan Alliance to Transform the Health Professions.

US Census Bureau. (2015) *State & county quick facts: Guilford County, North Carolina.* Retrieved from http://quickfacts.census.gov/qfd/states/37/37081.html

Voti, L., Richardson, L. C., Reis, I., Fleming, L. E., Mackinnon, J., & Coebergh, J. W. (2006). The effect of race/ethnicity and insurance in the administration of standard therapy for local breast cancer in Florida. *Breast Cancer Research and Treatment, 95,* 89–95.

Williams, D. R., & Rucker, T. D. (2000). Understanding and addressing racial disparities in health care. *Health Care Financing Review, 21,* 75–90.

Yonas, M. A., Aronson, R. E., Coad, N., Eng, E., Jones, N., Petteway, R., Schaal, J., & Webb, L. (2013). Infrastructure for equitable decision-making in research. In B. A. Israel, E. Eng, A. J. Schultz, & E. A. Parker (Eds.), *Methods for community-based participatory research for health* (2nd ed.). San Francisco, CA: Jossey-Bass.

Yonas, M. A., Aronson, R., Schaal, J., Eng, E., Hardy, C., & Jones, N. (2013). Critical incident technique: An innovative participatory approach to examine and document racial disparities in breast cancer healthcare services. *Health Education Research, 28*(5), 748–759.

Yonas, M. A., Jones, N., Eng, E., Vines, A. I., Aronson, R., Griffith, D. M., White, B., & DuBose, M. (2006). The art and science of integrating undoing racism with CBPR: Challenges of pursuing NIH funding to investigate cancer care and racial equity. *Journal of Urban Health, 83*(6), 1004–1012.

CHAPTER 9

SOUTH VALLEY PARTNERS FOR ENVIRONMENTAL JUSTICE

A STORY OF ALIGNMENT AND MISALIGNMENT

MAGDALENA AVILA, SHANNON SANCHEZ-YOUNGMAN, MICHAEL MUHAMMAD, LAURO SILVA, AND PAULA DOMINGO DE GARCIA

AS THE ORIGINAL settlement of Albuquerque, New Mexico, the South Valley has been home to generations of Chicano-Hispanic farmers and more recent Mexican immigrants. The South Valley is composed of many historic sub-neighborhood communities that have a long-established legacy of community organizing for social justice. Much of this history is rooted in the culture and tradition of New Mexican land grants and their long-term influence on the lives of residents. Faced with many economic and health disparities encountered by downstream communities, South Valley residents have also historically struggled with institutional and environmental racism, including no public services for multiple Mexican colonias and contamination from heavy industrial development within residential neighborhoods. Industries, such as wrecking yards and petrochemical storage, over the last several decades, have generated brownfields and two Superfund sites.

The South Valley Partners for Environmental Justice (SVPEJ) originated as a CBPR partnership among community-based organizations, the county environmental health department, and the University of New Mexico. This project received two cycles of National Institute of

Environmental Health Sciences (NIEHS) funding to map conditions and empower residents to address environmental justice issues. SVPEJ achieved multiple grant goals, including the training and empowerment of a cadre of research promotores (lay health workers) to provide environmental education within some of the most economically, socially, and politically vulnerable neighborhoods.

Despite this longevity, SVPEJ stakeholders identified multiple challenges for reaching their policy goals. These included the historical context, an inhospitable policy environment, and the impact of these contexts on issues of alignment and misalignment among the different partners and between the partnership and the community. Alignment is defined here as the ethical adjustments of a partnership to fit with the perspective of community partners about their sociocultural, historical, and political context to ensure the maximum potential for collectively producing knowledge for equity. This chapter demonstrates that different, and sometimes clashing, perspectives of key community leaders, promotores, academics, and policy makers toward their context, the purpose of the research, group decision making, governance, and community authority can impede CBPR efforts to achieve environmental justice. However, even when partnerships falter, effective community leadership can seed differential consciousness among activists. Although possibly not intended, differential consciousness, defined by Sandoval (1991) as an empowering mental state that prepares members of an oppressed group to undermine, reform, or overthrow a dominant system, became one of its most important accomplishments.

ENVIRONMENTAL JUSTICE IN THE UNITED STATES

The environmental health justice movement and CBPR are tightly linked in practice and through their institutional development (Brugge & Hynes, 2005; Corburn, 2005; Minkler et al., 2010; O'Fallon & Dearry, 2002). This approach fuses academic and community insights to define problems and research questions enabling collaboration to gather and analyze data and use grassroots organizing strategies to advocate for health justice issues. Through a process of coproduction of research and community action, CBPR and environmental health partnerships have the potential to reveal the contingency of knowledge and expertise and offer an innovative platform to influence community and political transformation. Importantly, the environmental justice movement preceded CBPR, with the NIEHS being the first institute to fund community-based research projects incorporating CBPR in 1995. At the federal level NIEHS initiated an innovative research approach that brought together environmental health, CBPR, and social justice.

The civil rights movement of the sixties was the precursor to the mainstream environmental justice movement that crystalized in the mid-1980s (Brown, 2015; Brulle & Pellow, 2006). Adopting an expansive view of equity, young leaders of color mobilized on toxic contamination, substandard housing, access to green space, land use and smart growth policy, food justice, and jobs (Faber & McCarthy, 2003). Using street science to advance their claims, lay community leaders made observations of health effects and pollutants, hypothesized connections, organized community groups, and brought in legal experts for advocacy and policy reforms. With a clear sense of structural determinants, movement groups typically framed their concerns in individual and collective terms. Battles about land use, for example, were not just about individual impacts but also stressed the impact on social cohesion and the well-being of communities of color. In sum, those communities experiencing the greatest environmental and health inequities asserted that their lived experiences, coping strategies, and cultural traditions qualified them as coproducers of environmental and health decision making (Corburn, 2007).

Alongside these developments, mainstream environmental organizations, predominantly representing interests of white, upper-middle-class liberals, fought to protect wilderness, endangered species, clean air and water, and often ignored the structural inequalities faced by people of color (Schlosberg & Carruthers, 2010). In 1991, the first People of Color Summit of Environmental Justice challenged these mainstream environmentalists by establishing seventeen environmental justice principles. In an act of differential consciousness, people of color and vulnerable communities named the issue of environmental racism, using their own oral histories, and identified siting of toxic waste in communities of color. Citing multiple conditions of oppression faced by people of color, these activists also called for new and multiple strategies to achieve equity. This critical act of resistance redefined environmental justice as a civil right and a social justice and human rights issue in the eyes of governmental funding agencies such as the NIH (Brulle & Pellow, 2006).

Building on these efforts, the environmental justice health movement also began to call for "recognition" as another crucial element of environmentalism (Gibson-Wood & Wakefield, 2012). In effect, Indigenous activists called for the inclusion of alternative ways of knowing in defining and solving environmental problems to promote broader environmental justice (Corburn, 2007; Haluza-Delay, 2008). They asserted that ignoring alternative ways of naming and framing environmental problems was unjust because it denied equal voice to those whose understandings and experiences of "the environment" were outside of dominant experiences.

Indigenous calls for a politics of recognition presented a natural fit for one of CBPR's major strategies to recognize the critical role of local culture and context in designing and implementing interventions with local ways of knowing (Belone et al., 2016; Wallerstein & Duran, 2010; Wallerstein et al., under review). For CBPR practitioners, lived experiences provide crucial venues to understand environmental health concerns from multiple vantage points. Further, the coproduction of knowledge disrupts power imbalances among academics, policy makers, and lay people, and alternative ways of knowing problematize the origins and substance of policy issues by highlighting that scientific legitimacy is a social, political, and material phenomena. Most critically, local ways of knowing give communities the agency to transform the social, political, and ethnoracial stratification systems that have subjugated their community knowledge (Dutta, 2008).

SOCIOCULTURAL RELATIONS AND ENVIRONMENTAL ACTIVISM IN THE SOUTH VALLEY

The South Valley (SV) is a vibrant, culturally rich community that intersects urban and rural living with pockets of neighborhoods that still have livestock in the backyard with those that are a bit trendier in their modernization. Latinos of New Mexican heritage and Mexican immigrants comprise the biggest percentage of SV residents. Although the majority of its residents are socioeconomically disadvantaged, there is also a long history of land-based ownership among the many New Mexican families who have made the SV home for generations.

The sociopolitical history of the SV is one that is deeply immersed, similar to the rest of New Mexico, in a history of community empowerment and the struggle for social justice related to land grant status, going back to the Treaty of Guadalupe in 1848. Through land grants, native

New Mexican community identities have been rooted in a long legacy of land-based people's struggles for the right to their lands, their water rights, and their perceived cultural inheritance. SV community leadership is also an attribute of generations of families who have spoken up for their rights as political activists and as elected officials at the county and state levels. More recent organizing related to environmental contamination has brought together local predominantly Latino advocacy organizations in formal and informal coalitions to advocate for the cleanup of two Superfund sites. With the increase of Mexican low-income immigrants in the SV over the last twenty years, the differences between immigrants and politically powerful native New Mexicans have created a complex constellation of cultural factors and values and principles that are often confusing to outside researchers and public health officials.

The SVPEJ originated as a research group in 2000 as a response to a request for proposals from NIEHS. Consisting of four partners—the University of New Mexico, Bernalillo County's Office of Environmental Health, the Rio Grande Community Development Corporation (RGCDC), and South Valley promotores—SVPEJ was successfully funded for two NIEHS grant cycles (2000–2004, 2005–2009). The research partnership came together to seek reductions of environmental health hazards and risks in the South Valley by bridging communication gaps among community residents, health care providers, policy makers, and environmental health researchers. In the first grant, the county was the principal investigator (PI) and worked in collaboration with the community to identify, define, and assess the disproportionate burden of environmental health risks and health inequities faced by Latino families. In the second grant, the community became the PI after community members challenged aspects of the first grant cycle. In the second phase, the goals were to develop a communication model, identify venues to better inform and engage SV residents on local land-use zoning and planning issues, and seek greater community participation in decision making on these zoning and policy issues. Key grant outcomes included increased understanding of the local land use zoning and policy process, the update and revision of a dated neighborhood sector plan that was decades old, and a communication model to better inform residents as part of an informed policy-making process. This increased capacity building among promotores, but after ten years of multiple fractures, the partnership dissolved.

These fractures, which emerged through conscious and unconscious practices, deepened throughout the ten-year project period. In the beginning, they emerged as almost invisible hairline cracks. Although seemingly unnoticed, they cumulatively contributed to misalignment between community and the academic and county partners. As these fractures expanded, they led to a major dissention and disagreements about how the research and advocacy was carried out in the SV.

METHODS

In 2012, the SVPEJ research project was selected as a case study from a larger National Institute of Health investigation known as the Research for Health (RIH) Project, led by the University of New Mexico (UNM) Center for Participatory Research. RIH sought to test a CBPR conceptual model, assess the variability of CBPR partnerships nationwide, and identify associations between contexts, partnering characteristics, research, and health outcomes (Hicks et al., 2012; Pearson et al., 2015). Data collection for the SV as part of the RIH case study took twelve months and included fifteen semi-structured individual interviews, one focus group, a document review, and a historical time-line exercise with case study partners (see Chapters 6 and 17 for more discussion of RIH case study methods).

DISCUSSION: TENSIONS AND FRACTURES

Environmental justice research and advocacy is a complex and challenging area—especially when collaborative partnerships are composed of such a unique constellation of interests, aims, and motivations. The SVPEJ partnership reveals how conflicting ways of knowing and divergent social justice tactics contributed to a series of fractures that ultimately eroded the partnership. As the next sections illustrate, the SVPEJ project represents an example in which academics and county policy makers missed several opportunities to recognize and build on the layers of community understandings of water and land use in New Mexico. These community understandings are critical sources of survival, political, and cultural identity, nation-state making, and become central metaphors that encapsulate generations of struggle(s) against stratification systems that continue to ripple on the basis of class, citizenship, ways of living, and ethno-racial dynamics.

Divergent Worldviews on Environmental Problems and Solutions

Seeding the development of these fractures, interviews with academic and county partners showed they approached the aims of the project through a distributive justice lens, which was informed by white, liberal environmentalism and their obligations as county officials. Academics and county representatives shared the community's values of reducing environmental racism. For them, the project presented the opportunity to fold in community member participation into ongoing struggles to promote equitable land use. They suggested that the project would use traditional tactics of agenda setting and policy advocacy at the county level to alleviate environmental ills.

A second aim was to cooperate with community members to achieve a unified vision of environmental justice. Academic and county partners imagined a process in which experts would develop the community's skills to identify environmental risks to advocate and inform community residents about how to build safer neighborhoods. Building community capacity meant teaching promotores to take air and water samples, develop their leadership skills, and use storytelling to influence formal policy reform. When reflecting on the major aims of these policy efforts, one county person said, "I think the purpose was developing skills amongst the community around land use issues. For instance, we did a training on when somebody submits a permit, what's the process that it goes to before becoming approved."

These county-driven aims were largely a response to their own bureaucratic constraints that limited their political advocacy. Guided, therefore, by technical approaches to policy advocacy, academic and county partners assumed that their role was to educate the community to become active participants in their local advocacy efforts. The shortcoming of this approach was that it implied that experts would provide information to vulnerable communities to create policy change.

Academics and policy makers also viewed the grant as a mechanism to provide resources to the community to improve local environmental conditions. For instance, the county leveraged funds to initiate several cleanup projects as part of the project. According to a local county official, "we wrote a grant to provide containers to do a community cleanup on Pajarito Mesa. But then of course, the community used them for gas and other things. So we did a training—all in Spanish and they learned how to use them." The presumption here is that the partnership provided the opportunity to promote individual behavior change in the community through culturally sensitive trainings. Although the resources provided were valuable for environmental cleanup, they downplayed the necessity to resist the unhealthy structures faced by community residents.

In the political sphere, academic and county partners often situated their analysis of local power relations on political corruption and sexism. According to county and academic partners, some major obstacles to their partnership's success were embedded in the "machismo" of Latino political leadership in the area and entrenched patronage politics between old New Mexican families and business owners. From their point of view, the partnership would leverage the perspectives of Chicano community leaders to fight against patronage politics and to fight against male control of the political agenda. One county official noted the following:

> Historically, a lot of the organizations that worked in the South Valley were male dominant. I think that there is some bias from attitudes like "you females, you are trying to change us and our power." And, I'm sorry, the Bernalillo County at that time was very male dominant in power. I don't think there was one female who had a leadership role in the county.

The community's vision of social justice, however, was premised on harnessing the lived experiences of immigrant and Chicano-Latino communities to fight for multiple reforms. Informed by oral stories passed on through generations, community members described water and land use struggles as multilayered issues embedded within deep historical struggles of community identity, distribution of material resources, and communal ways of living. One community member interviewee described the SV acequia (irrigation ditches) movement:

> For me, the acequia movement is another movement of struggle altogether that is currently happening. There is the association of acequias, because with a water problem, it's a movement based on tradition, and dealing with tradition. It's a New Mexican movement; the struggle for water, and that water is life, "se defiende no se vende," "Water is to defend, not to sell."

As this quote suggests, the community's struggle over water not only sought to preserve and reproduce a way of life but also entailed a struggle for political voice and autonomy for successful community functioning and independence.

Representing a movement premised on the decolonization of knowledge and political advocacy, community activists in the SV drew from the political skills of women and men of color that emanated from their everyday resistance. For community partners, a major aim of the project was to build from community resilience rooted in cultural practices to fight against environmental racism. One activist scholar stated the following:

> I think my approach and how I saw the project is first of all, it's certainly not a deficit model of knowledge from a community perspective, but rather a capacity model. There's already tremendous knowledge from what I call organic venues within the community. So when we're going to tap into those venues it's which one are we going to tap? How are we going to tap it? How do we acknowledge the depth and width of expertise? So it always comes from a model that acknowledges the foundation of knowledge that comes from a community . . . It's like constantly mapping. Always mapping the movement with the community.

Community partners did not envision their work as simply demanding formal legal equality through a multisector plan. Rather, a central task was to facilitate critical consciousness among community members and their academic and county allies to advocate for rights. A key community project leader saw educating the community as an exercise in "deconstructing a policy manual and working to educate the community about what a sector plan does and by taking it apart informing people of their rights."

Divergent Tactics for Environmental Justice

Community activists advocated for strategies encompassing a more holistic vision of social justice that promoted social, political, and economic actions that linked solutions to broader social change. For community leaders, this involved having the flexibility to read multiple situations and consciously choose strategies best suited to push against multiple forms of oppression. For these folks, organizing for change was neither linear nor utilitarian, and the goal was to mobilize community members to adopt a variety of organizing tactics, ranging from advocating for formal legal reforms to mobilizing against a broader field of unequal conditions that produced environmental injustices in the South Valley.

Informed by a more radical lens compared to academic and county partners, community residents felt that a bias existed in favor of industrial investment supported by elected policy officials. They argued that this conflicted with the traditional land use among Indigenous community members, placing community residents at greater health risks. As a result, community partners saw the community PI as a *champion* who would adopt a more hard-line position against perceived encroachments to SV self-determination. Promotores especially felt that researchers and county-level bureaucrats who preferred top-down approaches ultimately upheld the status quo of public health institutions:

> Well, I think it was real beneficial for me to be a promotor and to be a part of this process; and I think the leadership, the principal investigator of the promotores, I think he was one of these elders of the community that was connected, and that he did have a lot of knowledge of the community, a lot of knowledge about the university and with the county. He had a lot of experience, and I think that was really important. I don't think the community partners, as the principal investigators, would have been successful had it not been for somebody, for an elder that knows, that's been part of the community.

In contrast to the promotores who viewed the community PI as a powerful elder, academic and county partners suggested that the community PI's advocacy strategies were conflictual and ignored the science of public health. They argued that his conflictual advocacy-based approach ultimately decreased their participation in the project. A member from the academic team stated the following:

> The trust actually disintegrated towards the end. The promotores weren't trustful of me, because I was representing the university. I wasn't trustful of the community PI because he was pulling this power thing. And it really disintegrated quite a lot. We tried talking to the community PI about wanting to really have it be participatory. He was a guy that really held things close to his chest. And so it really wasn't a partnership towards the end. I think that we were ready to bag it and just call it a day.

For academic and community partners, advocating against environmental racism would have been more straightforward if community members had agreed to set timely goals with measurable outcomes. For them, CBPR offered the space to include community members in the process of linking science to policy. In fact, academic and county partners suggested that a major shortcoming of the project was its lack of linearity:

> I'm not a process person. And I'm a very structural person. So like I have "to do" lists. So this was a bit different for me, very different for me. And I had a difficult time seeing the end result, and I was impatient with some of the very loose dynamics that occurred, which I think are part of community work. And I recognize that. I think it wasn't as well-defined as it could have been. And to me that was a huge frustration . . . we didn't have time lines . . . we didn't have measurements . . . And I think without those time lines and without the structural components . . . we didn't achieve as much as we could have.
>
> Why? I think it was learning curve of the community people. They had done some community organizing, but did not have an academic base in public health or CBPR.

This quote highlights that some of the county or academic participants privileged results over process and ultimately felt that more structured approaches provided a better framework to produce policy change.

Ruptures in Ways of Knowing

A comparison of community, academic, and county partners' ways of naming, framing, and addressing environmental justice revealed important differences and misalignments among members of the SVPEJ project. Though CBPR as a field depends on the valuing of coproduction of knowledge, this case study reveals ways in which coproduction faltered throughout the ten-year period, reducing the partnership's effectiveness, in two primary ways.

As said previously, the county public health professionals and academics implicitly held a deficit-based approach to the community by believing that their technical resources and trainings would provide the necessary skill building for policy change. Indeed, this top-down approach was established by academic and county members in the initial design and early implementation of the grant. When promotores were recruited to participate, the first county leadership did not fully explain the aims of the project in an inclusive manner. This created early tensions because promotores perceived this omission as condescending. Academic and county partners also excluded promotores from research meetings, organized antiracism trainings for promotores without academic and county participation, and used promotores as interpreters among stakeholders. These actions discredited them as community knowledge holders. According to the community PI of the second grant,

> I think it's a question of basically community partners not having the respect that they deserve and the trust that they deserve. The academics didn't trust the community. And it's hard for academics to trust community. Community distrusts academics because they come in and mine the resources of the community and run away with it and don't leave anything behind.

By contrast, academic and county partners repeatedly expressed their frustration with the lack of "professionalism" and focus among the community partners. This skeptical view of community knowledge perpetuated the notion that science was the primary mechanism to speak truth to power.

Academic and policy partners also missed crucial opportunities to create meaningful dialogue with community partners about broader solutions that promoted social, political, and economy integration in the SV. By focusing on the narrower objectives of distributive environmental justice, they inadvertently didn't understand the deep and multifaceted politics of water and land in the Rio Grande region. In short, their proposed solutions adhered to mainstream conceptions of environmentalism that were individual and consumption based. This subtly reflected the biases of liberal environmentalism and ignored the reality that community members often lacked the basic infrastructure to meet their everyday living needs. As the community partners pointed out, the danger of tinkering with zoning laws did not necessarily change the key conditions of vulnerability in the South Valley.

This top-down approach had far-reaching consequences. Academic and county partners reproduced a mainstream science narrative that linked traditional forms of advocacy with progress and social transformation. From the community's perspective, the partnership failed to foster spaces for social change and structural transformation because academic and county participants did not leverage Indigenous knowledge to understand problems and solutions. By refusing to relinquish their control of the research process, promotores and community leaders argued that the process became paternalistic. According to one promotora,

> Towards the end of partnership you could see the true colors of the organizations when the community had the chance to be in the driver seat; and I don't think the partners—the university and the academic partners—were comfortable with it and I think their egos were hurt because these uneducated people were talking about publishing papers and having their names put on these publications that these professors need to have tenure . . . and that the county needs to show that they're doing something for the community. And so it is a very paternalistic relationship that is like, "We are taking care of you guys. We'll take care of this." And we're like, "No, we can put our names on the papers too we're doing the research or whatever else."

Community leaders also described how the partnership reproduced power asymmetries between structural positions of the white feminists and community members. For community activists, the project ultimately reinforced the status quo in academic-community interactions because the power to name, frame, and organize remained in the hands of the academy and in public health county bureaucratic institutions. According to one female academic,

> The PIs are white, the assistant PIs are white, everybody's white for the most part. And then what do you have? Again that, what do you call it? . . . that sister relationship, but the Great White Hope is holding the hand. It can't be that way. I'm just tired of seeing that. You cannot be afraid to give up your power. And I think for me that's my greatest test. I ask myself, "Am I afraid to be replaced or am I afraid to be questioned?" We need the community to challenge us. They're going to know stuff we don't know. Yeah, we have to develop more Indigenous experts. That's what's going to change the pendulum.

Community Resilience

In spite of the partnership's dissolution, community leaders were successful in empowering a cadre of research promotores that reappropriated the term of *environmentalism* and redefined it according to their lived realities at ground zero. Promotores and other community members did not agree with how the county and academic environmentalism was mirroring their struggle, so they took charge and completely redefined the aims of the project. This is an example of differential consciousness when communities of color experience, perceive, define, and advocate an environmentalism that was not aligned with the perceptions and social norms of mainstream environmentalism. Through their differential consciousness and struggles within the partnership and through the leadership of community leaders, promotores expressed an awakening of deep and profound knowledge that included shaking off oppressive practices that they saw and experienced through the research process. Through consciousness raising in dialogue with community leaders, promotores said that their critical lens changed on a daily basis as they became more confident in operational research methods. In the words of a key facilitator of this process,

> The SVPEJ started like a ripple when you throw the pebble into the pond and then it became a tsunami of intellectual and political force that left in its stead an infinite amount of ripples that hit at the mind, the soul, the spirit, the heart, the feet, and the legacy of each and every one of the promotores. Those are the elements of critical thinking in our communities that shift the alignment and that shocks those benevolent minds who have absolutely no understanding of its force and whence it comes. CBPR is an awakening from a total different point of consciousness and intellect than it is for the academic partners. The seed was planted and it came to fruition regardless of what anyone thinks; this was the success that can't be empirically measured. It is a seed of a movement. To me this is the greatest gift or seeding of what CBPR research can bring—such a degree of reflexivity that it opens the doors that oppression has closed. It reignites the spark. It's more than data . . . it's a social movement.

LESSONS LEARNED

Although these fractures and tensions challenged the success of the SV partnership, they also raised important lessons for other CBPR partnerships.

Establish structural mechanisms that promote mutuality from the outset. A fundamental principal of CBPR is to leverage the research process to bring everyone forward and create venues that equalize power differentials between academics and community members. Key to promoting a successful and equity-based partnership is demystifying and deconstructing the research process. A first step is for academics and community members to coproduce research documents, beginning with the research proposal. Most proposals consist of professional and technical language that is unfamiliar to community-based partners. Rather than confining proposal writing to academics, cowriting grants (or creating agreements) can seed the possibilities for meaningful change, and it establishes an equity-based framework from the outset.

Enter communities with humility. Academic partners must avoid entering communities with a "follow me and learn" attitude. They should listen, observe, and adopt a "let's walk together" approach to foster collaborative learning and collective empowerment. As the SV case study demonstrates, community partners do not see activities such as translating and interpreting as a newly acquired research skill but rather as part of their existing culturally based skill set. Effective partnerships promote community capacity by recognizing and building from community assets rather than appropriating cultural knowledge as a form of research skill development.

Embrace tensions. Working in a collaborative research partnership may give the impression that relational processes are always healthy and that all members should strive to maintain partnership perfection. Partnerships, similar to any relationship, often fall victim to maintaining the false perception that all is well. Yet, fractures and tensions may present some of the most valuable lessons for collaborative research processes. Genuine collaborations require continual collective reflexivity among all partners. This includes providing the space for members to reflect on and revise their roles and levels of input throughout the project. It means being conscious of institutional positions and the limitations and opportunities within each. It is imperative to recognize that the partnerships' configuration will not stay the same for the duration of the research project. If anything, the partnership pendulum will swing back and forth, and it should be accepted and perceived as a healthy indicator of a collaborative partnership process.

Differential consciousness is a catalyst for community-based research and social transformation. In a collaborative research partnership, it is critical that equal value be given to multiple ways of knowing to produce decolonized research and social transformation. This provides the intellectual engine for the team. Valued scholarship must be equally based and not anchored in condescending or patronizing approaches that are masked to pass as genuine. Community-based partners (i.e., promotores) did not want to be written about, but they wanted to participate in dissemination of knowledge by being treated and approached as scholarly partners. Promotores found out about project articles being discussed for publication that they were never invited to participate in. They felt they were not valued, and their perspective was seen as outside the dominant norm.

CBPR is like a prism that encourages different and changing viewpoints. It is a continuum that provides different anchor points to the research among the different partners. CBPR grows in its value and importance as communities take more ownership of the process and can change the merits of the research outcomes. Academic partners must be flexible and be prepared to accommodate this changing lens. Inflexibly forcing a linear research approach can produce unexpected levels of challenges, including partnership fractures, punctures, and tensions.

CONCLUSION

This case study demonstrates the issues that arise as a result of partnership alignment and misalignments. All research partnerships have challenges and, even when those challenges turn into tensions, fractures, and ruptures that derail the initial goals of the project, there are still lessons to be learned and successes to be gained. CBPR is a research orientation that promises equity and equanimity. Those who use this approach will be held to a higher standard from a community perspective than other traditional research approaches. Research can produce differential consciousness at a grassroots community level. CBPR therefore has within its very foundation the essential constructs to go beyond a canned approach and to give greater voice to organic narratives and knowledge.

QUESTIONS FOR DISCUSSION

1. All research partnerships will face challenges along the way, with larger and more diverse partnerships perhaps facing a more challenging journey. Given this reality, how would you as a research team member identify and address potential threats based on your perception of tensions and fractures? How would you differentiate perceived problems from actual problems?
2. What strategies would you develop to address tensions, fractures, and ruptures within a partnership? What strategies would you use to communicate this to community and academic team members, including identifying indicators of tensions early on?

ACKNOWLEDGMENTS

The authors of this chapter would like to acknowledge NIEHS for the two grants that they funded (2001–2009, #1r25eso14347-03), the NIEHS program officer, Liam O'Fallon, the South Valley Partners for Environmental Justice (SVPEJ), and the South Valley Community. Thanks also to the promotoras, and the many other partners who remain committed to health equity work from Bernalillo County, the University of New Mexico and the Rio Grande Community Development Corporation. Environmental justice will not be possible without all the collaboration and shared work. Thank you to all.

REFERENCES

Belone, L., Lucero, J., Duran, B., Tafoya, G., Baker, E., Chan, D., Chang, C., Greene-Moton, E., Kelley, M., & Wallerstein, N. (2016). Community-based participatory research conceptual model: Community partner consultation and face validity, *Qualitative Health Research,* pp. 1–19.

Brown, P. (2015). Integrating medical and environmental sociology with environmental health: Crossing boundaries and building connections through advocacy. *Journal of Health and Social Behavior, 54,* 145–164.

Brugge, D., & Hynes, P. (2005). *Community research in environmental health: Studies in science, advocacy and ethics.* Burlington, MA: Ashgate Publishing.

Brulle, R., & Pellow, D. (2006.) Environmental justice: Human health and environmental inequalities. *Annual Review of Public Health, 27,* 103–123.

Corburn, J. (2005). *Street science: Community knowledge and environmental health justice.* Cambridge, MA: MIT Press.

Corburn, J. (2007). Community knowledge in environmental health science: Coproducing policy expertise. *Environmental Science and Policy, 10,* 150–161.

Dutta, M. J. (2008). *Communicating health: A culture-centered approach.* Malden, MA: Polity Press.

Faber, D., & McCarthy, D. (2003). Neoliberalism, globalization and the struggle for ecological democracy: Linking sustainability and environmental justice. In J. Agyeman, R. D. Bullard, & B. Evans (Eds.), *Just sustainabilities: Development in an unequal world.* Cambridge, MA: MIT Press.

Gibson-Wood, H., & Wakefield, S. (2012). Participation, white privilege and environmental justice: Understanding environmentalism among Hispanics in Toronto. *Antipode, 45,* 641–662.

Haluza-DeLay, R. (2008). A theory of practice for social movements, environmentalism and ecological habitus, *Mobilization: An International Quarterly, 13,* 205–218.

Hicks, S., Duran, B., Wallerstein, N., Avila, M., Belone, L., Lucero, J., Magarati, M., Mainer, E., Martin, D., Muhammed, M., Oetzel, J., Pearson, C., Sahota, P., Simonds, V., Sussman, A., Tafoya, G., & White Hat, E. (2012). Evaluating community-based participatory research to improve community-partnered science and community health. *Progress for Community Partnerships, 6,* 289–311.

Minkler, M., Garcia, A. P., Williams, J., LoPresti, T., & Lilly, J. (2010). Si se puede: Using participatory research to promote environmental justice in a Latino community in San Diego, California. *Journal of Urban Health, 87,* 796–812.

O'Fallon, L. R., & Dearry, A. (2002). Community-based participatory research as a tool to advance environmental health sciences. *Environmental Health Perspectives, 110*(Supp 2), 155–159.

Pearson, C. R., Duran, B., Oetzel, J., Margarati, M., Villegas, M., Lucero, J., & Wallerstein, N. (2015). Research for improved health: Variability and impact of structural characteristics in federally funded community engaged research projects. *Progress in Community Health Partnerships: Research, Education, and Action, 9,* 17–29.

Sandoval, C. (1991). *Methodology of the oppressed.* Minneapolis, MN: Minnesota University Press.

Schlosberg, D., & Carruthers, D., (2010). Indigenous struggles, environmental justice, and community capabilities, *Global Environmental Politics, 10*(4), 12–35.

Wallerstein, N., & Duran, B. (2010). Community-based participatory research contributions to intervention research: The intersection of science and practice to improve health equity. *American Journal of Public Health, 100,* S40–S46.

Wallerstein, N., Oetzel, J., Duran, B., Margarati, M., Pearson, C., Davis, J., DeWindt, L., Lucero, J., Ruddock, C., Sutter, E., Villegas, M., & Dutta, M. (under review). Culture-centeredness in community-based participatory research: Implications for psycho-social health interventions. *Social Science and Medicine.*

PART 4

PROMISING PRACTICES: INTERVENTION DEVELOPMENT AND RESEARCH DESIGN

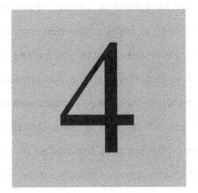

The impacts of context and partnering processes and practices are most often seen on the development of interventions and research designs. Stated most directly, if there is no or minimal engagement with key community stakeholders, intervention and research methodologies suffer isolation from critical community knowledge, priorities, and input on what would succeed for any particular geographic, policy, organizational, and cultural context. NIH has acknowledged the importance of community engagement for precisely ensuring that data

instruments, intervention components, and understanding of local implementation contexts can be recognized and incorporated into the research in order to make a difference in reducing health inequities.

CBPR takes engagement further than just input and looks to shared leadership, coproduction, and community-driven theories and interventions in these all-important knowledge appraisals. Judgements about the usefulness or validity of knowledge are increasingly recognized (by academics and communities) as being embedded in community contexts, not simply as images or beliefs but as dynamic processes of social and cultural reproduction. Communication scholar Mohan Dutta, as noted in Chapters 1 and 2, has proposed the language of "culture-centeredness" to represent community voice, agency, decision making, and reflexivity as key for creating interventions and research designs to transform top-down academic assumptions and other inequitable conditions. Coproducing knowledge not only improves intervention or research method fit within the community but also facilitates greater community ownership, research capacity, and program sustainability after grant funding might end. Valuing community culture and knowledge is also key to promoting the goal of knowledge democracy, which recognizes and celebrates the importance of multiple knowledge systems, such as organic, organizational, land-based, and spiritual systems, and frameworks emerging from social movements, and knowledges of the marginalized and excluded.

The four chapters in this section beautifully illustrate the opportunities for integrating CBPR principles and processes, with community knowledge, cultural agency, understanding of implementation contexts, and academic evidence in creating successful interventions. Case studies and vignettes are provided as examples and as inspiration for others.

In Chapter 10, Margarita Alegría and colleagues provide guidance for applying CBPR to the growing arena of health services research, with its diverse stakeholders of health care providers, payers, patients, patient advocacy groups, families, and other caregivers. They start with challenges, including limited CBPR training for health service researchers, and present useful implementation strategies for incorporating CBPR principles at different research stages. Three vignettes are presented: Community Partners in Care (CPIC), a randomized comparative effectiveness trial of two interventions to support depression quality improvement across health care and community-based agencies in Los Angeles; a PCORI-funded trial at Massachusetts General Hospital and thirteen clinics examining effectiveness of improved patient-provider behavioral health shared decision making through encouraging patients to ask questions and providers to be more receptive; and efficacy of a community health worker intervention to improve type 2 diabetes within the Bangladeshi American community in New York City. All three had extensive partnerships and illustrate how to better integrate CBPR within health care and agency settings.

In Chapter 11, Steven Barnett and colleagues present their experience at the National Center for Deaf Health Research, in Rochester, New York, a city with a large, vibrant, and diverse Deaf population. They showcase how they've developed and sustained CBPR research with members of the Deaf community, who are defined as having a Deaf culture and sign language and not by hearing acuity. The chapter starts with an overview of the cultural dimensions and context of this overlooked population and provides multiple examples of CBPR research with Deaf and hearing researchers, staff members, students, and community members on how they select health research priorities; adapt research methods, measures, and interventions to be language and culturally accessible and appropriate while maintaining scientific rigor; and translate and disseminate their findings to broad stakeholder audiences. Their lessons learned in terms of deeply connecting to the knowledge, values, language, and culture of the community within CBPR are applicable to other minority populations.

In Chapter 12, Nadia Islam and colleagues discuss CBPR with Asian Americans, the fastest growing racial-ethnic group in the United States. CBPR approaches are well suited for Asian American populations, whose contexts vary greatly by subgroup, who often reside in concentrated ethnic enclaves, and who possess rich cultural knowledge integral to conducting quality research and developing effective interventions. The authors present two case studies. The first case study focuses on a national-level, multiethnic approach based at the Center for the Study of Asian American Health at New York University and shares principles and lessons learned from sustaining multiple CBPR partnerships over many years. The second case study focuses on a study of health and working conditions in San Francisco Chinatown restaurants involving immigrant workers as key community researchers, with a local community-activist organization, university, and the local health department. Lessons are shared for building community capacity and successfully advocating for a major municipal worker protection policy.

In Chapter 13, Scott D. Rhodes and colleagues describe the development and refining of a thirteen-step ENGAGED for CHANGE strategy that provides a collaborative framework for CBPR intervention development. ENGAGED for CHANGE is a process that incorporates the lived experiences and decision making of community members and service practitioners working in these communities to ensure culture-centered and contextually appropriate interventions. Based on their fifteen-year experiences as a CBPR collaborative creating sexual health and HIV-prevention interventions for Latino gay and bisexual men, men who have sex with men (MSM), transgender persons, and Latina women, they provide examples for each step of how to incorporate community knowledge with evidence-based strategies in the design, piloting, implementation, and evaluation of their interventions. They hope others can benefit from this approach to maximize the potential for reducing and eliminating health disparities.

CHAPTER

10

CBPR IN HEALTH CARE SETTINGS

MARGARITA ALEGRÍA, CHAU TRINH-SHEVRIN, BOWEN CHUNG, ANDREA AULT, ALISA LINCOLN, AND KENNETH B. WELLS

DESPITE SCIENTIFIC ADVANCES since the 1990s, the translation of evidence-based research into clinical and community practice has been limited (Committee on Quality of Health Care in America, 2001; Pearson, Jordan, & Munn, 2012). Understanding what works in these settings requires moving beyond controlled research designs and settings into community and practice-embedded research partnerships. In the context of health care system research in communities experiencing health disparities, genuine community engagement throughout the research process is required to ensure improved translation of efficacy and effectiveness findings into adoption and practice (Mullins, Abdulhalim, & Lavallee, 2012; Wallerstein & Duran, 2010). Community-based participatory research (CBPR) can elucidate the mechanisms and strategies to support this translation and generate the practice-based evidence to disseminate and scale clinically proven strategies, particularly in under-resourced communities and vulnerable populations (D'Alonzo, 2010; Wallerstein & Duran, 2010).

In recent years, new directions and renewed interest in CBPR approaches have emerged with a focus on patient-centered outcomes research that emphasizes reaching out to patients for their perspectives and the perspectives of caregivers in the research process. With the recent movement toward patient-centered research, the application of CBPR to health services (HS) research has expanded to include health care providers and payers as well as patients, patient advocacy groups, families, and other caregivers and community members as stakeholders (Concannon et al., 2012).

Further, national efforts and discussions about patient-centered research have emphasized authentic stakeholder engagement (Woolf, Zimmerman, Haley, & Krist, 2016), supporting processes and mechanisms that ensure that stakeholder perspectives are integrated throughout the health care system research process and are reflective of CBPR principles. Although interest in patient and family engagement in HS and clinical effectiveness research has increased, there is a dearth of information related to appropriate tools for the measurement and evaluation of engagement in such research, including economic analyses of associated costs of engagement (Domecq et al., 2014; Mockford, Staniszewska, Griffiths, & Herron-Marx, 2012) as well as best practices for engagement. The dearth of information results from a general lack of comparisons of engagement approaches (Domecq et al., 2014) and the limited availability of CBPR training for HS researchers (Mockford et al., 2012).

This chapter proposes that rigorous HS interventions and research can incorporate CBPR principles and practices to better embrace patient and stakeholder engagement. CBPR can help address the preferences of these multiple stakeholders to accelerate implementation and problem-solve challenges. This chapter summarizes three case studies and uses examples from each study to offer guidance for scholars and practitioners in CBPR implementation within HS research.

USING CBPR PRINCIPLES TO ADVANCE HEALTH SERVICES RESEARCH

The Patient-Centered Outcomes Research Institute (PCORI), funded through the Affordable Care Act, seeks to improve the relevance of comparative effectiveness research for patient-prioritized outcomes and interventions. As such, it has explicit grant requirements to include patients, family, community members, and health care stakeholders in all aspects of study development, governance, implementation, and dissemination (Hickam et al., 2013).

Much like other forms of community-engaged research (see Chapter 1), traditional HS research has varied in the level of community engagement—from conducting focus groups and interviews with patients regarding outreach and recruitment strategies (minimal involvement), to stakeholders serving as advisors for research design and evaluation (medium involvement), to stakeholders driving the research questions and strategies as part of the decision-making team (high involvement). Several core CBPR principles (see Table 10.1, with full description in Chapter 3) address the importance of community-framed and community-driven identification of issues for study at the local level and balancing data generation and research with action-oriented solutions and programming efforts in HS research. Understanding patient barriers and facilitators for health improvement includes not only a comprehension of the disease but also the social ecology that predisposes vulnerability and enables disease prevention, treatment adherence, support to tackle comorbid health and social factors, as well as an attention to community preferences and cultural context for health. Dimensions such as social position, race, English language proficiency, or immigration status have substantial impact on the identification of patient priorities and outcomes. By drawing on the core CBPR theme of stakeholders determining priorities, HS studies have the opportunity to advance our understanding of "patient-driven" outcomes beyond those that are clinical or physiological in nature. For example, the National Institute of Mental Health Affective Disorders Work Group developed and validated the Individual Burden of Illness Index for Depression and found that the inclusion of

TABLE 10.1 CBPR Principles, Strategies, and Examples in Health Services Research

CBPR Principle	Strategies in Health Services Research	Examples from the Literature
Create collaborative, equitable partnerships in all research phases.	■ Include patients, caretakers, and patient advocacy group as research coleads. ■ Partner with patient stakeholders in study decision-making and dissemination processes.	■ PatientsLikeMe (Fourie, Biller-Andorno, & Wild, 2014) ■ Disease-specific foundations, particularly for rare conditions, can be important partners (Ginsberg, 2017; Sharpe, 2013).
Community is the unit of identity—focus is on the community.	■ Create a stakeholder board representing diverse patient and caretaker perspectives. ■ Use multiple strategies (Islam et al., 2012) to include diverse constituent and stakeholder perspectives.	■ The DREAM Project coalition involved patients, providers, and other multisector stakeholders serving the New York City Bangladeshi American community.
Build on strengths of community.	■ Use an asset-based approach to develop interventions with patients, their families, and providers.	■ Use community health workers: Positive Minds-Strong Bodies Project (Alegría et al., 2016).
Foster co-learning and capacity building.	■ Conduct learning exchanges in which researchers *and* stakeholders contribute to the research process.	■ Patient testimonials and narratives were tools in community mobilization around hypertension: Project AsPIRE (Trinh-Shevrin, 2014).
Focus on problems of local relevance.	■ Conduct a multi-method formative assessment to incorporate stakeholder perspectives in the study design, analysis, and interpretation.	■ A cancer screening study (Woolf et al., 2016) used formative assessments and ongoing stakeholder engagement to increase acceptability and reach.

(Continued)

TABLE 10.1 (CONTINUED)

CBPR Principle	Strategies in Health Services Research	Examples from the Literature
Balance knowledge generation and benefit.	■ Explore study designs that balance scientific rigor with benefits to participants and perceived community concerns.	■ Such designs include comparative-effectiveness trials that compare two or more relevant strategies, cross-over control, or wait-list control designs so no one is denied a beneficial strategy.
Use a cyclical and iterative process of improving the study.	■ Work with stakeholders to identify challenges and potential solutions.	■ In Projects AsPIRE and DREAM, coalitions met monthly to ensure progress and address challenges.
Partners are involved in dissemination.	■ Disseminate findings through multiple vehicles and strategies, ranging from patient narratives and forums, newspapers, policy briefs, community forums, and peer-reviewed articles.	■ Cancer survivors' narratives about treatment choices can be more compelling than reviewing recommended guidelines for patients grappling with similar decisions (Dohan et al., 2016).
Embrace a commitment to sustainability.	■ Prioritize sustainability from project inception.	■ Commitment to the sustainability of the community's capacity to remain engaged in research increases investment (Hacker et al., 2012).

functioning, perceived suffering, and quality of life indicators along with symptom severity more comprehensively captured patient perspectives of the impact of treatment on depressive symptoms (Cohen, Greenberg, & IsHak, 2013).

The idea of reciprocal capacity building is an essential component of CBPR and stems from the notion that as equal partners, community and academic partners have unique strengths and contributions that can be harnessed as well as learning needs that must be addressed (Minkler, 2010; Trinh-Shevrin et al., 2007). In the context of HS, and particularly in light of "big data" initiatives driven by PCORI and the Agency for Healthcare Research and Quality, patient stakeholders may benefit from capacity building in the use of big data initiatives (Fleurence et al., 2014), whereas researchers may need a better understanding of contextual factors, such as familial, neighborhood, and cultural influences that affect patient health and caregiving negatively and positively (Wallerstein & Duran, 2010).

IMPLEMENTING CBPR IN HEALTH CARE SETTINGS: CHALLENGES AND OPPORTUNITIES

Implementing community-partnered approaches in the design of health care interventions poses opportunities and inherent challenges. Populations engaged in research may be more committed to its use, particularly for HS (Chung et al., 2008). Engagement may increase attention to participants' life circumstances and cultures when designing interventions, which could yield more acceptable interventions for minority populations (Schensul, 2009). Research may be more feasible if community members are engaged in its development (Halpern, Johnson, Miranda, & Wells, 2004).

Potential challenges to the application of CBPR principles in HS research can arise when implementing evidence-based practices. These practices may or may not have been developed with community input; the treatments and language to describe them may not be familiar to stakeholders; they may compete with alternative practices in the community; or, they may raise concerns about addressing health issues that are stigmatized and difficult to discuss. Overall, there may be a greater risk that researchers will approach implementation from a top-down or expert-driven approach.

A CBPR approach would emphasize a two-way knowledge exchange within equitable partnerships, in which the clinical practice and research expertise is balanced with community expertise in lived experience, cultural adaptation, and context. Given genuine engagement, the system or research expert becomes part of the community of equal stakeholders, who then can incorporate local ecology and community values in the partnership and interventions (Trickett, 1998).

Research partnerships that aim to develop new interventions or adapt existing, evidence-based interventions for translation and dissemination to eliminate health disparities often contend with practical constraints in under-resourced communities that have important implications for study design and methods. Innovative research methods need to be used to address the numerous methodological challenges to ensure the rigorous design and analysis of interventions in the health field, which are appropriate to the community:

- Decisions to randomize at levels above the individual (e.g., clinic, community) require attention to potential cross-contamination effects and the feasibility of including a sufficient number of units to achieve adequate precision in cluster randomized designs (Murray, 2015).
- Improving the validity, reliability, and efficiency of measurement means attention to multiple levels in diverse populations and low resource settings (Charns et al., 2012)
- A CBPR process may require pre-specifying a participatory process to finalize a design protocol, even when there has been substantial stakeholder input into developing the initial research proposal.
- High attrition or poor adherence to study protocols can bias standard intent-to-treat analyses and especially affect racial-ethnic minorities living in under-resourced communities (Honas, Early, Frederickson, & O'Brien, 2003; Zeller et al., 2004).

Table 10.2 presents a brief summary of these challenges, research designs, and potential solutions.

TABLE 10.2 Types of Study Designs and Pros and Cons for the Community

Study Design	Randomized Controlled Trials	Stepped Wedge (or Lagged) Design	Pragmatic Randomized Trials	Randomized Encouragement Design
Design description	May involve random assignment to usual care or no care condition, strict inclusion or exclusion criteria, controlled setting, rigid interventions	Tested intervention is rolled out randomly to participants over a number of time periods so that everyone eventually gets the intervention.	Tests the effectiveness of an intervention in a broad range of settings in order to examine "if and how an intervention works," controlling for "all known biases and confounders," so that the intervention's effect is maximized	An encouragement trial randomizes participants to the control group or to an opportunity or encouragement to receive an intervention. Participants randomized to the opportunity or encouragement can then decide whether to engage and adhere to the intervention (West et al., 2008).
Strengths	Strong internal validity	All participants will receive intervention; they can model the effect of time on an intervention as a variable in assessing the effectiveness.	Strong external validity because of flexible inclusion or exclusion criteria and testing interventions in diverse, real-world settings	Strong internal and external validity; addresses practical and ethical challenges associated with participants engaging in interventions inconsistent with their preferences and evaluates the acceptability to engage in diverse interventions

Challenges	Control condition group receives no intervention or an enhanced control condition; limited external validity because of likelihood study will be limited to participants with one health condition (e.g., hypertension alone versus hypertension, depression, and diabetes) or limited to one setting (e.g., primary care only versus primary care, church, social services settings)	Participant groups may face delay in receiving intervention; contamination and extended learning effects in participants receive intervention later. Participants could be exposed to the general idea of interventions, and the single-blind approach may lead to diminished internal validity.	Potential difficulty drawing causal inferences; involves randomization of participants to different interventions that may be unacceptable for ethical reasons and difficult to implement	Study data collection costs may be higher because of requiring larger number of participants caused by smaller effect sizes and greater within-group variance, as well as needing qualitative and quantitative data on compared intervention implementation.

(Continued)

TABLE 10.2 (CONTINUED)

Study Design	Nonrandom Quantitative Intervention Assignment	Quasi-Experimental Designs	Observational Studies
Design description	Assigns participants to particular groups based on a numerical rank (e.g., community, household income, level of risk); the quantitative variable used to assign groups and the outcome variable of interest used for causal modeling, with separate modeling for the different groups to enable inferences regarding treatment effect to be made	Participants are not randomly assigned to intervention or control groups but are compared to the intervention groups. Matching methods (e.g., using propensity scores) to select controls can improve the design validity, but it requires significant details on relevant sociodemographic and clinical characteristics of a large population of individuals in a comparison condition. Examples of studies include natural experiments in which a policy or an intervention is given to one community or group of individuals while another similar group does not receive an intervention, such as public insurance benefits or unconditional cash transfers (Costello, Erkanli, Copeland, & Angold, 2010).	Observes an aspect of interest among a group of participants over time
Strengths	Addresses practical and ethical concerns of randomized studies; intervention can be assigned based on meaningful variables such as level of risk	Leverages existing differential policy implementation in demographically equivalent groups for evaluation purposes	Addresses practical and ethical challenges of randomized designs
Challenges	May be difficult to interpret study outcomes because of the challenge of discerning the precise relationship between the quantitative assignment variable and the outcome variable of interest	Funding to respond in real time to evaluate natural experiments may be difficult. Systematic or unmeasured differences between compared groups, such as secular trends or neighborhood or community characteristics, may make it difficult to interpret results and determine the impact of policy or program.	Difficult to draw causal inferences

SHARED ANALYSIS, INTERPRETATION, AND DISSEMINATION OF RESULTS

For more traditional HS or clinical researchers not familiar with CBPR processes, inclusion of nonscientists or community partners in data analyses may seem particularly challenging. Researchers may worry about compromised scientific integrity because of the limited capacity of community partners to contribute meaningfully to the technical aspects of data analysis, or the lack of "efficiency" of data analysis with partners unfamiliar with statistical or qualitative analyses. However, community members might be concerned about the lack of contextual and historical knowledge that researchers bring to these partnerships.

What are the options to structure complementary roles and skills for academic and community partners to work together in data analysis? Similar to all processes in a participatory research project, community partners' roles in data analysis and interpretation should be determined collaboratively, and, depending on the partnership, these roles may vary. For example, if a partnership is new, expanding resources to cover partners' participation may improve the overall quality of the shared data. Multiple institutions have developed "Research 101" trainings or resources for nonscientists that provide an easy-to-understand overview of different research methods. For example, PCORI's "Methodology 101 Training Booklet and Resource Guide" reviews study design, analysis, and interpretation for comparative effectiveness research (PCORI, 2014). Training and resource manuals have also been created for clinicians on collaborating with researchers in HS research (Potter et al., 2010). Less has been done to train researchers on how to learn about the ecology of lives in community settings.

Often if the technical data analyses are conducted by university partners, then data interpretation can be done collaboratively. This generates trust and understanding of the research process and findings and further develops health care research that has greater external validity by virtue of being more relevant and reflective of partners' perspectives and priorities.

Another potential benefit of including community partners in data analysis and interpretation is the increased capacity of the partnership to conduct more effective research over time through the augmentation of research skills. As one community partner in the Community Partners in Care project noted, "Even though I didn't completely understand all of the statistical programming and numbers the first time around, I felt that taking the time to have all of us work together was important in building trust and making sure that we could do the work more quickly the next time around." In CBPR, it can be helpful to view research as two-way capacity building in a shared process of exchanging expertise. For example, while sharing and training community or patient stakeholders in analysis principles, it may be effective to have stakeholders train academic partners on the meaning of concepts in community context or share information on community resources and culture. In this way, all participants are valued in an ongoing process of development, using a strength-based paradigm. Developing such a strategy for partnered analysis can benefit from intentional planning for inclusion of CBPR principles into all phases of research design, including budgeting activities.

Partnered analysis goes hand-in-hand with partnered research presentations and publications, which also require preparation and anticipation of budgets (e.g., for travel to meetings). In addition to traditional peer-reviewed approaches to dissemination, participatory research projects in health care require approaches that share findings and lessons learned with groups directly affected by the results (e.g., patients, community members), who might not read or have easy access to academic journals or conferences. In developing a dissemination approach with community collaborators, researchers must be open to a diversity of different partnerships. For example, the Los Angeles health advocacy organization Healthy African American Families (HAAF) II has partnered with hundreds of researchers over the last twenty-five years and holds all-day conferences in local community settings, such as churches or in the meeting rooms of local community agencies for the local population. All events are free and invitations are sent to nearly fifty thousand individuals on their e-mail list. Individuals attending these conferences range from the general public to policy makers, representatives of local community agencies, health care clinics, mental health clinics, and churches. In order to incentivize attendance, audience members are offered free food or raffled prizes, such as gift cards, computer equipment, or televisions. Continuing education credits are offered for the wide array of professionals in attendance. The events often cover a particular health condition, such as cancer, depression, diabetes, or autism, and the content of each conference is reflective of the stage of implementation that HAAF II has reached with a research institution at the time. For conferences devoted to disseminating the results of a recently completed research study, presentations range from traditional academic style presentations that summarize design, goals, outcome measures, results, and interpretation of study findings to small-group discussions on how attendees would interpret the study findings and what the potential implications for the findings may be for community members. This has been the case for a PCORI-funded study, DECIDE (Alegría, Grant ID 4187).

Other approaches include printed or e-mailed newsletters, presentation of study results in local media (e.g., newspapers, radio, television), social media reports, or even through the art initiatives. For example, one researcher supported adolescent patients' work by collaborating with a professional drama teacher to disseminate study findings on improving hospital care for adolescents with chronic health conditions. "A group of nine young people worked with a professional drama teacher to create the play, using role-play and improvisation . . . Their self-created rap urged the hospital board to listen to young people and adjust care to their needs" (Van Staa, Jedeloo, Latour, & Trappenburg, 2010). The key for ensuring appropriate dissemination is to actively collaborate on all aspects of dissemination so that the approaches, format, and language used in the dissemination of results will be understood by and accessible to the intended recipients.

VIGNETTES

In the following sections, we present three vignettes to illustrate the ideas we elaborate on in this chapter.

Community Partners in Care (CPIC)

Community Partners in Care (CPIC) was a program-level randomized comparative effectiveness trial of two interventions to support depression quality improvement across health care and community-based agencies in Los Angeles. To our knowledge, CPIC is the first randomized US-based study of the added value of community engagement and planning beyond a traditional approach to implementing depression collaborative care (Ngo et al., 2016). According to a Cochrane Collaborative Review, it is one of the few such comparative studies internationally in any field of health (Anderson et al., 2015) that uses a community engagement intervention that was implemented using a community-partnered participatory research (CPPR) approach, a manualized form of CBPR developed in South Los Angeles, with community and academic partners coleading under equal authority in all aspects of research. CPPR emphasizes principles such as equal partnership and power sharing between partners, which are reinforced in a memorandum of understanding in all research phases. The study was designed and implemented by the CPIC Council, co-led by UCLA, RAND, HAAF II, Behavioral Health Services, Queens Care Health, Faith Partnership, and fifty other agencies providing safety-net services. The monthly meetings of the CPIC Council and working groups were supplemented as needed by telephone, text, online, or e-mail voting to facilitate timely decision making in all phases of research, following principles of CBPR (trust building, strength based, two-way knowledge exchange, inclusive partnerships with full and equitable participation). Larger decisions were discussed for further input with larger community groups in an open forum, such as a church, museum, or movie theater. This reinforced that the community or patient representatives were viewed as the primary stakeholders for major decisions. In these presentations, community and academic partners as well as patients or family members presented what the council and work groups had deliberated and provided their synthesized opinions and outlined pros and cons. This process was used in finalizing the design for CPIC, developing the final plan for interventions, and presenting study findings.

Both interventions were based on evidence-based depression quality improvement (QI) tool kits, using a stepped-care approach with case management tool kits. Community engagement and planning (CEP) supported networks of programs in tailoring tool kits to local communities in a four- to six-month planning period followed by training in depression QI; resources for services (RS) offered each program the opportunity to participate in twelve webinars and primary care site visits on depression collaborative care. Health care providers received training on treatment (including assessment, therapy, and medication) and case managers and non-licensed staff members received training on screening, referral, education, and behavioral management skills. This approach could support patient engagement in evaluation and treatment regardless of the door of entry to services.

The active inclusion of partners at all levels, but especially community and policy partners, led to the rapid dissemination of the CPIC approach and findings into health care policy in two large urban areas: the County of Los Angeles (LAC) and city of New York's public health care systems. In Los Angeles, the Department of Mental Health with the Departments of Public Health and Health Services proposed the Health Neighborhood Initiative to increase service capacity for behavioral health homes under expanded Medicaid services. The Health Neighborhood Initiative was added to the LAC Strategic Plan by the LAC board of supervisors in 2014 and proposes to coordinate county services for shared behavioral health clients while engaging neighborhood coalitions to address one or more locally prioritized social determinants of mental health. This project is currently being supported by a $100 million investment through the California Mental Health Services Act. Similarly, the city of New York's Office of Health and Mental Health has been actively exploring using the CPIC model as an approach to integrate health care, mental health, and non-health-care community agencies to address depression as part of their mental health road map or ThriveNYC initiative. This illustrates the potential of CBPR to generate stakeholder engagement and support sustainability.

PCORI

The PCORI-funded "Effectiveness of DECIDE in Patient-Provider Communication, Therapeutic Alliance & Care Continuation" examined the combined effectiveness of a patient and provider intervention designed to improve shared decision making (SDM), the working alliance, and communication between patients with behavioral health issues and their providers. The patient intervention (DECIDE-PA) was designed to encourage patients to ask questions in their clinical sessions and increase their level of involvement in the management of their own care. This project was the result of a partnership among Massachusetts General Hospital, the Disparities Research Unit, thirteen clinics, and the community advisory board (CAB) of the overall study. The provider intervention (DECIDE-PC) coached providers on how to be more receptive to their patients' questions and concerns. The study took place in thirteen outpatient behavioral health clinics in the Northeast region of the United States. Patient participants were between the ages of eighteen and eighty; spoke English, Spanish, or Mandarin Chinese; and received behavioral health care (e.g., psychotherapy, psychopharmacology, or counseling) from behavioral health providers (e.g., psychiatrists, psychologists, social workers, addiction counselors, and mental health nurse practitioners) enrolled in the study. The study recruited 312 patients and 74 providers.

Guided by principles of CBPR, the study was committed to involving patients, providers, and other stakeholders throughout the course of the study, ensuring that they had a purposeful and equal voice in the research. Stakeholder engagement efforts were led by the CAB, which was composed of a patient, a patient caregiver or patient advocate, behavioral health clinicians, and a community-academic liaison. CAB members met with the PI and leaders of the research team on a bimonthly (sometimes monthly) basis throughout the course of the study and were all equally compensated for their time helping design and implement the study.

First-year CAB activities included identifying strategies for clinic, provider, and patient recruitment and reviewing and editing the provider's and patient's assessment questionnaires. CAB members were also instrumental in shaping the patient and provider assessments so that the data gathered could help produce findings more relevant to diverse stakeholder groups. For example, the CAB identified the need to add questions related to patient stigma about seeking mental health care and issues related to continuity of care. The CAB also helped ensure the comprehension of our assessment measures and other study materials, such as patient recruitment flyers.

In year 2, the CAB began to think about how best to disseminate study findings, with many suggesting peer conferences they could attend to present study findings as well as ideas for papers they wanted to write (in addition to helping with writing the main paper for the study). The engagement of the CAB in paper writing started off with a formal introduction of writing research papers from the study's PI and project director, because some members of the CAB had no prior experience in writing research papers. Beginning in year 3, CAB members played a major role in planning focus groups to help disseminate preliminary study findings, allowing the study to get feedback from provider and patient stakeholders on their respective interpretation of the findings. Overall, the engagement of the CAB helped to make the study successful in recruiting a wide range of clinics, providers, and patients. It facilitated the creation of assessment questionnaires that were more relevant to diverse stakeholder groups and dissemination activities that provided contextual, real-world feedback on how to make the intervention practical and effective for patients, providers, and other key stakeholders.

DREAM (Diabetes, Research, Education, and Action for Minorities) Project

The DREAM Project, established in 2009, was a CBPR study developed in a partnership between the NYU Center for the Study of Asian American Health (CSAAH) and a community coalition serving the Bangladeshi American community in New York City (NYC). The overall goal of the DREAM Project was to develop, implement, and test the efficacy of a community health worker (Tomfohr, Schweizer, Dimsdale, & Loredo, 2013) intervention designed to improve type 2 diabetes mellitus control and management in the Bangladeshi community. The DREAM Coalition played a critical role in informing intervention design—selecting a community health worker (CHW) approach as a strategy to build on community assets and strengthen community leadership for diabetes prevention and control. In developing this approach, community partners agreed to use a rigorous methodology that balanced their concerns regarding the ethics of research design with an understanding of the need for scientific rigor. This approach helped support the development of an evidence base and policies for CHW integration in health care for underserved populations.

Using a two-arm randomized controlled trial (RCT) design, study participants were recruited from hospitals, community health centers, primary care practices, and community settings, including faith-based organizations (FBOs) and community-based organizations (CBOs). Participants were randomly assigned to either the control or treatment group. In a six-month intervention program, treatment group participants received five monthly educational sessions with an overview of diabetes, nutrition, physical activity, complications of diabetes, and stress management and family support. In addition, CHWs conducted two one-on-one meetings with treatment group participants to develop and implement individualized goal-setting plans.

CBPR principles were integrated into all phases of the DREAM study and operationalized through a coalition partnership. This coalition included a diverse stakeholder group of those with lived experiences as members of the community, as members living with or having family members who have diabetes, FBOs, CBOs, health providers, ethnic media, and academic partners serving the Bangladeshi community. The coalition, which met on a monthly basis, ensured that the study maintained a delicate balance between academic research, community interests, and the linguistic and cultural appropriateness of the research. A key participatory feature of DREAM has been the integration of CHWs into the coalition and study team. The DREAM Project intervention was delivered by four trained bilingual Bangladeshi CHWs who were trusted community members and leaders with shared ethnicity, language, culture, and life experiences as study participants. They served as a vital source of community knowledge and were closely involved in all aspects of the study, including the development of study instruments, data collection, informing research design, and interpreting study results. Throughout the intervention period, CHWs not only worked with the participants but also with the participants' care providers, family members, support groups, and others to assist participants with diabetes control and management. CHWs also played a key role in dissemination of the intervention through community forums and the ethnic media. In addition to reporting results of the intervention back to the community, community forums were also conducted in response to the community's concerns and questions, regarding new policies and initiatives (e.g., Affordable Care Act). Finally, CHWs also played a capacity-building role in clinical settings by conducting cultural competency trainings with medical students, residents, and health care providers at clinical sites to enhance knowledge and understanding about unique religious and cultural practices that might influence diabetes management among Bangladeshi Americans.

By employing CBPR approaches, the DREAM Project was able to ensure cultural and social relevance for the community and facilitated linkages to the health care system in meaningful ways that built on community assets and addressed concerns related to diabetes control. The DREAM Project is now an established, trusted, and recognized community resource with a high level of popularity in the New York City Bangladeshi community.

CONCLUSION AND RECOMMENDATIONS

There have been multiple calls for the increased involvement of community members in research addressing health and well-being. Patient and consumer groups have long advocated for their inclusion in the research process across multiple health outcomes including HIV/AIDS, mental illness, diabetes, and environmental health concerns. These efforts often grew from those who felt marginalized and disengaged from the research being conducted on their communities. Later, researchers and policy makers joined these efforts because the benefits to the quality of the research process and the scope and impact of the research were seen to be improved by increased community participation and the use of CBPR.

This chapter addressed the benefits to HS research, particularly those engaged in clinical trials, to broaden their research strategies and designs by using methods to increase community involvement through the addition of patients or service users, their families and caretakers, clinicians and administrators, and the communities within which research occurs. In fact, CBPR is an effective tool for generating knowledge and developing models of care and treatment programs as well as policies to meet the needs of traditionally under-resourced and marginalized populations. Through community partnerships, the design and conduct of research is strengthened and the impact of findings on policy and practice is bolstered. Community involvement in the development of research questions can increase the study's relevance to patients and service users and help researchers to be confident that they are addressing areas of real concern to communities.

This chapter presented illustrative case studies for reflecting on the inclusion of the community in multiple study designs as well as the challenges these study designs could present. We have described how community partners can contribute in meaningful and critical ways to the development of research, ensuring that assessment tools are appropriate and respectful to patients in HS studies. In addition, we have shown how community involvement in design, such as choosing appropriate recruitment strategies, can be critical to successful research, because patients' lived experiences of engaging with our health care systems can help to identify appropriate points of interface with researchers at clinical sites; but more important, bringing the voice of diverse stakeholders ensures that research is meaningful for the different stakeholders.

As we continue to explore innovative models for the delivery and financing of health care services, we must be vigilant in ensuring that these services and approaches to deliver them meet the needs of our most vulnerable populations. Inclusion of stakeholders in the research process through CBPR may be one of our most powerful tools for this endeavor. This work is not without its challenges, and efforts to increase community involvement in research should draw on the success and challenges identified by previous HS researchers to improve our capacity for integrating CBPR within health systems research.

QUESTIONS FOR DISCUSSION

1. How do community partners benefit from being included in the analysis and interpretation of study results? How do academic partners benefit from their inclusion?
2. Using Table 10.1 as a reference, can you comment on the CBPR principles each vignette portrays and any similarities or differences you see between CBPR in health care settings versus community settings?

REFERENCES

Alegría, M., Alvarez, K., Ishikawa, R. Z., DiMarzio, K., & McPeck, S. (2016). Removing obstacles to eliminating racial and ethnic disparities in behavioral health care. *Health Affairs, 35*(6), 991–999.

Anderson, L. M., Adeney, K. L., Shinn, C., Safranek, S., Buckner-Brown, J., & Krause, L. K. (2015). Community coalition-driven interventions to reduce health disparities among racial and ethnic minority populations. *Cochrane Database of Systematic Reviews, 6,* 1–189.

Charns, M. P., Foster, M. K., Alligood, E. C., Benzer, J. K., Burges s, J. F., Jr., Li, D., Mcintosh, N. M., Burness, A., Partin, M. R., & Clauser, S. B. (2012). Multilevel interventions: Measurement and measures. *Monographs: Journal of the National Cancer Institute, 2012*(44), 67.

Chung, B., Jones, L., Campbell, L. X., Glover, H., Gelberg, L., & Chen, D. T. (2008). National recommendations for enhancing the conduct of ethical health research with human participants in post-disaster situations. *Ethnicity & Disease, 18*(3), 378–383. Retrieved from www.ncbi.nlm.nih.gov/pubmed/18785455

Cohen, R. M., Greenberg, J. M., & IsHak, W. W. (2013). Incorporating multidimensional patient-reported outcomes of symptom severity, functioning, and quality of life in the Individual Burden of Illness Index for Depression to measure treatment impact and recovery in MDD. *JAMA Psychiatry, 70*(3), 343–350.

Concannon, T. W., Meissner, P., Grunbaum, J. A., McElwee, N., Guise, J.-M., Santa, J., Conway, P. H., Daudelin, D., Morrato, E. H., & Leslie, L. K. (2012). A new taxonomy for stakeholder engagement in patient-centered outcomes research. *Journal of General Internal Medicine, 27*(8), 985–991.

Costello, E. J., Erkanli, A., Copeland, W., & Angold, A. (2010). Association of family income supplements in adolescence with development of psychiatric and substance use disorders in adulthood among an American Indian population. *JAMA Psychiatry, 303*(19), 1954–1960.

D'Alonzo, K. T. (2010). Getting started in CBPR: Lessons in building community partnerships for new researchers. *Nursing Inquiry, 17*(4), 282–288.

Dohan, D., Garrett, S. B., Rendle, K. A., Halley, M., & Abramson, C. (2016). The importance of integrating narrative into health care decision making. *Health Affairs, 35*(4), 720–725.

Domecq, J. P., Prutsky, G., Elraiyah, T., Wang, Z., Nabhan, M., Shippee, N., Brito, J. P., Boehmer, K., Hasan, R., Firwana, B., & Erwin, P. (2014). Patient engagement in research: A systematic review. *BMC Health Services Research, 14*(1), 1.

Fleurence, R. L., Beal, A. C., Sheridan, S. E., Johnson, L. B., & Selby, J. V. (2014). Patient-powered research networks aim to improve patient care and health research. *Health Affairs, 33*(7), 1212–1219.

Fourie, C., Biller-Andorno, N., & Wild, V. (2014). Systematically evaluating the impact of diagnosis-related groups (DRGs) on health care delivery: A matrix of ethical implications. *Health Policy, 115*(2–3), 157–164.

Ginsberg, S. (2017). *Arthritis Patient Partnership with Comparative Effectiveness Researchers (AR-PoWER).* Retrieved from www.pcori.org/research-results/2013/arthritis-patient-partnership-comparative-effectiveness-researchers-ar-power

Hacker, K., Tendulkar, S. A., Rideout, C., Bhuiya, N., Trinh-Shevrin, C., Savage, C. P., Grullon, M., Strelnick, H., Leung, C., & DiGirolamo, A. (2012). Community capacity building and sustainability: Outcomes of community-based participatory research. *Progress in Community Health Partnerships: Research, Education, and Action, 6*(3), 349.

Halpern, J., Johnson, M. D., Miranda, J., & Wells, K. B. (2004). The partners in care approach to ethics outcomes in quality improvement programs for depression. *Psychiatric Services, 55*(5), 532–539.

Hickam, D., Totten, A., Berg, A., Rader, K., Goodman, S., & Newhouse, R. (2013). *The PCORI methodology report.* Washington, DC: Patient-Centered Outcomes Research Institute.

Honas, J. J., Early, J. L., Frederickson, D. D., & O'Brien, M. S. (2003). Predictors of attrition in a large clinic-based weight-loss program. *Obesity Research, 11*(7), 888–894.

Institute of Medicine (US) Committee on Quality of Health Care in America. (2001). *Crossing the quality chasm: A new health system for the 21st century*. Washington, DC: Author.

Islam, N. S., Tandon, D., Mukherji, R., Tanner, M., Ghosh, K., Alam, G., Haq, M., Rey, M., & Trinh-Shevrin, C. (2012). Understanding barriers to and facilitators of diabetes control and prevention in the New York City Bangladeshi community: A mixed-methods approach. *American Journal of Public Health, 102*(3), 486–490.

Meade, C. D., Menard, J. M., Luque, J. S., Martinez-Tyson, D., & Gwede, C. K. (2009). Creating community-academic partnerships for cancer disparities research and health promotion. *Health Promotion Practice, 12*(3), 456–462.

Minkler, M. (2010). Linking science and policy through community-based participatory research to study and address health disparities. *American Journal of Public Health, 100*(S1), S81–S87.

Mockford, C., Staniszewska, S., Griffiths, F., & Herron-Marx, S. (2012). The impact of patient and public involvement on UK NHS health care: A systematic review. *International Journal for Quality in Health Care, 24*(1), 28–38.

Mullins, C. D., Abdulhalim, A. M., & Lavallee, D. C. (2012). Continuous patient engagement in comparative effectiveness research. *JAMA Psychiatry, 307*(15), 1587–1588.

Murray, D. M. (2015). Design and analysis of studies to evaluate multilevel interventions in public health and medicine. National Institutes of Health. Retrieved from https://prevention.nih.gov/docs/programs/mind-the-gap/mtg2015-murray-presentation.pdf

Ngo, V. K., Sherbourne, C., Chung, B., Tang, L., Wright, A. L., Whittington, Y., Wells, K., & Miranda, J. (2016). Community engagement compared with technical assistance to disseminate depression care among low-income, minority women: A randomized controlled effectiveness study.*American Journal of Public Health, 106*(10),1833–1841.

Patient-Centered Outcomes Research Institute (PCORI). (2014). *Methodology 101: Training for patients and stakeholders* [training booklet and resource guide]. Retrieved from www.pcori.org/sites/default/files/PCORI-Methodology-101-Training-Booklet-and-Resource-Guide.pdf

Pearson, A., Jordan, Z., & Munn, Z. (2012). Translational science and evidence-based healthcare: A clarification and reconceptualization of how knowledge is generated and used in healthcare. *Nursing Research and Practice, 2012,* 1–6.

Potter, M., Handley, M., Goldstein, E., Abrams, D., Alvarez, R., Benson, M., Benton, L. D., Bird, W., Fischer, D., & Raine-Bennett, T. (2010). *Community-engaged research with UCSF researchers: A resource manual for community-based clinicians*. Retrieved from https://accelerate.ucsf.edu/files/CE/manual_for_clinicians.pdf

Schensul, J. J. (2009). Community, culture and sustainability in multilevel dynamic systems intervention science. *American Journal of Community Psychology, 43*(3–4), 241–256.

Sharpe, R. (2013). Establishing a patient-centered research community for cystic fibrosis. Retrieved from www.pcori.org/research-results/2013/establishing-patient-centered-research-community-cystic-fibrosis

Tomfohr, L. M., Schweizer, C. A., Dimsdale, J. E., & Loredo, J. S. (2013). Psychometric characteristics of the Pittsburgh Sleep Quality Index in English-speaking non-Hispanic whites and English and Spanish-speaking Hispanics of Mexican descent. *Journal of Clinical Sleep Medicine, 9*(1), 61.

Trickett, E. J. (1998). Toward a framework for defining and resolving ethical issues in the protection of communities involved in primary prevention projects. *Ethics & Behavior, 8*(4), 321–337.

Trinh-Shevrin, C. (2014). Community health workers offer culturally tailored interactive workshops and counseling to Filipino Americans, leading to improvements in medication adherence and cardiovascular risk factors. Retrieved from https://innovations.ahrq.gov/profiles/community-health-workers-offer-culturally-tailored-interactive-workshops-and-counseling

Trinh-Shevrin, C., Islam, N., Tandon, S. D., Abesamis, N., Hoe-Asjoe, H., & Rey, M. (2007). Using community-based participatory research as a guiding framework for health disparities research centers. *Progress in Community Health Partnerships: Research, Education, and Action, 1*(2), 195–205.

Van Staa, A., Jedeloo, S., Latour, J. M., & Trappenburg, M. J. (2010). Exciting but exhausting: Experiences with participatory research with chronically ill adolescents. *Health Expectations, 13*(1), 95–107.

Wallerstein, N., & Duran, B. (2010). Community-based participatory research contributions to intervention research: The intersection of science and practice to improve health equity. *American Journal of Public Health, 100*(S1), S40–S46.

West, S. G., Duan, N., Pequegnat, W., Gaist, P., Des Jarlais, D. C., Holtgrave, D., . . . Clatts, M. (2008). Alternatives to the randomized controlled trial. *American Journal of Public Health, 98*(8), 1359–1366.

Woolf, S. H., Zimmerman, E., Haley, A., & Krist, A. H. (2016). Authentic engagement of patients and communities can transform research, practice, and policy. *Health Affairs, 35*(4), 590–594.

Zeller, M., Kirk, S., Claytor, R., Khoury, P., Grieme, J., Santangelo, M., & Daniels, S. (2004). Predictors of attrition from a pediatric weight management program. *The Journal of Pediatrics, 144*(4), 466–470.

CHAPTER 11

NATIONAL CENTER FOR DEAF HEALTH RESEARCH

CBPR WITH DEAF COMMUNITIES

STEVEN BARNETT, JESSICA CUCULICK, LORI DEWINDT, KELLY MATTHEWS, AND ERIKA SUTTER

DEAF SIGN LANGUAGE users and people with hearing loss comprise health disparity populations overlooked by most public health research, surveillance, and programs (Barnett, McKee, Smith, & Pearson, 2011). The mission of the Rochester Prevention Research Center (RPRC) is to promote health and prevent disease with populations of Deaf sign language users and people with hearing loss through community-based participatory research (CBPR). These two populations differ in many aspects, including language, culture, and lived experience. Three similarities are risk for health inequities, barriers to health care communication, and limited engagement with public health. In this chapter, we focus on research conducted with Deaf sign language users in Rochester, New York, by RPRC's National Center for Deaf Health Research (NCDHR).

INTRODUCTION TO DEAF COMMUNITIES

Deaf communities. The word *Deaf* refers to identity and culture, not hearing acuity. This distinction is sometimes indicated with an uppercase *D*. Use of sign language is a prime characteristic of being Deaf. An individual's audiogram is not relevant. For example, hearing children with Deaf parents are often also Deaf. Most Deaf sign language users were born deaf or became deaf in early childhood. Deaf culture, mores, and folkways come from a worldview shaped by common experiences and a shared understanding of those experiences. Sign language is part of that shared experience.

Language. American Sign Language (ASL) is the primary language used in US Deaf communities. ASL is indigenous to the United States and is not universally used by Deaf people around the world. ASL is a natural, living language that evolved with US Deaf communities over time. ASL and English are different languages; ASL is not a form of English. Similar to other languages, ASL has "accents" and other regional variations, variations by social groups (such as age), and jargon, such as specialized technical terminology used by Deaf professionals in a particular field.

Diversity. The broad range of human diversity is expressed within Deaf populations, including race, ethnicity, gender, sexual orientation, age, educational attainment, income, and presence of physical disabilities and health conditions. The distribution of that diversity in Deaf populations differs from the distribution in the US general population.

Early experiences. Most deaf children have hearing parents, and most hearing parents with a deaf child do not become ASL fluent. Many hearing people view being deaf in the context of a medical model that wants to fix being deaf. The attempts to "fix" the child often occur in health care settings and in school settings. These early experiences likely influence a Deaf adult's perception of health care institutions and educational institutions. These perceptions, in turn, likely influence a Deaf person's willingness to engage with health researchers, who are often from university medical centers (a health care and educational institution).

Communities of Deaf ASL users are in some ways similar to, though also different from, other language minority populations (Barnett, 1999; Steinberg et al., 2006). Familiarity with these similarities and differences is relevant to doing community-based participatory health research with Deaf ASL users (Table 11.1).

TABLE 11.1 Comparison of Deaf ASL-Using Communities and Some Other Language Minority Groups

	Similarities	CBPR Relevance
Social	▪ Use of a non-English language ▪ Socialize and partner or marry within community ▪ Sociocultural norms different than those of the majority community ▪ Children often become bicultural and bilingual.	▪ Language minority model (cultural model) approach fits better than a medical model or disability model.
Health care	▪ Infrequently encounter a doctor from their own cultural group ▪ Language differences and health knowledge limitations are often barriers to appropriate health care. ▪ Many have poorer health than those in the general population. ▪ Less likely to visit a physician than those in the general population	▪ Inclusion of Deaf people on the research team will be welcomed and appreciated by community members. ▪ Low health literacy is common. ▪ Research recruitment from community settings will likely work better than recruitment from health care settings.

	Similarities	CBPR Relevance
Opportunity	■ Lower education level, socioeconomic status, and English literacy than the general population ■ Often encounter prejudices that limit opportunities ■ Limited access to English language–based information	■ Written English recruitment materials may have limited reach; consider direct person-to-person interactions in ASL; consider videos in ASL.
Assimilation	■ Children forbidden to use their language ■ Children taught that their language is inferior	■ Some research terms (e.g., *community voice*) are reminders of social and institutional oppression.
Research	■ History of oppression and mistreatment influences perceptions of research ■ Limited experience with survey research and public health surveillance	■ Negative experiences in health care during childhood (to "fix" being deaf) may explain some of the adult suspicions of health researchers. ■ Common research practices (e.g., randomization, repeated measures) may be unfamiliar and will likely need explanation.
Biology	■ Biology sometimes used to justify bias, barriers, and the existence of social inequalities	■ Health research with deaf people often focuses on ears and hearing, rather than health.
	Differences	**CBPR Relevance**
Expectations	Unlike members of other language minority groups, Deaf people are expected to do the following: ■ Have fluency in written English ■ Communicate with clinicians by writing notes in English ■ Communicate with clinicians by speech-reading in English	■ Language-congruent approaches will be welcomed and will enhance connection and recruitment. ■ Research teams that include Deaf community members will be welcomed and will enhance connection and recruitment.
Cultural transmission	■ Deaf culture and ASL are usually transmitted horizontally (from peers) rather than vertically (from parents).	■ Health information (e.g., about breastfeeding) likely comes from Deaf peers and community leaders, rather than hearing parents and grandparents.

(*Continued*)

TABLE 11.1 (CONTINUED)

	Similarities	CBPR Relevance
Language deprivation	■ Many Deaf children experience limited exposure to accessible language during the critical period for language development.	■ Cognitive and interpersonal consequences of early language deprivation are associated with health risks, conditions, and outcomes. ■ Cognitive and interpersonal consequences of early language deprivation are relevant to the relationship building required for CBPR.
Legal	■ Guidelines for health care communication with Deaf people come from the Department of Justice (DOJ). ■ Guidelines for health care communication with others who have low English proficiency come from the Department of Health and Human Services.	■ Legal guidelines from the DOJ apply to health research. ■ There is no standard approach used by funders regarding budgets for communication access services.

Source: Adapted from Barnett (1999) and Steinberg et al. (2006).

CBPR FOR HEALTH WITH ROCHESTER DEAF COMMUNITIES

Rochester, New York, has a large, vibrant, and diverse Deaf population with deep local historical roots. The Rochester School for the Deaf (RSD), established in 1876 and still operating today, works with deaf and hard-of-hearing children and their families. RSD also employs Deaf teachers and staff members and has an active alumni association. The National Technical Institute for the Deaf (NTID) was established as one of the colleges of Rochester Institute of Technology (RIT) in 1966 to provide postsecondary technical education to people who are Deaf or hard of hearing. NTID is the largest technical college for Deaf and hard-of-hearing students in the United States, with about 1,400 NTID students included in the more than fifteen thousand RIT students. NTID and RIT employ faculty and staff members who are Deaf, and a number of NTID/RIT graduates remain in Rochester. The critical mass of Deaf people influences the local Rochester economy, and many local companies hire qualified Deaf people for blue- and white-collar jobs, and local service industries, such as restaurants, are comfortable with Deaf customers. University of Rochester research and clinical training programs include Deaf graduate students, medical students, and fellows. Deaf people migrate to Rochester, attracted by the economic, social, and educational opportunities.

The Rochester Deaf Health Task Force (RDHTF) is the immediate precursor to the community-academic collaboration that became RPRC/NCDHR. The RDHTF was a diverse stakeholder group formed in 2003 to identify local health and health care priorities with Rochester's large Deaf population (Rochester Deaf Health Task Force, 2004). RDHTF included representatives from Deaf communities, community-based organizations, health care (including clinicians and insurers), public health, and academic institutions.

The RDHTF identified the absence of health data from Deaf communities as a major limitation to identifying priorities. RDHTF members decided to address this lack of data and submitted a proposal to CDC to establish RPRC/NCDHR, with an initial core research project to develop accessible health surveillance to collect basic health data from Deaf ASL users. The CDC Prevention Research Centers (PRC) Program funded RPRC/NCDHR in 2004, and many from the RDHTF became members of the RPRC/NCDHR Deaf Health Community Committee (DHCC) or one of the other RPRC/NCDHR committees.

With the establishment of RPRC/NCDHR and a focus on creating accessible surveillance, community-academic collaboration grew. Researchers and DHCC members worked together to prioritize topics to include in the Rochester Deaf Health Survey, translated English language survey questions (Graybill et al., 2010) and developed new survey questions, recruited community members to help RPRC/NCDHR evaluate and improve the survey, recruited community members to take the survey, interpreted preliminary findings, disseminated research findings to local and national stakeholder audiences, and chose next steps in the research process. RPRC/NCDHR dissemination includes coupling RPRC/NCDHR academic journal articles (Barnett, Klein, et al., 2011; Barnett, McKee, et al., 2011) with videos that present in ASL the content of the written English article (Table 11.2; at the end of the chapter).

With data from the first Rochester Deaf Health Survey, Rochester's Deaf communities could, for the first time, select health research priorities based on their own data. RPRC/NCDHR and DHCC members hosted community forums to share findings of the 2008 Rochester Deaf Health Survey, discuss interpretation of findings, and identify next steps. Deaf community members selected three health priorities based on findings from the 2008 Rochester Deaf Health Survey: obesity, partner violence, and suicide risk (Barnett, Klein, et al., 2011). RPRC/NCDHR successfully obtained research funding for all three priorities. RPRC/NCDHR's second core research project focused on obesity: the Deaf Weight Wise clinical trial.

CBPR, INTERVENTION DEVELOPMENT, AND RESEARCH DESIGN

For the RPRC/NCDHR Deaf Weight Wise (DWW) clinical trial, we adapted for use with Deaf adult ASL users a healthy lifestyle intervention (Weight Wise) previously demonstrated to be effective with a different population (rural women in North Carolina) (Samuel-Hodge et al., 2009). Deaf and hearing researchers and community members worked together to adapt interventions materials, measures, and methods to be culturally appropriate and language congruent. Key to the success of the two-year DWW clinical trial are the Deaf people on the research team, including as research coordinators and other research staff members.

Deaf and hearing RPRC/NCDHR research team members worked with DHCC members to make important decisions on research trial design. Following are three examples.

DWW intervention. Researchers and community members agreed that all DWW intervention leaders must be Deaf and not hearing people working with interpreter services or hearing people who are ASL fluent. Team members felt strongly that having DWW group meetings consist only of Deaf people, including a Deaf person as the intervention group leader, would be a benefit to the intervention. Designing the trial with Deaf people as intervention leaders provided another opportunity for RPRC/NCDHR to "give back" to the community by providing training and employment. RPRC/NCDHR trained and employed ten Deaf people to be DWW counselors during the two-year clinical trial.

Delayed-start design. Researchers and community members discussed the need to compare those who received the DWW intervention with those who did not. Randomization to "usual care" would mean that half the people enrolled in the trial would not receive an intervention at all. Whereas hearing people have access to myriad healthy lifestyle interventions, there are no healthy lifestyle interventions designed for use by Deaf people. RPRC/NCDHR researchers and community members agreed that the DWW randomized trial design would assign people to either immediate intervention or intervention delayed one year. This approach permitted research comparison, at the trial midpoint, of those who participated in the DWW intervention and those who had not yet. The delayed-start design also meant that everyone in the trial would participate in the DWW intervention, important because there are no accessible alternative interventions.

Informed consent information. Research informed consent information presented in written English is often challenging to understand for many people. It is best to present research consent information in the primary language of the person considering research participation. Prior to DWW, RPRC/NCDHR presented research study information in a video monologue in ASL. The study information video for the 2008 Rochester Deaf Health Survey was seven minutes long, and many Deaf Health Survey participants complained about the video length. Researchers and DHCC members discussed informed consent processes for the DWW clinical trial. The research detail required to make an informed decision about participation in a two-year clinical trial would result in an ASL video that was twice as long as the video for the 2008 Rochester Deaf Health Survey. The group decided to use a video novella approach to presenting research consent information. The video novella has been used to present health information in ASL to Deaf audiences (Pollard, Dean, O'Hearn, & Haynes, 2009) and in spoken Spanish to Hispanic audiences (US Food and Drug Administration, 2014). RPRC/NCDHR worked with the University of Rochester institutional review board (IRB) to adapt the video novella approach for use in research informed consent. The DWW consent video novella was successful in terms of presenting information needed for viewers to make a decision about DWW participation and in terms of the viewers' experience of the video. The DWW consent video was eighteen minutes long, and no one complained that the video was too long (see Table 11.2).

RPRC/NCDHR growth and success during this period meant that RPRC/NCDHR was conducting multiple research projects simultaneously. Some research participants found it difficult to keep track of which RPRC/NCDHR research projects they had already participated in, in part because the computer-based surveys looked similar. A project-specific logo, developed in collaboration with Deaf artists, became a communication aid to help RPRC/NCDHR research staff members to identify the different projects with participants and to provide a visual memory aid to help research participants remember whether they had participated in a specific project. The logo development process enhanced the feeling of shared project ownership by community and research team members and provided an opportunity for RPRC/NCDHR to employ Deaf artists and graphic designers (Figure 11.1).

NCDHR National Center for Deaf Health Research

General NCDHR logo. The image depicts the ASL sign for "health."

DWW

Logo for the Deaf Weight Wise (DWW) clinical trial with Deaf people ages 40–70. The person is showing the ASL sign for "success."

FIGURE 11.1 *Examples of RPRC/NCDHR Logos Designed by Deaf Community Partners*

RPRC/NCDHR CAPACITY BUILDING

Building relationships is essential for successful CBPR. RPRC/NCDHR facilitates this by bringing together community members with researchers and Deaf people with hearing people. The process of learning about each other builds trust needed for CBPR.

Deaf people work in RPRC/NCDHR in a variety of roles, including as faculty and staff members, trainees, teachers, community members, advisors, and RPRC/NCDHR committee members, including the executive committee. RPRC/NCDHR community committees bring together Deaf and hearing individuals and organizations that would otherwise not interact. RPRC/NCDHR community engagement with DHCC focused primarily on collaboration with individuals. We created the local partner advisory board (LPAB) to better engage with community organizations and institutions, such as Rochester School for the Deaf, the local county health department, and health insurers. Center-wide retreats include diverse stakeholders and encourage dialogue and feedback to inform RPRC/NCDHR development.

Relationship building is one facet of growing capacity; research training is another. RPRC/NCDHR worked with DHCC to create a training program to teach Deaf community members about research ethics and to develop together the Cross-Cultural Research Competencies Curriculum (Table 11.2) to teach hearing researchers about CBPR with Deaf communities. Summer internship programs foster the interest of deaf and hearing college students in CBPR and public health research. RPRC/NCDHR summer interns have subsequently gone on to medical and nursing schools and research PhD programs. Deaf and hearing graduate students, postdoctoral fellows, faculty members with research career development awards, and community members do research training with RPRC/NCDHR.

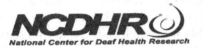

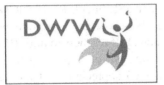

Communication is vital to RPRC/NCDHR capacity building, as is the funding to support communication access services. Interpreter services are needed for all communication that includes Deaf ASL users and people who do not know ASL. This includes communication during weekly RPRC/NCDHR staff meetings, RPRC/NCDHR committee meetings and retreats, trainings that include Deaf teachers or Deaf students with people who do not know ASL, professional conferences and research networking opportunities, and telephone calls and other interactions with funders. If the costs of communication access come from core program budgets, accessible programs will have fewer resources for research or programs, and this perpetuates disparities. RPRC/NCDHR continues to explain to funders and other audiences the necessity of communication access services and has successfully advocated with some funders to provide budget supplements to support communication access services.

Capacity building related to communication also includes supporting the development of ASL skills among faculty and staff members who are not ASL fluent. RPRC/NCDHR includes Deaf people as staff members, trainees, and faculty members, working alongside hearing people with a range of ASL skills. RPRC/NCDHR hires qualified Deaf teachers to tutor RPRC/NCDHR faculty and staff members who are interested in learning ASL or improving their ASL skills. RPRC/NCDHR's commitment to tutoring demonstrates an appreciation of the value of ASL, important for relationships and trust. The tutoring program supports *informal* communication that builds relationships and trust, in the workplace and with communities. Clear communication is paramount, and RPRC/NCDHR works with interpreter services for formal workplace communication that includes people not ASL fluent and for RPRC/NCDHR-sponsored events.

RPRC/NCDHR growth and capacity building also requires collaboration with IRBs. CBPR health research with Deaf adult ASL users was new for the University of Rochester IRB, and standard IRB-required training was not accessible to some Deaf ASL users. RPRC/NCDHR researchers, DHCC members, and the University of Rochester IRB agreed to an approach to adapt the content of existing written English-language CITI training modules into ASL. This process enabled RPRC/NCDHR to include more DHCC members as research team members.

To ensure appropriate IRB review of ASL materials, RPRC/NCDHR met with IRB leadership to develop ways to ensure that research participants were safe and that informed consent information was accessible. We discussed approaches to evaluating the ASL measures and certifying the accuracy of the translations. The University of Rochester IRB agreed to assign one IRB specialist to all RPRC/NCDHR research; the continuity was helpful for relationship building and efficiency and added a level of cultural awareness to the University of Rochester IRB team. The University of Rochester IRB and RPRC/NCDHR worked together to develop mutually agreeable approaches to documenting informed consent that did not require Deaf adult ASL users to sign their names to written English consent forms (See Figure 11.2 below).

RPRC/NCDHR sometimes needed to navigate potential conflicts between research needs and relationship needs. One example from the DWW clinical trial involved inclusion criteria. DWW had strict parameters regarding eligibility for the clinical trial, including age range (40–70) and BMI (25–45). Some Deaf individuals wanted to enroll in the trial but were ineligible because of age or BMI. It was a challenge for RPRC/NCDHR to turn people away, especially because there were no accessible alternative programs to refer people to. Some RPRC/NCDHR faculty and staff members also work as clinicians in the University of Rochester Department of Psychiatry's Deaf Wellness Center (DWC). RPRC/NCDHR and DWC worked together to create an accessible alternative to DWW, called the *Mindful Eating Group*. The DWC Mindful Eating Group was led by ASL-fluent therapists who used psychotherapeutic techniques to encourage healthy choices, and the cost to participate was covered by some health insurance policies. This solution was good for relationships, research, and institutional and community capacity building.

Deaf Weight Wise Research Study: Consent Form with Signatures

Documentation of Consent

- I have watched a video about Deaf Weight Wise. I was given a copy of the video.
- I understand what it means to be involved in the Deaf Weight Wise research study.
- I agree that it is my choice to participate in the Deaf Weight Wise research study.
- I will get a signed copy of this form and information letter.

Research Subject:

____

Print Name

____

Signature

Person Obtaining Consent (Research Staff)

- The person watched a video in sign language about the Deaf Weight Wise study.
- The person was able to ask questions and all questions were answered.
- The person understands the Deaf Weight Wise study.
- I will provide the person with a copy of this consent form.

____

Print Name and Title

____

Signature

__________ Research subject watched video no.: __________

Date

FIGURE 11.2 *Documentation of Consent Signature Form*

CULTURE-CENTEREDNESS APPROACH

The RPRC/NCDHR experience of CBPR with Rochester Deaf communities fits the culture-centeredness approach (CCA) (see Chapter 2; Dutta, 2008; Wallerstein et al., under review). The collaboration creates space for and encourages *agency* through shared decision making and acknowledging the expertise in communities. The Rochester collaboration values and fosters the trust necessary for *critical reflection* that occurs during retreats, committee meetings, and community forums. Working together, the Rochester collaboration *transformed* some dominant practices in research culture, such as the IRB changing processes and academic journals publishing ASL videos to accompany written English articles about Deaf communities. Clear communication and safe, bidirectional sharing of knowledge has been essential to our collaboration.

LESSONS LEARNED

We have learned a great deal about community-researcher collaboration to do CBPR with Rochester Deaf communities, and those lessons inform non-research collaborations and research with other communities. We have listed some key lessons that contributed to our growth and success.

Work with Deaf people. RPRC/NCDHR conducts research *with* Deaf people, not *for* Deaf people, and not *on* Deaf people. The collaboration is a partnership with shared decision making. The collaborative process begins early in a project, with research topic selection and research project design. Each project provides opportunities to learn, strengthen relationships, and build trust. New projects build on the foundation created by prior projects; the investment in the current project contributes to the current project and to future projects. We list this lesson first because of its paramount importance. This lesson also permeates other lessons listed in the following paragraphs.

Shared ownership. RPRC/NCDHR research works best when Deaf and hearing people, working together, feel shared ownership for the project. Having *you* work on *my* project, or having *me* work on *your* project, does not work as well as having *us work together on our project.* Achieving shared ownership often requires early collaboration and mutual development of a project, which builds trust and meaningful relationships.

Cultivate relationships. The infrastructure of RPRC/NCDHR is built on relationships. We recognize that relationships are the primary resource for our CBPR work. Relationships require attention. One way we nurture relationships is by working *with* Deaf communities, and acknowledging the value they add to our research together. Clear, accurate, and accessible communication is vital to relationships. RPRC/NCDHR commits resources for communication access services, including sign language interpreter services and tutoring in ASL, to support an environment that nurtures relationships. Experiences of present-day collaborations have roots in history. Knowing about the historical context can help build relationships (Table 11.3; at the end of the chapter).

Find common values. A goal of RPRC/NCDHR research is to promote health and well-being. This is consistent with a value in Deaf communities to "give back," such as to provide a needed service. RPRC/NCDHR research "gave back" with a breastfeeding project (see Box 11.1), providing accessible information and support to Deaf mothers. RPRC/NCDHR "gave back" with the Mindful Eating Group, providing an accessible alternative program to Deaf Weight Wise for those who did not qualify for the research trial. For some researchers, "giving back" initially felt outside of their scope as researchers, but when viewed in the frame of "common values," the process of "giving back" was recognized as being consistent with "promoting health and well-being."

Box 11.1 Deaf Moms and Infant Care Project

RPRC/NCDHR research topics are selected in collaboration with communities. Some research topics are identified from community forums to share and discuss RPRC/NCDHR research data, other topics come from discussions during community meetings, and some are selected based on recent events or experiences. The Deaf Moms and Infant Care project came about from the last category.

During an RPRC/NCDHR executive committee meeting, the chair of the Deaf Health Community Committee (DHCC), a Deaf woman who was currently pregnant, wondered about the infant care knowledge and experiences of other Deaf women and their sources of information. The RPRC/NCDHR director and the rest of the RPRC/NCDHR executive committee agreed that this was a great topic for research. The DHCC chair began attending the weekly meetings of the RPRC/NCDHR research committee to learn more about research. RPRC/NCDHR devoted resources to the project and facilitated a connection with hearing faculty mentors with related research interests and relevant research expertise to work with the DHCC chair and other Deaf women who joined the project. Communication during these project team meetings was facilitated by interpreter services funded by RPRC/NCDHR. The project team adapted qualitative research methods to be accessible for use in research with Deaf people. The DHCC chair presented findings from the project at national public health conferences and an international Deaf conference. The project findings were published in written English in a peer-reviewed health journal (Chin et al., 2013). The project team and research participants also shared findings with other Deaf women through the production of informational videos in ASL regarding breastfeeding. RPRC/NCDHR provided video-editing support and facilitated posting the completed videos online to make them broadly available (Table 11.2).

Recognize community strengths. RPRC/NCDHR researchers and community members work together to identify and prioritize disparities for research and intervention. Although RPRC/NCDHR grant proposals often emphasize disparities to successfully compete for grants, RPRPC/NCDHR research also seeks to identify community strengths. These strengths, and sharing information about these strengths, have inherent value, cultivate relationships, empower individuals and communities, and support a sense of self-worth. Sometimes collaborative discussions of community strengths identify strategies and resources that will help address disparities.

These lessons learned reinforce RPRC/NCDHR's commitment to the values of CBPR and help ground us in our efforts to work together with communities to promote shared ownership of health research in order to achieve our mutual goal to improve health and well-being with and within Deaf communities.

QUESTIONS FOR DISCUSSION

1. Think about the following two true statements:

   A. Throughout history (including today), hearing people routinely have developed and still use visual communication systems in situations in which sound is inadequate, inappropriate, or unavailable for clear and accurate communication. Some examples:

- Hand and body signals used in baseball by umpires, coaches, and players
- Signal mirrors used by hikers, militaries, and others
- Hand signals used by underwater divers

B. Throughout history (including today), some deaf people have been forbidden to use sign language, even though sound is unavailable and inadequate for clear and accurate communication. Speech reading, a form of visual communication, is visually limited compared with the visual range available in American Sign Language.

How do you explain the two different approaches to visual communication?

How would you feel if society prevented you from using a communication modality that worked for you?

How likely would you be to engage with health researchers from that society?

When you answered that question, did you assume the "health researchers" were hearing?

What do the assumptions about "health researchers" teach us about bias?

Do you think whether a health researcher is Deaf or hearing would make a difference in terms of Deaf community members' willingness to engage? What other factors might influence that engagement?

2. Personal experiences of discrimination can influence an individual's trust. Historical events, such as the Tuskegee Syphilis Study and the slow US response to the AIDS epidemic in the 1980s (predominantly affecting gay communities and other minority communities), can influence a community's trust for generations.

In what ways do you think this is true with Deaf communities?

In what ways do you think Deaf communities might be different than some other minority communities? What about minority Deaf communities, such as African American Deaf communities or LGBT Deaf communities?

TABLE 11.2 Online Resources Related to CBPR for Health with Deaf Communities

Resource	Link
General Information about RPRC/NCDHR	
Rochester Prevention Research Center: National Center for Deaf Health Research (RPRC/NCDHR) website	www.urmc.edu/ncdhr
RPRC/NCDHR Cross-Cultural Research Competencies Curriculum	www.urmc.rochester.edu/ncdhr/information/training/cross-cultural-competency.aspx
National Center for Deaf Health Research YouTube Channel	www.youtube.com/user/NCDHResearch

Resource	Link
General Information about RPRC/NCDHR	
American Sign Language Video-Blogs ("vlogs") about Research Concepts, Produced by RPRC/NCDHR	
How do I become a research volunteer?	www.youtube.com/watch?v=AB5ULOxpPhI
What is a randomized controlled trial?	www.youtube.com/watch?v=9MRKgdXiOP8
What is informed consent?	www.youtube.com/watch?v=uqobwRzqiLg
What is a cognitive interview?	www.youtube.com/watch?v=vGyBEitJvS0
Peer-driven recruitment	www.youtube.com/watch?v=lFDm1Q4TLlM
American Sign Language Video Adaptions of Published Academic Articles	
Barnett, S., Klein, J. D., Pollard, R. Q., Jr., Samar, V., Schlehofer, D., Starr, M., . . . Pearson, T. A. (2011). Community participatory research with deaf sign language users to identify health inequities. *American Journal of Public Health, 101*(12), 2235–2238. An American Sign Language video adaption of this article was also created by RPRC/NCDHR and the Deaf Health Community Committee. The video is available in the journal's online appendix.	Full article: www.ncbi.nlm.nih.gov/pmc/articles/PMC3222424/pdf/2235.pdf ASL video adaption of article available in online appendix (scroll to bottom of page): http://ajph.aphapublications.org/page/VideoArchive ASL video adaptation also posted here: www.urmc.rochester.edu/ncdhr/research.aspx
Barnett, S., McKee, M., Smith, S. R., & Pearson, T. A. (2011). Deaf sign language users, health inequities, and public health: Opportunity for social justice. *Preventing Chronic Disease, 8*(2), A45. An American Sign Language video adaption of this article was also created by the RPRC/NCDHR and community partners. The two-part video is posted on the journal's web page along with the article.	Full article: http://cdc.gov/pcd/issues/2011/mar/10_0065.htm ASL video adaption of article: www.cdc.gov/pcd/issues/2011/mar/10_0065.htm#Appendix ASL video adaptation also posted here: www.urmc.rochester.edu/ncdhr/research.aspx
Community-driven Health Information in ASL	
Deaf Breastfeeding Project Breastfeeding facts and stories from the Deaf community Breastfeeding facts: Information for Deaf moms	Main page: www.youtube.com/channel/UChEfH47LLsnrgRdV3WgjN_A Video 1: www.youtube.com/watch?v=m36FCJLQLGs Video 2: www.youtube.com/watch?v=P53LvHkJrYE

(*Continued*)

TABLE 11.2 (CONTINUED)

Resource	Link
General Information about RPRC/NCDHR	
Research Informed Consent in ASL	
The Deaf Weight Wise Study: informed consent in American Sign Language	www.youtube.com/watch?v=ZVGSOGcQRNU
American Sign Language Video-Blogs ("vlogs") about the Importance of Public Health Surveillance with Deaf Communities	
Deaf Health Survey 2013 movie	www.urmc.rochester.edu/ncdhr/research/deaf-health-survey-2013.aspx
Deaf Health Survey 2013 vlog in American Sign Language	www.youtube.com/watch?v=gggDQm4DaRw
Education and Training Programs	
Rochester Bridges to the Doctorate program	http://deafscientists.com/
Rochester Postdoc Partnership: Rochester Partnership for Research and Academic Career Training of Deaf Postdoctoral Scholars	www.deafpostdoc.urmc.edu

TABLE 11.3 Significant Historical Events Relevant to Community-Based Participatory Research for Health with Deaf Communities

Year	Event	Relevance to CBPR for Health with Deaf Communities
1817	American School for the Deaf: The first permanent school for Deaf people in the United States established in Hartford, Connecticut (now called the American School for the Deaf). The founders include Laurent Clerc, a Deaf man and a graduate of and teacher at the Royal Institute for the Deaf in Paris, and Thomas Hopkins Gallaudet, a hearing American from Hartford who visited Paris to learn about educating Deaf children.	■ Acknowledges and demonstrates the value of specific programs developed by and for Deaf people ■ Social determinants of health: access to education and employment ■ Successful collaboration of deaf and hearing people

Year	Event	Relevance to CBPR for Health with Deaf Communities
1864	Gallaudet College: The first college for Deaf people in the world established in Washington, DC (now Gallaudet University).	▪ Social determinants of health: access to education and employment ▪ Many past and current Deaf community leaders are Gallaudet graduates. ▪ Successful collaboration of deaf and hearing people
1876	Rochester School for the Deaf established.	▪ One institution that led to the rise of Rochester's Deaf communities ▪ Social determinants of health: access to education and employment
1876	Telephone invented. The telephone connected hearing people with other hearing people. Deaf people did not communicate directly over telephone lines until the development of the teletypewriter (TTY) and acoustic coupler nearly one hundred years later.	▪ Amplified the separation of hearing and Deaf people and institutions
1880	Milan Conference: endorses spoken language over sign language for education of Deaf students. Of the 164 participants, from the United States and some European countries, one was Deaf. The conference's endorsement of spoken language was not unanimous.	▪ Social determinants of health: changes in education approach associated with worsening of educational attainment, literacy, and employment, still evident today ▪ Loss of Deaf role models, including Deaf teachers and other successful Deaf adults ▪ Hearing people not valuing ASL ▪ Hearing people making decisions for Deaf people, especially for Deaf children ▪ Some research terms (e.g., *community voice*) are reminders of social and institutional oppression.
1880	National Association of the Deaf (NAD) is established by Deaf Americans "to deliberate on the needs of the deaf as a class." NAD continues to advocate today for the needs of Deaf communities, including opposing the suppression of sign language.	▪ Self-determination ▪ Self-advocacy ▪ Community leadership

(Continued)

TABLE 11.3 (CONTINUED)

Year	Event	Relevance to CBPR for Health with Deaf Communities
1966	National Technical Institute for the Deaf (NTID) established at Rochester Institute of Technology (RIT). NTID is the largest technical college for Deaf and hard-of-hearing students in the United States.	■ One institution that contributed to the rise of Rochester's Deaf communities ■ Social determinants of health: access to education and employment ■ Many Deaf community leaders are NTID/RIT graduates. ■ Successful collaboration of deaf and hearing people
1960s	Teletypewriter (TTY) invented. The TTY, developed by a Deaf engineer, made it possible for Deaf people to communicate directly over telephone wires via typing.	■ Access to information ■ Access to community ■ Telecommunication led to changes in in-person communication ■ Led to changes in the roles of local Deaf clubs
1973	Rehabilitation Act: federal law that forbids discrimination and mandates access in programs that receive federal funding; as with other civil rights laws, societal change was not immediate	■ Social determinants of health: acknowledges barriers to access to education, health care services, and employment
1988	Deaf President Now (DPN): Gallaudet students led a movement that successfully advocated that one of the qualified Deaf candidates be selected as the first Deaf president of Gallaudet University.	■ Self-determination ■ Self-advocacy ■ Successful broad collaboration
1990	Americans with Disabilities Act (ADA): federal law that forbids discrimination and mandates access across a variety of societal entities (public and private) and infrastructure; mandates telecommunication relay services to make telephone networks accessible; as with other civil rights laws, societal change was not immediate	■ Social determinants of health: acknowledges barriers to access to education, health care services, and employment

Year	Event	Relevance to CBPR for Health with Deaf Communities
2004	National Center for Deaf Health Research (NCDHR) is established in Rochester, New York.	■ CBPR for health applied to work with Deaf communities ■ Engages, trains, and employs Deaf people in health research and programs ■ Raises awareness with agencies in the US Department of Health and Human Services regarding disparities ■ Successful broad collaboration

ACKNOWLEDGMENTS

The work described here was funded in part by the CDC Prevention Research Centers Program (U48 DP000031, U48 DP001910, and U48 DP005026), a CDC Community Transformation Grant (U58 DP003599), and a grant from the Association of Teachers of Preventive Medicine (ATPM) in collaboration with CDC (TS-0817). The findings and conclusions in this chapter are those of the authors and do not necessarily represent the official position of the funders.

Thank you to the staff and faculty members, students, Deaf Health Community Committee (DHCC) members, research participants, other community members, other stakeholders, and funders who contributed to the success of the Rochester Prevention Research Center: National Center for Deaf Health Research. We also thank our partners, including the National Technical Institute for the Deaf at the Rochester Institute of Technology. With deep gratitude we thank Thomas A. Pearson, the founding director of RPRC/NCDHR.

REFERENCES

Barnett, S. (1999). Clinical and cultural issues in caring for deaf people. *Family Medicine, 31*(1), 17–22.

Barnett, S., Klein, J. D., Pollard, R. Q., Jr., Samar, V., Schlehofer, D., Starr, M., . . . Pearson, T. A. (2011). Community participatory research with deaf sign language users to identify health inequities. *American Journal of Public Health, 101*(12), 2235–2238.

Barnett, S., McKee, M., Smith, S. R., & Pearson, T. A. (2011). Deaf sign language users, health inequities, and public health: Opportunity for social justice. *Preventing Chronic Disease, 8*(2), A45.

Chin, N. P., Cuculick, J., Starr, M., Panko, T., Widanka, H., & Dozier, A. (2013). Deaf mothers and breastfeeding: Do unique features of deaf culture and language support breastfeeding success? *Journal of Human Lactation, 29*(4), 564–571.

Dutta, M. J. (2008). *Communicating health: A culture-centered approach*. Malden, MA: Polity Press.

Graybill, P., Aggas, J., Dean, R., Demers, S., Finigan, E., & Pollard, R. (2010). A community-participatory approach to adapting survey items for deaf individuals and American Sign Language. *Field Methods, 22*(4), 429–448.

Pollard, R. Q., Dean, R. K., O'Hearn, A., & Haynes, S. L. (2009). Adapting health education material for deaf audiences. *Rehabilitation Psychology, 54*(2), 232–238.

Rochester Deaf Health Task Force. (2014, August). *Deaf Health Task Force report*. Rochester, NY: Finger Lakes Health Systems Agency. Retrieved January 30, 2017, from www.urmc.rochester.edu/ncdhr/information/documents/FLHSARDHTFreport2004.pdf

Samuel-Hodge, C. D., Johnston, L. F., Gizlice, Z., Garcia, B. A., Lindsley, S. C., Bramble, K. P., . . . Keyserling, T. C. (2009). Randomized trial of a behavioral weight loss intervention for low-income women: The Weight Wise Program. *Obesity, 17*(10), 1891–1899.

Steinberg, A. G., Barnett, S., Meador, H. E., Wiggins, E. A., & Zazove, P. (2006). Health care system accessibility. Experiences and perceptions of deaf people. *Journal of General Internal Medicine, 21*(3), 260–266.

US Food and Drug Administration. (2014, December 2). ¡Nunca Más! Novelas. Retrieved January 31, 2017, from www.fda.gov/ForConsumers/ByAudience/ForWomen/ucm269846.htm

Wallerstein, N., Oetzel, J., Duran, B., Magarati, M., Pearson, C., Belone, L., Davis, J., DeWindt, L., Lucero, J., Ruddock, C., Sutter, E., Villegas, M., Dutta., M. (under review). Culture centeredness in community-based participatory research: Its impact on psycho-social health interventions. *Social Science and Medicine*.

CHAPTER

12

CBPR IN ASIAN AMERICAN COMMUNITIES

NADIA ISLAM, CHARLOTTE YU-TING CHANG, PAM TAU LEE, AND CHAU TRINH-SHEVRIN

ASIAN AMERICANS (AAs) COMPRISE 5.6 percent of the US population, and in metropolitan areas make up between 13 percent (New York City and Los Angeles) to 33 percent (San Francisco) (Hoeffel, Rastogi, Kim, & Shahid, 2012). The AA category includes East Asian (e.g., Chinese, Japanese, Korean); South Asian (e.g., Bangladeshi, Indian, Pakistani); Southeast Asian (e.g., Filipino, Cambodian, Thai, Vietnamese); and sometimes Pacific Islander Americans (e.g., Native Hawaiians, Chamorros, Marshallese), denoting a vastly diverse array of subpopulations with unique ethnic, cultural, linguistic, and historical profiles, stretching across the Asian continent and its millions of islands. The US AA population is projected to double in size to more than 43 million by 2050 and comprise approximately 40 percent of the country's immigrant population (Hoeffel et al., 2012). More than 65 percent of AAs are foreign-born immigrants and refugees who come from low-income, limited-English-proficient (LEP) backgrounds, compounding the unique challenges faced by these communities (Ortman & Guarneri, 2009).

Given the diversity of the AA community and a changing history of how racial and ethnic groups have been categorized, the use of consistent terminology regarding the AA community presents a challenge. AAs are defined here using the US Census 2000 classification as a race of "individual people having origins in any of the original peoples of the Far East, Southeast Asia, or the Indian subcontinent." In this chapter, we did not include Native Hawaiian and Pacific Islanders (NHPIs) because of their different political realities and major disparities that are masked when aggregated with the AA population and, as such, contend that CBPR efforts in NHPIs warrant exclusive attention.

CBPR'S RELEVANCE FOR AA COMMUNITIES

Tandon and Kwon's (2009) review of fifty-three articles on CBPR in AA communities highlighted key reasons why CBPR approaches are appropriate and relevant for AA communities.

AAs are subject to the "model minority myth." AAs have been unfairly portrayed as a "model minority" in many societal outcomes. From a broad perspective, this stereotype implies that Asian Americans are not an underprivileged racial-ethnic minority because of their economic success compared with other racial-ethnic groups; accordingly, Asian Americans merit neither resources nor attention as an ethnic minority group within the American population. The persistence of this myth is also reflected in continued portrayals of Asian Americans in the media as overachieving, successful, and without problems (Kristof, 2015; Murphy, 2011; Powell, 2011). In health, this is driven by and a result of a systematic lack of collection, reporting, and analysis of AA data (Islam et al., 2010; Yi, Kwon, Sacks, & Trinh-Shevrin, 2016). Prior to 2010, there were few epidemiologic studies of AA health in the United States, with most data part of studies examining multiple racial-ethnic groups. Recent large-scale AA studies have documented health status diversity, though analysis on any aggregated AA sample still masks disparities across and among subgroups. CBPR studies, with the principles of defining communities of identity and local context, have therefore played important roles in documenting these health disparities that traditional epidemiologic research fails to capture.

AAs represent many separate racial and ethnic groups. CBPR approaches enable researchers to take differences across Asian subgroups into account with each aspect of the research process. CBPR strategies involving community health workers (CHWs) have strengthened the ability to engage Bangladeshi and Korean populations in cardiovascular disease and diabetes prevention. Bangladeshi CHWs have leveraged the cultural value of *niyiom* ("rules to live by") to motivate community members' commitment to engaging in healthy behaviors. Korean American populations' preferences for health-promotion efforts delivered by health professionals led to the use of a team-based care approach with CHW-led diabetes prevention and control studies. Although cultural awareness is critical, CBPR approaches also call for reflexivity and cultural humility. This requires a balance between incorporating important cultural norms and beliefs into research and interventions while avoiding cultural stereotypes.

AAs often live in densely populated "ethnic enclaves." Asian ethnic groups often reside heavily in centralized geographic locations, particularly in urban areas, thereby creating ethnic enclaves. These communities' close geographical proximity lends itself to working within community contexts in CBPR.

CBPR is an asset-based and community-building approach that is particularly relevant for immigrant communities. Recent AA immigrants often feel disempowered by traditional top-down research and wary of research because of their immigration status. By contrast, CBPR validates community members' expertise and capabilities as researchers and agents for social change to engage the entire community. In our work in New York City and New Jersey Filipino communities, coalition development efforts focused on inclusion of a broad range of stakeholders organized around wellness (Aguilar et al., 2010). In immigrant communities, the role of storytelling and personal narratives (Trinh-Shevrin, 2014) have been compelling ways to engage communities already marginalized by their social position.

An updated literature search (2007–2015) found an additional 266 publications that described a CBPR or community-engaged framework in AA communities, with approximately half explicitly using a CBPR approach.

CBPR CASE STUDIES

First, we highlight a federally funded research center rooted in a CBPR approach with AA communities at local, regional, and national levels. Second, we highlight a local effort to demonstrate how a CBPR partnership involving Asian immigrant workers built community capacity, leadership, and equitable participation while also organizing the community toward policy change.

Case Study 1: National Research Center of Excellence in Asian American Communities: NYU Center for the Study of Asian American Health

In 2003, the NYU Center for the Study of Asian American Health (CSAAH) was established with funding from the National Center for Minority Health and Health Disparities (NCMHD) Project EXPORT initiative. In the following sections, we describe our evolution as a federally funded research center rooted in CBPR principles and our impact on improving the health of Asian Americans.

Phase 1 The funding of CSAAH in 2003 formalized a long-standing relationship among the New York University School of Medicine and several community partners that promote health research and access in underserved AA communities across New York City (NYC) (Trinh-Shevrin et al., 2007). CSAAH and its community partners were interested in conducting AA health disparities research using CBPR. Given the considerable cultural variations among AA ethnic groups, political dynamics among the community-based organizations (CBOs), fragmentation among the AA population, and paucity of pan-Asian CBOs, it was critical to nurture existing relationships and create new relationships with community partners during the establishment of the center.

Three key principles guided CSAAH's relationship building with NYC AA community partners: (1) creating and sustaining multiple partnerships, (2) promoting equity in partnerships, and (3) commitment to action as well as research (Trinh-Shevrin et al., 2007, 2015). Each of these principles aligned with a CBPR approach.

Creating and Sustaining Multiple Partnerships Building on the central CBPR tenet of engaging multiple and diverse stakeholders in the research process (see Chapter 1; Israel, Eng, Schulz, & Parker, 2013; Parker et al., 2010), one of CSAAH's guiding principles was to create and sustain partnerships with multiple CBOs and leaders serving NYC's AA community. First, CSAAH developed or participated in ethnic-specific and pan-Asian advisory groups. In developing advisory boards, we recruited stakeholders from health and non-health sectors (e.g., worker's rights, faith, arts and cultures) to ensure that members could provide nuanced and context-driven perspectives. We also developed operational norms, guidelines, and bylaws for each coalition that were driven by coalition members, particularly community stakeholders, to facilitate consensus building and communication and define partner roles, thus enhancing accountability among members. Partnership roles were further delineated through letters of support for grant applications and memoranda of understanding that formalized the roles, responsibilities, and activities of respective partners. Finally, outside of the work of the coalition, CSAAH staff members and investigators engaged in reciprocal support through participation in CBO activities, joining CBO advisory or executive boards, or cosponsoring health events. Engagement in CBOs, from the Chinatown YMCA, the Korean American Services of Metropolitan NYC, the DREAM Coalition, the Kalasugan Coalition, to pan-ethnic boards, such as Project CHARGE, strengthened our voices in community efforts and deepened the acceptance and legitimacy of our collective work to advance health and well-being. Together, these steps were important in demonstrating mutual understanding, respect, and reciprocity between CSAAH and its community partners and establishing processes and norms for the academic-community collaboration.

Promoting Equity in Partnerships A central strategy in building equity was to ameliorate negative stereotypes that stemmed from the historical lack of attention to immigrant and AA needs by academics, particularly in NYC. Using a multipronged approach, we built capacity within the center to understand diverse communities through the hiring of diverse staff members and investigators, as well as promoting institutional understanding through seminars, symposiums, and trainings for faculty members and leadership.

To establish equity in grants development and the distribution of resources, we undertook two action steps. First, we created spaces and mechanisms for partners to play an equal role in pursuing grants and research projects, including identifying the research priorities and methodologies. By engaging partners at the beginning to ensure their ownership of a research project through meetings, brainstorming sessions, and joint grant writing, we have successfully maintained the active participation of community partners throughout several CBPR projects they and CSAAH have initiated. For example, our research on the role of CHWs in reducing chronic disease disparities among AA populations was driven by community partners' desires to build on the strong history of community organizing and lay leadership in many Asian immigrant communities. We have, therefore, developed and tailored CHW interventions for the Chinese, Korean, Filipino, Bangladeshi, and Asian Indian communities in response to our partners' needs and perspectives. Second, we negotiated distribution of research funds depending on the roles and responsibilities by CSAAH and community partners. Because all partners helped develop research priorities and methods, they gained a greater appreciation for resources they would need to implement outreach, training, and research activities. Furthermore, to promote co-learning, academic and community partners received education and training on grant writing, budgeting, research design, and community engagement. As a result of learning exchanges, we have been able to more confidently and accurately estimate the funding partners need on an ongoing basis to engage in research activities.

Commitment to Action as Well as Research A key feature of CBPR is a commitment to turning research results into impactful action. To accomplish this, we maintained a strong commitment to community-level dissemination by engaging with ethnic media as a primary source of health and other information within AA communities. Second, CSAAH built advocacy efforts into our research platform early, including encouraging locally elected officials to attend CSAAH events, recognizing them for their support, educating them on AA health issues, and working with legislators directly to increase their awareness of AA health disparities. CSAAH also mobilized community partners to advocate for funding on specific health disparities issues to deepen coalition efforts to ensure sustainability beyond the research partnership.

Phase 2 In 2007, CSAAH received renewal funding from NIMHD to establish itself as a National Research Center of Excellence. Although this offered an opportunity to ensure AA health disparities were addressed at the national level, it also presented the challenge of balancing the evolving needs of a federal institutional stakeholder (NIH) with those of community and public health stakeholders and ensuring sustained community ownership of CSAAH research priorities and framework based on CBPR principles. In doing so, CSAAH used a population health equity framework to maximize the impact of our work in promoting population health while remaining grounded in participatory, context-driven approaches to address health disparities in AA communities (Trinh-Shevrin et al., 2015).

Apply a Social Determinants of Health Perspective to Research For community partners across all Asian subgroups and sectors, the social determinants approach for equity is especially relevant because they are confronted on a daily basis with the role that social inequities and position play, including immigration and refugee status, racism, and discrimination. For AA communities that are predominantly first- and second-generation immigrants, a transnational approach that integrates life course frameworks allows for greater elucidation of the role of migration, immigration, and acculturative experiences on health and how they differ across generations and are aligned with CBPR's focus on context-driven research and action (Acevedo-Garcia, Sanchez-Vaznaugh, Viruell-Fuentes, & Almeida, 2012; Spallek, Zeeb, & Razum, 2011). For example, CSAAH has supported pilot studies to understand the impact of early childhood–intervention programs in Chinese and Bangladeshi communities (Huang, Calzada, Cheng, & Brotman, 2012) and has initiated mixed-methods needs assessments in youth and older adult populations to better understand contextual factors affecting the health of these communities. Intergenerational strategies have been profoundly influential in mobilizing Filipino American community members to the Kalusugan Coalition and strengthening CSAAH's outreach, recruitment, and retention efforts for various studies (Aguilar et al., 2010).

Use a Multi-Sectorial (Health in All Policies) Approach With multi-sector coalitions, CSAAH was well positioned to consider a health in all policies approach that integrates health considerations into decision making on policies within health and other sectors. From 2012 to 2014, CSAAH co-led the innovative CDC-funded Strategies to Reach and Implement the Vision of Health Equity (STRIVE) program, which worked with fifteen CBOs serving AAs and NHPIs across the United States. Guided by a multi-sector coalition, each site led the development and implementation of culturally relevant and sustainable, high-impact, policy, systems, and environmental strategies to improve access to healthy food and increase physical activity within their local communities, reaching an estimated 1,472,373 people across the United States (Patel et al., 2014).

Invest in Asset-Based Approaches That Build Human and Social Capital We used a CBPR assets-based approach at the local level to recognize the role of lay leaders such as CHWs, frontline public health professionals who have a unique understanding of and are trusted members of the community. Several of CSAAH's NIH and CDC research studies have demonstrated the efficacy and effectiveness of a CHW model to improve access to health care and cardiovascular disease and diabetes-related outcomes for Filipino (Ursua et al., 2014), Bangladeshi (Islam, Wyatt, et al., 2013), Asian Indian (Islam et al., 2014), and Korean (Islam, Zanowiak, et al., 2013) populations. Using a CBPR framework, studies have elucidated the cultural and social mechanisms through which CHWs affect health outcomes. For instance, in their study of a CHW intervention on diabetes management among Bangladeshi individuals in NYC, Islam and colleagues found statistically significant increases in reported self-efficacy in accessing health care. Qualitative findings provided support by demonstrating specific mechanisms through which CHWs were able to enhance self-efficacy, such as assisting female participants with learning to access and navigate public transportation systems so that they were able to attend regular doctor visits without relying on family or friends (Islam, Wyatt, et al., 2013).

Build Sustainability through Internal Structures To ensure that research is action driven, CBPR calls for research partners to address and build in sustainability, including strengthening CBO infrastructure, from the outset of program development. Through a subcontract with the UNITED SIKHS, a major community partner serving the South Asian communities in NYC and nationally, CSAAH investigators invested approximately $198,000 over the course of five years to support the implementation and development of a CHW initiative housed within the organization. By enhancing the capacity of the organization to engage in health programming and evaluation efforts and supporting CHWs as part of the organization's staff, UNITED SIKHS has subsequently been successful in initiating new efforts to address oral health, policy, systems, and environmental strategies to improve access to healthy foods and access to care in the South Asian community. UNITED SIKHS acquired more than $600,000 in additional funding as either a lead or subcontracted agency. Similarly, of the fifteen funded CBO partners of the STRIVE program, six have gone on to successfully receive a CDC grant as the lead agency to implement, enhance, and strengthen existing policy, systems, and environmental strategies to address chronic disease-related risk factors affecting AA and NHPI local communities. In the case of several of our community partners, sustainability moved beyond the immediate interventions and also encompassed sustaining the core infrastructure to support organization's efforts independent of CSAAH funds.

Thus, though CSAAH experienced an evolution in terms of structure, scope, and purpose, a commitment to employing CBPR principles through all phases of our center's development enabled us to develop action-oriented research, programs, and policies across diverse AA communities at the local and national levels.

Case Study 2: Developing Worker Leaders, Adapting CBPR Principles, and Moving Policy Action at the Local Level: San Francisco Chinatown Restaurant Worker Health and Safety Study

The San Francisco Chinatown Restaurant Worker Health and Safety Study was conducted by a community-university–health department collaboration that undertook extensive efforts to facilitate equitable participation among its members, in particular with its immigrant worker partners. The partnership's experience underscored that participation of non-English-speaking immigrant community members cannot be taken for granted given the complex power dynamics at play within diverse partnerships. The "participatory starting points" (Chang et al., 2013) or "participatory readiness" (Belone et al., 2016) of immigrant communities, may be affected by members' language and civic skills as well as the larger "contexts of reception," or economic, social, and political opportunity structures and societal signals of inclusion or exclusion in which they are embedded (Bloemraad, 2006).

This case study describes the worker leadership development process and the application and adaptations of CBPR principles of the partnership that took into account the participatory starting points of immigrant worker partners. The research effort ultimately ended with groundbreaking policy change addressing wage theft at the city level and with the building of critical community capacity at multiple levels. It serves as an example of how efforts initiated in one immigrant community can have broader societal impact in helping to lift up conditions beyond the ethnic enclave.

Research Context: Setting and Partnership Restaurants are the largest employer of Chinese immigrants in San Francisco's Chinatown district. Health issues in restaurants include traditional occupational health concerns such as cuts, burns, falls, and on-the-job stress (Jayaraman, 2013; Webster, 2001) and also encompass serious economic and social risk when employers engage in "wage theft" by not paying the legal minimum wage or delaying or withholding payment of wages or benefits earned by employees (Minkler et al., 2014).

Building on previous collaborations, a partnership was formed in 2007 to carry out a CBPR study of working conditions and health among Chinatown restaurant workers. The research used an ecological approach and included focus groups with restaurant workers, a survey of working conditions and health among 433 Chinatown restaurant workers, observations of working conditions in 106 of the 108 neighborhood restaurants, and a mixed-methods evaluation of the partnership (Gaydos et al., 2011; Minkler et al., 2014).

Partners included the Chinese Progressive Association of San Francisco (CPA), a grassroots CBO; two universities (the University of California, Berkeley, School of Public Health and its Labor Occupational Health Program [LOHP] and the University of California, San Francisco, School of Medicine); and the Occupational and Environmental Health Section of the San Francisco Department of Public Health (SFDPH). Notably, in addition to the professional staff members participating at CPA, nine current and former immigrant Chinese restaurant workers provided on-the-ground community expertise to the research, analysis, and action components.

The study presented an important opportunity for each of the partners involved. Community-based partners would be able to leverage scientific research in their work to address the ongoing economic hardship workers in the Chinese immigrant community were facing and in the process build worker leadership capacity. And university and health department partners committed to community-driven research and action and focused on issues of work and health were able to collaborate with trusted community partners on the effort.

Contexts of Reception and Participatory Starting Points Contexts of reception were mentioned by worker partners in evaluation interviews as potentially affecting the "participatory starting points" of community participants in the project, for themselves in the partnership and for survey respondents. Relevant contexts included limited job opportunities, social marginalization, and discrimination, which worker partners tended to link to a lack of English language skills.

Work-related challenges were identified by worker partners as among their and their community's most pressing problems. They described how people often could not transfer their job skills from their countries of origin to the US labor market because of language barriers. Reflecting on the economic vulnerability of new immigrants in particular, they noted how seldom people questioned difficult or problematic working conditions as a result. Key among these was wage theft, which had been a critical issue in the community for years. Worker partners additionally described experiences of feeling not fully incorporated into broader society or of being actively rejected or discriminated against in public spaces and social interactions, again, primarily because of English language limitations.

Regarding challenges to their own participation in the project, worker partners again drew the connection to language, reflecting the relative positions of privilege within the partnership based on English language facility, though also on the basis of scientific training. One worker described feeling nervous and intimidated when joining in project meetings with the rest of the partners even after undergoing trainings with CPA staff members on the project and even when Chinese was the primary language used during meetings because she felt "everyone else's English was so good."

Worker Leadership Development Based on years of organizing in the community, CPA staff partners anticipated challenges that a research partnership in particular would present for worker participation. Together with the project director from LOHP, who played a critical bridging role having grown up in Chinatown and with deep ties to the community, CPA staff partners designed a worker partner recruitment and training plan to support worker engagement in the project as well as in CPA's longer term organizing efforts for preventing wage theft and increasing labor rights.

Workers partners engaged in an initial eight-week training followed by biweekly meetings with CPA staff members that facilitated their in-depth participation throughout the project. The trainings and leadership development component of the project used a popular education approach with interactive, participatory, and learner-centered activities that incorporated critical reflection and community action (Chang et al., 2012). Activities included risk mapping (Brown, 2008), power mapping (Ritas, Minkler, Ni, & Halpin, 2008), workshops on policy making, mock food inspections in a simulated kitchen, and the use of visual triggers for discussion (images of Chinese restaurant workers in various work-related situations). The exercises supported workers in drawing connections between their own lives and the study and CPA-organizing goals and helped to draw out their knowledge and expertise.

In addition to enhancing participation and building community capacity, the worker leadership development component provided critical co-learning opportunities for the entire partnership. Workers' active participation and contributions yielded rich information and insights throughout the research and action phases, from developing the survey and checklist tools and procedures to data interpretation and in planning for and taking action.

Application and Adaptations of CBPR Principles Acknowledging variations in local context, CBPR principles encourage individual partnerships to adapt their approaches to collaboration because "no one set of CBPR principles is applicable to all partnerships" (see Chapter 3).

One example of the partnership's adaptations was alterations to its collaborative structures, following the recommendations of CPA staff partners. They moved toward a more separate and parallel process in which there were meetings of the primarily English-speaking institutional partners (university, CPA staff members, DPH) and meetings of primarily Chinese-speaking partners (worker partners, CPA staff members, and university members). English-speaking university and health department partners would individually attend and participate in the worker partner meetings and trainings from time to time, and full "steering committee" meetings of all partners together occurred twice during the project.

This adaptation created space for community members to safely participate on their own terms and to develop skills and engage in transformative critical reflection and action, while forming their own relationships to the project and to each other. In this arrangement, trusted facilitators playing critical bridging roles, such as CPA staff members and the LOHP project director, became even more central to facilitating effective communication among all partners.

During the two full steering committee meetings when all project partners were present, the sessions were conducted in Cantonese with simultaneous translation provided to English-only speakers. Prior to the meetings, partners from CPA, the university, and the DPH also discussed and prepared for "stepping back" their own participation to make more space for worker partners.

Policy and Community Capacity Outcomes In addition to building worker leadership capacity, the Chinatown study from the beginning was focused on generating data for policy and practice that could help promote change (Minkler et al., 2014). DPH partners reached out to several key agencies with study results urging stronger enforcement of existing labor laws, began verifying workers compensation insurance when issuing new business licenses to restaurants (Gaydos et al., 2011), and later would coordinate with the Office of Labor Standards Enforcement to suspend health permits of food facilities across the city with outstanding labor law violations (Minkler et al., 2014). At the same time, CPA cofounded the Progressive Workers Alliance (PWA), which developed a "low-wage worker bill of rights" and pushed the San Francisco board of supervisors to pass an anti-wage theft ordinance in 2011, followed by a dedicated Wage Theft Ordinance Task Force in 2012. These actions would be pivotal to the success of several important campaigns in subsequent years, including one involving a $4 million settlement between a major Chinese restaurant and its workers in 2014 (Hua, 2015).

In addition to policy gains, a major outcome of the Chinatown study was the individual, organizational, and community capacity built through the training and active engagement of the worker partners and community members in the study. Worker partners described overcoming fear of engaging with new people, gaining experience speaking in public, and a generalized sense of "courage," confidence, and ability to think about social issues. They additionally reported learning about worker rights, labor laws, and Chinatown restaurant working conditions.

CPA acquired new grants and trained a new generation of worker leaders, several of whom remain active as the community leadership core with the organization. CPA has continued to organize on wage theft and other issues of importance to the community, while also forging alliances and expanding its national-level movement building efforts on other economic and racial justice issues. Through the project, critical transformation took place at the individual level for members of the partnership, including worker partners, as well as at the organizational, community, and the broader society levels through its contributions to policy change and continued organizing efforts.

CONCLUSION: OPPORTUNITIES AND FUTURE CONSIDERATIONS FOR CONDUCTING CBPR IN ASIAN COMMUNITIES

As demonstrated throughout this chapter, there are robust CBPR efforts in AA communities at national and local levels. Nationally, a growing commitment to the CBPR approach in AA communities, evidenced by the exponential growth in the published literature and the funding of research infrastructures to support community-engaged research in Asian communities, provides researchers, advocates, and funding agencies with key evidence that CBPR produces sustainable efforts that amplify and address the health needs of this growing population (Hoeffel et al., 2012; Ortman & Guarneri, 2009). As highlighted in our second case study, CBPR efforts at the local level require a deep commitment to multi-sector engagement that is iterative, multistep, and reflective in nature. Moreover, careful attention to integrating capacity-building efforts into all stages of the research process is crucial. Whereas the local CBPR effort focused on a single AA community of interest, the national example illustrates clearly the increased complexity of collaborating over time with multiple AA communities and the opportunities and challenges of pan-ethnic work. Community participation helps ensure that unique cultural perspectives and strengths are built into interventions. From national and local examples, practitioners have a wealth of best practices from which to draw in initiating CBPR in their own communities.

In addition to the benefits and strengths of CBPR, our case studies demonstrate some of the unique challenges faced in using this approach in AA communities, such as those related to inclusivity and addressing diversity across myriad AA ethnic groups, immigrant statuses, and language proficiencies.

We anticipate that these challenges and strategies used to address them will serve as a basis for key future considerations in conducting CBPR in AA communities, incorporating multilevel and equity-based strategies. Some of these considerations are highlighted in the following:

- The United States is facing the growth of new waves of emerging, smaller AA immigrant groups throughout the country (such as the Himalayan and Burmese communities). Many of these populations have migrated as refugees and have acute health needs, yet their relatively small size may mask their disparities and issues in regional and local research efforts. CBPR researchers working in AA communities must maintain a commitment to engaging and building capacity in new and emerging communities while continuing to engage with more established communities, which can be challenging in the context of limited resources. In doing so, there are opportunities to share best practices and capacity-enhancing models across communities, new and established.
- Particularly concerning may be the growth of discriminatory language and fears, such as Islamophobia, which will affect a growing number of refugees and immigrants with Islamic religious backgrounds. CBPR partnerships may have to strengthen our determination to raise sensitive issues and confront the norms and values as well as the structural inequalities that face diverse populations. CBPR may be more important than ever to systematically document the health risks and concerns these communities may be experiencing and allow

communities under attack to have voice and self-determination in understanding and acting on issues affecting them.

- Though first- and second-generation Asian immigrant populations will continue to grow, areas with long-term AA settlement will concurrently experience growth in third- and fourth-generation AA communities. Accounting for the multigenerational nature of AA citizenship and incorporating diverse perspectives into CBPR efforts will be critical. Similarly, the growth in multiracial communities will necessitate researchers and communities alike to challenge their notions of identity in initiating CBPR efforts.
- Finally, ongoing and future efforts should consider building alliances across communities of color. Given the emphasis of CBPR on equity promotion, there is a unique opportunity in the multiethnic context of the United States to recognize that justice denied for anyone is justice denied for all—and to build research programs accordingly.

As the diversity and attendant complexity of the AA population grow in the coming decades, CBPR principles will continue to provide an important means of ensuring research is meaningful, context driven, and action oriented for this community.

QUESTIONS FOR DISCUSSION

1. What were the different CBPR-related opportunities and challenges that CSAAH faced as it grew from a new initiative in 2003 to becoming an NIMHD National Research Center of Excellence? How did it address these? What other changes might occur in Asian American communities or among academic and other partners that have implications for using a CBPR approach?
2. Why might you need to make adaptations to CBPR principles when working with Asian American communities? Are there any adaptations that would not be acceptable for a CBPR approach? Why or why not?

ACKNOWLEDGMENTS

We sincerely thank Julie Kranick for her assistance with this chapter. The efforts of Drs. Islam and Trinh-Shevrin are supported by the National Institutes of Health National Institute on Minority Health and Health Disparities (NIH NIMHD) grants P60MD000538; National Institutes of Health National Center for the Advancement of Translational Science (NCATS) Grant UL1TR000038; and Centers for Disease Control and Prevention (CDC) Grants U48DP001904 and U58DP005621. The San Francisco Chinatown Restaurant Worker Health and Safety Study was supported by the National Institute for Occupational Safety and Health/Centers for Disease Control and Prevention Grant (R219081) and the California Endowment, with additional support from the Occupational Health Internship Program. We dedicate this chapter to the numerous community partners we have had the privilege of working with over the past two decades. Their commitment and dedication to improving the lives of Asian American communities is awe-inspiring.

REFERENCES

Acevedo-Garcia, D., Sanchez-Vaznaugh, E. V., Viruell-Fuentes, E. A., & Almeida, J. (2012). Integrating social epidemiology into immigrant health research: A cross-national framework. *Social Science Medicine, 75*(12), 2060–2068. doi:10.1016/j.socscimed.2012.04.040

Aguilar, D. E., Abesamis-Mendoza, N., Ursua, R., Divino, L. A., Cadag, K., & Gavin, N. P. (2010). Lessons learned and challenges in building a Filipino health coalition. *Health Promotion Practice, 11*(3), 428–436. doi:10.1177/1524839908326381

Belone, L., Lucero, J. E., Duran, B., Tafoya, G., Baker, E. A., Chan, D., . . . Wallerstein, N. (2016). Community-based participatory research conceptual model: Community partner consultation and face validity. *Qualitative Health Research, 26*(1), 117–135. doi:10.1177/1049732314557084

Bloemraad, I. (2006). Becoming a citizen in the United States and Canada: Structured mobilization and immigrant political incorporation. *Social Forces, 85*(2), 667–695.

Brown, M. P. (2008). Risk mapping as a tool for community-based participatory research and organizing. In M. Minkler & N. Wallerstein (Eds.), *Community-based participatory research for health: From process to outcomes* (pp. 453–457, 2nd ed.). San Francisco, CA: Jossey-Bass.

Chang, C., Salvatore, A., Lee, P., Liu, S. S., & Minkler, M. (2012). Popular education, participatory research, and community organizing. In M. Minkler (Ed.), *Community organizing and community building for health.* San Francisco, CA: Jossey-Bass.

Chang, C., Salvatore, A. L., Lee, P. T., Liu, S. S., Tom, A. T., Morales, A., . . . Minkler, M. (2013). Adapting to context in community-based participatory research: "Participatory starting points" in a Chinese immigrant worker community. *American Journal of Community Psychology, 51*(3–4), 480–491. doi:10.1007/s10464-012-9565-z

Gaydos, M., Bhatia, R., Morales, A., Lee, P. T., Liu, S. S., Chang, C., . . . Minkler, M. (2011). Promoting health and safety in San Francisco's Chinatown restaurants: Findings and lessons learned from a pilot observational checklist. *Public Health Reports, 126*(Suppl 3), 62–69.

Hoeffel, E. M., Rastogi, S., Kim, M. O., & Shahid, H. (2012). The Asian population: 2010 census briefs. Retrieved from http://census.gov/prod/cen2010/briefs/c2010-11.pdf

Hua, V. (2015). The dim sum revolution. *San Francisco Magazine, 62*(4).

Huang, K. Y., Calzada, E., Cheng, S., & Brotman, L. M. (2012). Physical and mental health disparities among young children of Asian immigrants. *Journal of Pediatrics, 160*(2), 331–336. doi:10.1016/j.jpeds.2011.08.005

Islam, N. S., Khan, S., Kwon, S., Jang, D., Ro, M., & Trinh-Shevrin, C. (2010). Methodological issues in the collection, analysis, and reporting of granular data in Asian American populations: Historical challenges and potential solutions. *Journal of Health Care for the Poor and Underserved, 21*(4), 1354–1381. doi:10.1353/hpu.2010.0939

Islam, N. S., Wyatt, L. C., Patel, S. D., Shapiro, E., Tandon, S. D., Mukherji, B. R., . . . Trinh-Shevrin, C. (2013). Evaluation of a community health worker pilot intervention to improve diabetes management in Bangladeshi immigrants with type 2 diabetes in New York City. *Diabetes Education, 39*(4), 478–493. doi:10.1177/0145721713491438

Islam, N. S., Zanowiak, J. M., Wyatt, L. C., Chun, K., Lee, L., Kwon, S. C., & Trinh-Shevrin, C. (2013). A randomized-controlled, pilot intervention on diabetes prevention and healthy lifestyles in the New York City Korean community. *Journal of Community Health, 38*(6), 1030–1041. doi:10.1007/s10900-013-9711-z

Islam, N. S., Zanowiak, J. M., Wyatt, L. C., Kavathe, R., Singh, H., Kwon, S. C., & Trinh-Shevrin, C. (2014). Diabetes prevention in the New York City Sikh Asian Indian community: A pilot study. *International Journal of Environmental Research and Public Health, 11*(5), 5462–5486. doi:10.3390/ijerph110505462

Israel, B. A., Eng, E., Schulz, A. J., & Parker, E. A. (2013). *Methods in community-based participatory research for health* (2nd ed.). San Francisco, CA: Jossey-Bass.

Jayaraman, S. (2013). *Beyond the kitchen door.* Ithica, NY: ILR Press.

Kristof, N. (2015). The Asian advantage. *New York Times* (October 10). www.nytimes.com/2015/10/11/opinion/sunday/the-asian-advantage.html?_r=1

Minkler, M., Salvatore, A. L., Chang, C., Gaydos, M., Liu, S. S., Lee, P. T., . . . Krause, N. (2014). Wage theft as a neglected public health problem: An overview and case study from San Francisco's Chinatown district. *American Journal of Public Health, 104*(6), 1010–1020. doi:10.2105/AJPH.2013.301813

Murphy, P. A. (2011). Tiger moms: Is tough parenting really the answer? *Time* (January 20). http://content.time.com/time/magazine/article/0,9171,2043477,00.html

Ortman, J. M., & Guarneri, C. E. (2009). *United States population projections: 2000 to 2050.* Washington, DC: US Census Bureau.

Parker, E. A., Chung, L. K., Israel, B. A., Reyes, A., & Wilkins, D. (2010). Community organizing network for environmental health: Using a community health development approach to increase community capacity around reduction of environmental triggers. *Journal of Primary Prevention, 31*(1–2), 41–58. doi:10.1007/s10935-010-0207-7

Patel, S., Kwon, S., Tepporn, E., Arista, P., Rideout, C., Linkin, F., . . . Trinh-Shevrin, C. (2014). Strategies to Reach and Implement the Vision of Health Equity (STRIVE) project: Qualitative findings about the process of implementing evidence-based strategies in local AANHPI communities. In A.P.H. Association (Ed.), *Strengthening communities through participatory research (APHA 142nd Annual Meeting* & Expo ed.). New Orleans, LA: Author.

Powell, B. (2011). An American dad on raising a tiger daughter. *Time* (January 20). http://content.time.com/time/magazine/article/0,9171,2043420,00.html

Ritas, C., Minkler, M., Ni, A., & Halpin, H. A. (2008). Using CBPR to promote policy change: Exercises and online resources. In M. Minkler & N. Wallerstein (Eds.), *Community-based participatory research for health: From process to outcomes* (2nd ed., pp. 459–463). San Francisco, CA: Jossey-Bass.

Spallek, J., Zeeb, H., & Razum, O. (2011). What do we have to know from migrants' past exposures to understand their health status? A life course approach. *Emerging Themes in Epidemiology, 8*(1), 6. doi:10.1186/1742-7622-8-6

Tandon, S. D., & Kwon, S. C. (2009). Community-based participatory research. In C. Trinh-Shevrin, N. S. Islam, & M. J. Rey (Eds.), *Asian American communities and health: Context, research, policy, and action* (pp. 464–503). San Francisco, CA: Jossey-Bass.

Trinh-Shevrin, C. (2014). Community health workers offer culturally tailored interactive workshops and counseling to Filipino Americans, leading to improvements in medication adherence and cardiovascular risk factors. Retrieved from https://innovations.ahrq.gov/profiles/community-health-workers-offer-culturally-tailored-interactive-workshops-and-counseling

Trinh-Shevrin, C., Islam, N. S., Nadkarni, S., Park, R., & Kwon, S. C. (2015). Defining an integrative approach for health promotion and disease prevention: A population health equity framework. *Journal of Health Care for the Poor and Underserved, 26*(2 Suppl), 146–163. doi:10.1353/hpu.2015.0067

Trinh-Shevrin, C., Islam, N., Tandon, S. D., Abesamis, N., Ho-Asjoe, H., & Rey, M. J. (2007). Using community-based participatory research as a guiding framework for health disparities research centers. *Progress in Community Health Partnerships: Research, Education, and Action, 1*(2), 195–205.

Trinh-Shevrin, C., Kwon, S. C., Park, R., Nadkarni, S. K., & Islam, N. S. (2015). Moving the dial to advance population health equity in New York City Asian American populations. *American Journal of Public Health, 105*(Suppl 3), e16–e25. doi:10.2105/AJPH.2015.302626

Ursua, R. A., Aguilar, D. E., Wyatt, L. C., Katigbak, C., Islam, N. S., Tandon, S. D., . . . Trinh-Shevrin, C. (2014). A community health worker intervention to improve management of hypertension among Filipino Americans in New York and New Jersey: A pilot study. *Ethnicity and Disease, 24*(1), 67–76.

Webster, T. (2001). Occupational hazards in eating and drinking places. *Compensation and Working Conditions* (Summer). Retrieved from www.bls.gov/opub/mlr/cwc/occupational-hazards-in-eating-and-drinking-places.pdf

Yi, S. S., Kwon, S. C., Sacks, R., & Trinh-Shevrin, C. (2016). Commentary: Persistence and health-related consequences of the model minority stereotype for Asian Americans. *Ethnicity and Disease, 26*(1), 133–138. doi:10.18865/ed.26.1.133

CHAPTER 13

ENGAGED FOR CHANGE

AN INNOVATIVE CBPR STRATEGY TO INTERVENTION DEVELOPMENT

SCOTT D. RHODES, LILLI MANN, FLORENCE M. SIMÁN, JORGE ALONZO, AARON T. VISSMAN, JENNIFER NALL, AND AMANDA E. TANNER

ALTHOUGH CBPR IS committed to equitable partnering practice and science to promote health equity within complex sociocultural, political, and economic contexts, the challenge remains for academics to engage with communities to develop, implement, and evaluate individual-, community-, system-, and policy-level interventions designed to reduce health disparities and increase health equity. Intervention development is difficult, and little guidance exists in terms of strategies and processes, especially in involving community members as experts in their own community and culture to co-develop interventions designed to promote health and prevent disease. The science behind intervention development remains largely underdeveloped, and there is a profound need for evidence-based strategies to guide the development of interventions (Bartholomew, Parcel, Kok, & Gottlieb, 2001; Hoddinott, 2015; Wallerstein & Duran, 2010; Yardley, Morrison, Bradbury, & Muller, 2015).

In this chapter, we outline the intervention research that our long-standing and well-established partnership has been conducting and describe a multistep process that we have developed to provide guidance to intervention development through CBPR. The process provides a framework for developing an intervention that is well informed by the lived experiences of community members, the experiences of representatives from service- and practice-based organizations, and sound science. The process ensures the culture-centeredness of interventions. Rather than an intervention that merely incorporates appropriate language, beliefs, and images, culture-centeredness locates culture at the center of the intervention including identities, meanings, and experiences, which are grounded in historical and social contexts (Dutta, 2008), as described in Chapter 2.

OUR CBPR PARTNERSHIP'S EXPERIENCE WITH INTERVENTION DEVELOPMENT

Our CBPR partnership is located in western North Carolina. North Carolina has one of the fastest growing Latino populations in the country. Members of our partnership focus on the health of ethnic-racial, sexual, and gender minorities and economically disadvantaged communities, with HIV incidence rates in North Carolina 40 percent higher than the national rate. Since the new millennium, our partnership has evolved to reflect demographic trends and the evolving impact of the HIV epidemic. Many of our CBPR studies focus on promoting sexual health and preventing HIV among Latino communities and gay, bisexual, and other men who have sex with men (MSM). Current partners include representatives from North Carolina public health departments (local and state level); AIDS service organizations; community-based organizations, including Latino soccer leagues and teams, a local lesbian, gay, bisexual, and transgender (LGBT) pride organization, and Latino-serving organizations; a local LGBT foundation; local businesses, including media organizations, Internet applications ("apps"), bars, and clubs, a video production company, and *tiendas* (Latino grocers); the Centers for Disease Control and Prevention (CDC); and three universities. Our partnership consists of a variety of members working on multiple projects. Members may be involved with and committed to different projects; however, our partnership is not study-specific. Members may join and leave, and be more or less involved, but despite transitions, the partnership remains.

Our partnership has developed multiple interventions designed to address community-identified health priorities:

- HoMBReS (Hombres Manteniendo Bienestar y Relaciones Saludables; Men Maintaining Well-being and Healthy Relationships), designed to promote sexual health and HIV prevention through social networks of Latino men who are members of recreational soccer leagues (Rhodes, Leichliter, Sun, & Bloom, 2016)
- CyBER/M4M (Cyber-based Education and Referral/Men for Men), designed to increase knowledge of HIV among gay and bisexual and other MSM who use online chat rooms for social and sexual networking (Rhodes et al., 2010)
- C-CAPRELA (Cervical Cancer Prevention for Latinas), designed to reduce cancer-related health disparities through social networks of Latina women living within the same housing communities (Rhodes, Kelley, et al., 2012)
- CyBER/testing, designed to increase HIV testing among gay, bisexual, and other MSM and transgender persons who use social media for social and sexual networking (Rhodes, McCoy, et al., 2016)
- MuJEReS (Mujeres Juntas Estableciendo Relaciones Saludables; Women United Establishing Healthy Relationships), designed to promote sexual health through social networks of Latina women (Rhodes, Kelley, et al., 2012)
- HoMBReS por un Cambio (Men for Change), designed to promote sexual health and advocate for social justice through mobilizing and organizing social networks of Latino men who are members of recreational soccer leagues (Rhodes, Leichliter, et al., 2016)

- HOLA, designed to reduce HIV-related health disparities among Latino gay, bisexual, and other MSM and Latina transgender women (Rhodes, Daniel, et al., 2013)
- HOLA en Grupos, designed to reduce HIV-related health disparities through social networks of Latino gay, bisexual, and other MSM and Latina transgender women (Rhodes, Alonzo, Mann, Freeman, et al., 2015)
- MAP'T (Mobile Apps to Promote Testing), designed to increase HIV testing through the use of mobile applications (e.g., A4A/Radar, Grindr, Jack'd, and SCRUFF) commonly used for social and sexual networking among gay, bisexual, and other MSM and transgender persons (Sun et al., 2015)
- weCare, designed to support the health and well-being of young racially ethnically diverse gay, bisexual, and other MSM and transgender persons with HIV through social media (Tanner et al., 2016)
- ChiCAS (Chicas Creando Acceso a la Salud; Girls Creating Access to Health), designed to promote the sexual and transition-related health of Latina transgender women

During the development, implementation, and evaluation of these interventions since the new millennium, our CBPR partnership developed a process for intervention development that evolved and became more sophisticated (Rhodes, Alonzo, Mann, Freeman, et al., 2015; Rhodes, Daniel, et al., 2013; Rhodes, Duck, Alonzo, Daniel, et al., 2013; Rhodes, Duck, Alonzo, Downs, et al., 2013; Rhodes et al., 2006, 2007).

Although our initial processes followed typical steps of partnership trust building, developing, adapting, pilot-testing, and launching interventions, we also created a grid of resources for intervention development (GRID). This GRID enabled us to outline existing interventions and related programs and documented how activities met intervention objectives; explored whether existing approaches or activities met local priorities; and began the process of thinking creatively about the intervention strategies, activities, theories, and logic model development.

Since the earlier processes, however, we have worked to better deconstruct, clarify, and codify our intervention development process throughout our ongoing intervention research. We do not assume that what worked in the past will work in the future; we are reflective and do not work on "auto-pilot." Furthermore, we wanted to support other partnerships that want to apply a systematic and engaged approach to intervention development and maximize the potential impact of their interventions.

STEPS IN INTERVENTION DEVELOPMENT THROUGH CBPR

We have developed a refined and enhanced thirteen-step process that is known as ENGAGED for CHANGE, with each letter signifying one step within the intervention development process. These steps are outlined in Table 13.1.

Expand the Partnership

The first step in the process involves expanding the partnership. Often CBPR partnerships lack sufficient representation of key community or academic partners. Our partnership has learned that we may not always have the expertise, connections, or other resources that are needed to move an intervention project forward. Although our partnership already had some Latino members, during our initial CBPR study focusing on Latino men's health, we realized that to be successful, we needed to expand participation by increasing representation of Latino men who

TABLE 13.1 ENGAGED for CHANGE: A Stepped Approach to Intervention Development

	Step	Objective
E	Expand the partnership.	To ensure that necessary key partners and perspectives are not missing from the partnership
N	iNtervention team established.	To assign responsibility to a small team representing the partnership and its diversity that will move the intervention development process forward
G	Gather existing literature and data.	To build on what is already known in terms of epidemiologic data; existing local, regional, national, and global data; and so on
A	Assess community needs, priorities, and assets.	To ensure that community needs, priorities, and assets are blended with existing data
G	Generate and refine intervention priorities.	To begin the process of focusing intervention goals based on community needs and priorities
E	Evaluate and incorporate appropriate and meaningful theory.	To apply theory when appropriate; to ensure the intervention is informed by theory
D	Design an intervention conceptual or logic model.	To describe the logic of the intervention (what is expected to happen)
for		
C	Create objectives and craft activities and materials.	To develop and refine intervention objectives and all necessary activities and materials, ensuring activities and materials are clearly linked to objectives
H	Hone and pretest all activities and materials.	To ensure activities and materials make sense for those for whom they are designed
A	Administer intervention pilot test.	To ensure intervention components fit together coherently
N	Note process of implementation during the pilot test.	To document challenges, problems, weaknesses, and successes identified through the pilot test
G	Gather feedback from the pilot and those who conducted and participated in the pilot.	To include all perspectives in the intervention editing step
E	Edit the intervention based on feedback.	To refine, enhance the intervention based on lessons learned from the pilot

were involved in local recreational soccer leagues. Of course, the expansion of representation is not easy. It can take months to identify potential members, build trust, and increase understanding of the rationale for CBPR partnerships and the relevant processes, history, and goals.

Although networking and building trust to expand a partnership is a challenge (Becker, Israel, & Allen, 2005), within some communities, networking and building trust can be particularly complicated. As we learned in our work with Latinos in North Carolina, some community members were hesitant to participate in a process they initially did not understand or trust; some were undocumented, others were not, but many shared a fear of engagement within a state in which there were high levels of racism and anti-immigration sentiment (Rhodes, Mann, et al., 2015; Rhodes et al., 2006). This is also true for working with sexual and gender minorities. Partnering with gay, bisexual, and other MSM and transgender persons requires careful consideration and effort given the intersectionality of identities and stigmas.

Intervention Team Established

The second step is establishing an intervention team, which is a smaller working group, tasked with overseeing the entire intervention development process. The team works collaboratively with the partnership, providing updates and brainstorming solutions to challenges faced. This team must have broad and diverse representation from the partnership; its work cannot be done in isolation and requires thorough involvement of members representing all partner types, including community members, organization representatives, and academic researchers.

Gather Existing Literature and Data

This next step allows for the intervention team and partnership to build on what is known through collection and interpretation of existing literature and data describing community needs, priorities, and assets. These may include community assessments that are regularly conducted by public health departments, hospitals, and local foundations; epidemiologic and disparities reports from state and national agencies; data collected and synthesized by community-based organizations used in their own service delivery and grant proposals; and other sources, including those from traditional academic research efforts (e.g., peer-reviewed publications). A partnership approach to this step is important because different members will be aware of and have access to different types of existing literature and data depending on their different roles (e.g., organization representatives and academics), and gathering information from a broad range of sources helps to have a more complete picture of the current community landscape and inequities.

Assess Community Needs, Priorities, and Assets

Because not all necessary literature and data may be readily available, the partnership also must examine the needs, priorities, and assets of communities themselves. For example, in the early 2000s, Latino communities in the southern United States, often referred to as "new Latino settlement states," were not well understood and remained relatively isolated (Gill, 2010). Thus, working with community members to understand community needs, priorities, and assets was a key component of our early work.

We used multiple research methodologies. One approach was photovoice, an empowerment-based qualitative method of inquiry that enables participants to record and reflect on their personal and community strengths and concerns through group discussions and photographs.

Not only does it provide images of lived experiences but also the space for participants and others who may be able to support action to collaboratively identify next steps (Hergenrather et al., 2009). Our partnership has successfully used photovoice with Latino adolescents (Streng et al., 2004), Latino men (Rhodes et al., 2009), persons living with HIV (Rhodes, Hergenrather, Wilkin, & Jolly, 2008), African American–Black men with HIV, and Latina transgender women (Rhodes, Alonzo, Mann, Sun, et al., 2015).

In our photovoice project with Latina transgender women, nine transgender women documented their daily experiences through photography, engaged in discussions about their photographs, and organized a bilingual community forum to move knowledge to action. From the participants' photographs and words, eleven themes emerged in three domains: daily challenges (e.g., health risks, uncertainty about the future, discrimination, and anxiety about family reactions); needs and priorities (e.g., health and social services, emotional support, and collective action); and community strengths and assets (e.g., supportive individuals and institutions, wisdom acquired through lived experiences, and personal and professional goals).

As an example of the health risks Latina transgender women often take, a participant took and shared with the group a photo (Figure 13.1) of hormones that she had purchased at a tienda (Mexican grocery store) and injected without the guidance of a medical professional. This resonated with other participants and triggered a discussion about health risks that many Latina transgender women take (e.g., unsafe hormone use), the reasons that they take these risks (e.g., barriers to care), and the need to increase access to affordable and culturally congruent transition-related health services.

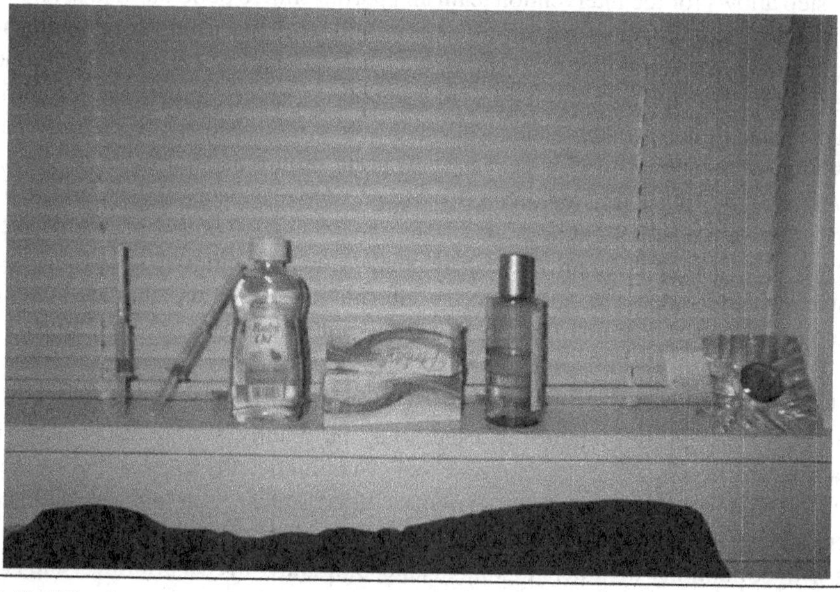

FIGURE 13.1 *Latina Transgender Women's Photovoice Project Photograph and Corresponding Quotation, "It Is Important to Go down the Right Path and to Not Just Inject Yourself with Whatever."*

At the community forum, sixty influential advocates, including Latina transgender women, community-based organization staff members, health and social service providers, and law enforcement, reviewed findings and developed ten recommended actions. These included educating staff members at the Mexican Consulate in Raleigh about the lives of Latina transgender women in order to reduce discrimination they felt when seeking consulate services; increasing health promotion programming in specific priority areas, that is, linking HIV, sexual health, and transition-related services; and raising consciousness about negative experiences with police about intimate partner violence. Overall, photovoice served to obtain rich qualitative insight of Latina transgender women that was then shared with local leaders and agencies to help address priorities (Rhodes, Alonzo, Mann, Sun, et al., 2015).

Gaps can also be filled by collecting data using innovative quantitative methods, such as respondent-driven sampling, which uses chain referrals or initial respondents as "seed" to yield representative samples and prevalence estimates for populations that may be considered "difficult to reach" by researchers or other outsiders or for which no sampling frame exists (Rhodes, McCoy, et al., 2012; Song et al., 2012).

Generate and Refine Intervention Priorities

Based on existing data and data uncovered by the previous step, the intervention team generates priorities, presents them to the entire CBPR partnership, and iteratively refines intervention priorities based on feedback. For example, our photovoice project in partnership with Latina transgender women uncovered the need for more access to sexual health information and services, a finding that aligns with the literature on high rates of HIV among transgender women, especially among racial-ethnic minorities. However, access to transition-related health care services, including safe hormone use, emerged as a more salient and urgent priority for photovoice participants, particularly given existing barriers because of high un-insurance and limited English, much less culturally congruent and transgender-specific services. Thus, our partnership developed the ChiCAS intervention to focus jointly on sexual health and transition-related health based on these qualitative data and on our enhanced understanding that transition-related needs must be met first. In addition, the community forum that was the culmination of the photovoice project identified community organizations, which already offered low-cost hormone therapy, where future intervention participants could be referred for transition-related health care.

Evaluate and Incorporate Appropriate and Meaningful Theory

Discussions of theory enable partners to understand processes of change, at whatever level, from a systematic perspective and identify where and how theory fits into their lived experiences. Understanding theory and integrating it with community member perspectives on the lived experiences of community members is critical to making informed decisions about interventions. This blending of perspectives and integration of theory reflects knowledge democracy as described in Chapter 2.

For example, through the exploration of theory and its uses, our partnership determined that to support sexual health of Latino gay, bisexual, and other MSM and Latina transgender women, two theories "fit" our desired approach: social cognitive theory (Bandura, 1986) and empowerment education (Freire, 1970, 1973; Wallerstein, 1994). We also decided that using a lay health advisor model would enable us to reach a larger number of Latino gay, bisexual, and other MSM and Latina transgender women with an approach that was authentic to how these communities convene. Thus, our HOLA intervention was designed to train members from the community across North Carolina to promote sexual health through their naturally existing social networks (i.e., through their friends), and our approach to training and supporting these lay health advisors drew on constructs from both theories. This approach also enables the knowledge to live in the community (in this case through the lay health advisors) even after a project is complete.

Design an Intervention Conceptual or Logic Model

Designing an intervention conceptual or logic model helps partnership members visually depict the links among determinants of health (e.g., HIV risk and use of unsafe transition-related practices among Latina transgender women); the intervention strategies designed to address these determinants; and expected immediate, intermediate, and long-term outcomes. The conceptual or logic model enables partnership members to visually depict and see the logic in their thinking, discuss their assumptions, and engage in a process of blending perspectives, insights, and experiences with science while keeping an eye on outcomes. Table 13.2 provides an abbreviated logic model from our HOLA en Grupos HIV prevention intervention for gay, bisexual, and other MSM and Latina transgender women.

During these discussions, community members may describe their real-world experiences and perspectives on health and risk within contexts and evaluate what might and might not work to reach expected outcomes. Service providers, including representatives from community-based organizations, may provide insights based on their rich experience in service provision, and academic researchers will synthesize the literature and provide expertise in health behavior theory and health promotion. During development of the logic model, new variables may be identified for measurement, including mediating and moderating variables and outcomes.

Create Objectives and Craft Activities and Materials

Intervention team members collaboratively draft objectives and craft activities and materials. In this step, the team develops a general outline for the intervention including goals, objectives, key messages, and theoretical underpinnings. Intervention activities are then outlined, refined, and developed. Necessary culturally congruent materials (e.g., use of penis models for practicing condom use) also are developed at this stage. This process is iterative with multiple opportunities for intervention team and partnership members to provide feedback.

Hone and Pretest All Activities and Materials

We have learned that over time, partnership members, even those who represent the community, become more alike others within the partnership (including organization representatives and academic researchers) and may become out of touch with their peers in the community. Thus, we have found it critical to pretest intervention activities and materials with community members outside of the partnership who may be naive to the research and the partnership.

For example, we developed a condom tips card designed to support proper condom use among Latino gay, bisexual, and other MSM. Our partnership debated how "real" to make the illustrations, with the partnership deciding that the illustrations of the receptive partner should be unclear so that the gender was vague. Our rationale was that we did not want to put at risk anyone who might forget the tips card in his pants pocket or car, as examples, for someone else

TABLE 13.2 An Abbreviated, Sample Logic Model from Our Partnership's HOLA en Grupos Intervention

Problem statement: The US South carries disproportionate HIV burden compared to other parts of the United States. Spanish-speaking Latino gay, bisexual, and other MSM and Latina transgender women in the South are at increased risk for HIV. Unfortunately no efficacious culturally congruent behavioral interventions exist to reduce risk among these communities. HOLA en Grupos is designed to increase consistent condom use and HIV and STD testing among Spanish-speaking Latino gay and bisexual men, MSM, and transgender persons ages eighteen years and older.

Behavioral Determinants *Factors that affect risk and protective behaviors*	**Activities** *To address behavioral determinants*	**Outcomes** *Expected changes as a result of activities targeting behavioral determinants* — *Immediate Outcomes*	*Intermediate Outcomes*
1. Knowledge of HIV and STDs (including magnitude and impact on communities); the types of infections; modes of transmission; signs; symptoms; and prevention strategies 2. Knowledge of available health care services and eligibility 3. Perceived access to available health care and related services 4. Condom use skills and self-efficacy 5. Sexual communication skills and self-efficacy 6. The sociocultural environment (e.g., reactions to machismo, fatalism, homophobia, and discrimination)	Module 1: General information about the intervention and an introduction to sexual health Activities: 1. Icebreaker, introduction to the intervention, and group introductions; 2. Ground rules; 3. Magnitude of HIV and STDs; 4. "Find someone who" game; 5. HIV/STD presentation and discussion, distribution of STD and health department brochures; 6. HIV/STD vocabulary game *Activities correspond to determinants 1 and 2.* Module 2: Protecting Yourself and Your Partners Activities: 1. Discussion of module 1; 2. Demonstrating and practicing correct condom use; 3. Practical advice about condoms; 4. Putting condom use steps in correct order; 5. Condom use DVD and discussion; 6. Internal condom use DVD and discussion; 7. Why some people use and some do not use condoms activity in pairs; 8. Condom negotiation role-plays; 9. Homework (learning about different types of condoms) *Activities correspond to determinants 3, 4, and 5.*	Increased knowledge of HIV and STDs Increased levels of correct knowledge about HIV and STDs: the types of diseases, modes of transmission, signs, symptoms, and prevention strategies Increased condom use skills, self-efficacy, and intention Increased sexual communication and safer sex negotiation skills and self-efficacy	Increased consistent condom use during anal and vaginal sex Increased communication with sexual partners about condom use Increased HIV and STD testing and receipt of test results

(Continued)

TABLE 13.2 (CONTINUED)

Behavioral Determinants *Factors that affect risk and protective behaviors*	**Activities** *To address behavioral determinants*	**Outcomes** *Expected changes as a result of activities targeting behavioral determinants*	
		Immediate Outcomes	***Intermediate Outcomes***
	Module 3: Cultural Values That Affect Our Health Activities: 1. Discussion of module 2; 2. Group discussion of what it means to be Latino/a and gay or transgender; 3. How Latino cultural values influence behavior; 4. Confronting health-compromising attitudes and beliefs; 5. Overcoming sociocultural obstacles to accessing medical services discussion and accessing health department HIV and STD testing services DVD. *Activities correspond to determinants 2, 3, 5, and 6.* Module 4: Review activities: 1. Group discussion of previous module; 2. Review of HIV and STD transmission and prevention; 3. Distinguishing between HIV and STD myths and realities; 4. Living with HIV DVD and group discussion; 5. Discussion about abstinence; 6. Conclusions *Activities correspond to determinants 1, 2, 3, 4, 5, and 6.*	Decreased negative and increased positive attitudes toward condoms Reduced adherence to traditional notions of masculinity and fatalism Decreased homo-negativity Increased ethnic group pride Reduced perceived barriers to HIV testing	

to find. However, when pretesting the card, Latino gay, bisexual, and other MSM reported that the clearer images spoke to them. They were less worried about safety and prioritized the card's meaningfulness.

Administer Intervention Pilot Test

Pilot testing is essential to analyzing activities and materials for attention, comprehension, personal relevance, credibility, and acceptability by those for whom the activities and materials are developed (Bartholomew et al., 2001; National Cancer Institute, 1989; Rhodes et al., 2006, 2007). Questions include (1) Do activities and materials motivate and sustain the participants' attention and interest? (2) Are activities and materials perceived as they were intended? (3) Is there anything offensive in them? (d) Do the participants recognize and identify with the activities and materials? (Rhodes, Kelley, et al., 2012; Rhodes et al., 2006, 2007). Results of this step are used in the last step (editing of intervention).

Note Process of Implementation during the Pilot Test

It is critical to learn as much as one can from the pilot test. For this reason, it is recommended that, in addition to those partnership members who are involved directly in implementing the intervention during the pilot test, other partnership members be present to observe the process of implementation. They may complete observer's logs to capture details of implementation in a systematic way. These details may identify where the intervention curriculum is vague, unclear, or confusing for those who are delivering the intervention. Instructions may need to be refined, for example.

Gather Feedback from the Pilot and Those Who Conducted and Participated in the Pilot

Discussions with those who implemented the pilot are vital to explore how they felt about the process, what worked well, and what did not from their perspectives. We have conducted qualitative interviews with pilot participants to better understand what worked and what did not work well. With participants for whom the intervention worked well, we conducted interviews that we referred to as "stories of success," and with participants for whom the intervention did not work well, we conducted interviews that we referred to as "stories of learning." This process ensured that we explored the strengths and weaknesses of the intervention during the pilot phase.

Edit the Intervention Based on Feedback

Based on the feedback and results from the pilot test, the intervention team edited and revised intervention activities, strategies, and implementation processes. This may be an iterative process with the intervention team revisiting previous steps of the ENGAGED for CHANGE model. This editing process is crucial to ensure that the most-promising intervention—based on science and the unique needs of the community—is used and evaluated.

CONCLUSION

There continues to be profound need to move from knowledge generation to the translation of knowledge into interventions designed to promote community health. The strategy outlined in this chapter can serve as a guide for other CBPR partnerships. Each step is complex, and our partnership's work has not been without challenges. Members face the realities of health disparities and inequities every day and know that something must be done for the communities we each belong to. The slow pace of securing research funding and conducting sound research is an ongoing frustration. Furthermore, communities themselves are not infallible; community members and members of research partnerships may have strongly held prejudices about one another that require ongoing attention and work highlighting the need to return to trust building throughout the course of the partnership. Although there has been much literature on approaches to address differences among partners, we have used team-building exercises, regular in-person meetings to develop and nurture relationships, and celebrations of partnership successes as well as life events (e.g., birthdays and births of babies).

Of course, the thirteen steps that we outline rely on a foundation of trust, transparency, clear communication, and ongoing commitment by partnership members. Partnership principles were not outlined in this chapter, but there are multiple places to find examples of these principles (including Chapter 3 and Appendices 2 to 4), which are designed to support processes that facilitate equal participation in research among community members, organization representatives, and academic researchers (Rhodes et al., 2011, 2014; Seifer & Maurana, 2000). Moreover, the steps may overlap and be iterative.

It is also essential that once partnerships develop interventions, they rigorously evaluate those interventions. Though there are strong arguments for why using a CBPR approach to develop interventions may help increase intervention efficacy, outcome evaluation to measure the effectiveness of interventions, as well as process evaluation, are essential for having an impact on community and population health. Evaluation findings can inform dissemination and adaption of those interventions that are found to be effective and help ensure intervention fidelity. Strong collaborations and diverse perspectives among partnership members are important in evaluation also, including development of instruments; data collection, analysis, and interpretation; and dissemination of findings (Cashman et al., 2008; Schaal et al., 2016).

We are committed to this innovative CBPR approach to intervention development because it maximizes the probability that our work as a partnership is based on what community members identify as priorities; is more informed because of the sharing of broad perspectives, insights, and experiences; builds capacity of all partners to solve community problems, harness community assets, and conduct meaningful research; and promotes sustainability. We also think that working together in partnership and building on the strengths of communities, organization representatives, and academic researchers is ethical. Health disparities, such as HIV, for example, require that we develop interventions that have the highest likelihood of success to ensure the reduction and elimination of disparities over time. We must maximize our potential for change.

QUESTIONS FOR DISCUSSION

1. What are the strengths of using ENGAGED for CHANGE as a strategy for intervention development?
2. What challenges do you see with applying this strategy to developing interventions, and how could these challenges be overcome?

REFERENCES

Bandura, A. (1986). *Social foundations of thought and action: A social cognitive theory*. Englewood Cliffs, NJ: Prentice-Hall.

Bartholomew, L. K., Parcel, G. S., Kok, G., & Gottlieb, N. H. (2001). *Intervention mapping: Designing theory- and evidence-based health promotion programs*. New York, NY: McGraw-Hill.

Becker, A. B., Israel, B. A., & Allen, A. J. (2005). Strategies and techniques for effective group process in CBPR partnerships. In B. A. Israel, E. Eng, A. J. Schulz, & E. A. Parker (Eds.), *Methods in community-based participatory research for health* (pp. 52–72). San Francisco, CA: Jossey-Bass.

Cashman, S. B., Adeky, S., Allen, A. J., Corburn, J., Israel, B. A., Montaño, J., . . . Eng, E. (2008). The power and the promise: Working with communities to analyze data, interpret findings, and get to outcomes. *American Journal of Public Health, 98*(8), 1407–1417.

Dutta, M. J. (2008). *Communicating health: A culture-centered approach*. Malden, MA: Polity Press.

Freire, P. (1970). *Pedagogy of the oppressed*. New York, NY: Herder and Herder.

Freire, P. (1973). *Education for critical consciousness*. New York, NY: Seabury Press.

Gill, H. (2010). *The Latino migration experience in North Carolina: New roots in the old north state*. Chapel Hill, NC: University of North Carolina.

Hergenrather, K. C., Rhodes, S. D., Cowan, C. A., Bardhoshi, G., & Pula, S. (2009). Photovoice as community-based participatory research: A qualitative review. *American Journal of Health Behavior, 33*(6), 686–698. doi:10.5555/ajhb.2009.33.6.686 [pii]

Hoddinott, P. (2015). A new era for intervention development studies. *Pilot and Feasibility Studies, 1*(36), doi:10.1186/s40814-40015-40032-40810.

National Cancer Institute. (1989). *Making health communications work: A planner's guide*. Bethesda, MD: US Department of Health and Human Services.

Rhodes, S. D., Alonzo, J., Mann, L., Freeman, A., Sun, C. J., Garcia, M., & Painter, T. M. (2015). Enhancement of a locally developed HIV prevention intervention for Hispanic/Latino MSM: A partnership of community-based organizations, a university, and the Centers for Disease Control and Prevention. *AIDS Education and Prevention, 27*(4), 312–332.

Rhodes, S. D., Alonzo, J., Mann, L., Sun, C. J., Simán, F. M., Abraham, C., & Garcia, M. (2015). Using photovoice, Latina transgender women identify priorities in a new immigrant-destination state. *International Journal of Transgenderism, 16*(2), 80–96.

Rhodes, S. D., Daniel, J., Alonzo, J., Duck, S., Garcia, M., Downs, M., . . . Marsiglia, F. F. (2013). A systematic community-based participatory approach to refining an evidence-based community-level intervention: The HOLA intervention for Latino men who have sex with men. *Health Promotion Practice, 14*(4), 607–616.

Rhodes, S. D., Duck, S., Alonzo, J., Daniel, J., & Aronson, R. E. (2013). Using community-based participatory research to prevent HIV disparities: Assumptions and opportunities identified by The Latino Partnership. *Journal of Acquired Immunodeficiency Syndromes, 63*(Supplement 1), S32–S35.

Rhodes, S. D., Duck, S., Alonzo, J., Downs, M., & Aronson, R. E. (2013). Intervention trials in community-based participatory research. In D. Blumenthal, R. J. DiClemente, R. L. Braithwaite & S. Smith (Eds.), *Community-based participatory research: Issues, methods, and translation to practice* (pp. 157–180). New York, NY: Springer

Rhodes, S. D., Hergenrather, K. C., Duncan, J., Ramsey, B., Yee, L. J., & Wilkin, A. M. (2007). Using community-based participatory research to develop a chat room-based HIV prevention intervention for gay men. *Progress in Community Health Partnerships: Research, Education, and Action, 1*(2), 175–184.

Rhodes, S. D., Hergenrather, K. C., Duncan, J., Vissman, A. T., Miller, C., Wilkin, A. M., . . . Eng, E. (2010). A pilot intervention utilizing Internet chat rooms to prevent HIV risk behaviors among men who have sex with men. *Public Health Reports, 125*(Supplement 1), 29–37.

Rhodes, S. D., Hergenrather, K. C., Griffith, D., Yee, L. J., Zometa, C. S., Montaño, J., & Vissman, A. T. (2009). Sexual and alcohol use behaviours of Latino men in the south-eastern USA. *Culture, Health & Sexuality, 11*(1), 17–34.

Rhodes, S. D., Hergenrather, K. C., Montano, J., Remnitz, I. M., Arceo, R., Bloom, F. R., . . . Bowden, W. P. (2006). Using community-based participatory research to develop an intervention to reduce HIV and STD infections among Latino men. *AIDS Education and Prevention, 18*(5), 375–389.

Rhodes, S. D., Hergenrather, K. C., Vissman, A. T., Stowers, J., Davis, A. B., Hannah, A., . . . Marsiglia, F. F. (2011). Boys must be men, and men must have sex with women: A qualitative CBPR study to explore sexual risk among African American, Latino, and white gay men and MSM. *American Journal of Men's Health, 5*(2), 140–151.

Rhodes, S. D., Hergenrather, K. C., Wilkin, A. M., & Jolly, C. (2008). Visions and voices: Indigent persons living with HIV in the southern United States use photovoice to create knowledge, develop partnerships, and take action. *Health Promotion Practice, 9*(2), 159–169.

Rhodes, S. D., Kelley, C., Simán, F., Cashman, R., Alonzo, J., Wellendorf, T., . . . Reboussin, B. (2012). Using community-based participatory research (CBPR) to develop a community-level HIV prevention intervention for Latinas: A local response to a global challenge. *Women's Health Issues, 22*(3), 293–301.

Rhodes, S. D., Leichliter, J. S., Sun, C. J., & Bloom, F. R. (2016). The HoMBReS and HoMBReS Por un Cambio interventions to reduce HIV disparities among immigrant Hispanic/Latino men. *MMWR, 65*(1), 51–56.

Rhodes, S. D., Mann, L., Alonzo, J., Downs, M., Abraham, C., Miller, C., . . . Reboussin, B. A. (2014). CBPR to prevent HIV within ethnic, sexual, and gender minority communities: Successes with long-term sustainability. In S. D. Rhodes (Ed.), *Innovations in HIV prevention research and practice through community engagement* (pp. 135–160). New York, NY: Springer.

Rhodes, S. D., Mann, L., Simán, F. M., Song, E., Alonzo, J., Downs, M., . . . Hall, M. A. (2015). The impact of local immigration enforcement policies on the health of immigrant Hispanics/Latinos in the United States. *American Journal of Public Health, 105*(2), 329–337.

Rhodes, S. D., McCoy, T. P., Hergenrather, K. C., Vissman, A. T., Wolfson, M., Alonzo, J., . . . Eng, E. (2012). Prevalence estimates of health risk behaviors of immigrant Latino men who have sex with men. *Journal of Rural Health, 28*(1), 73–83.

Rhodes, S. D., McCoy, T. P., Tanner, A. E., Stowers, J., Bachmann, L. H., Nguyen, A. L., & Ross, M. W. (2016). Using social media to increase HIV testing among gay and bisexual men, other MSM, and transgender persons: Outcomes from a randomized community trial. *Clinical Infectious Diseases, 62*(11), 1450–1453. doi:10.1093/cid/ciw127

Schaal, J. C., Lightfoot, A. F., Black, K. Z., Stein, K., White, S. B., Cothern, C., . . . Eng, E. (2016). Community-guided focus group analysis to examine cancer disparities. *Progress in Community Health Partnerships, 10*(1), 159–167. doi:10.1353/cpr.2016.0013

Seifer, S. D., & Maurana, C. A. (2000). Developing and sustaining community-campus partnerships: Putting principles into practice. *Partnership Perspectives, 1*(2), 7–11.

Song, E. Y., Vissman, A. T., Alonzo, J., Bloom, F. R., Leichliter, J. S., & Rhodes, S. D. (2012). The use of prescription medications obtained from non-medical sources among immigrant Latinos in the rural southeastern US. *Journal of Health Care for the Poor and Underserved, 23*(2), 678–693.

Streng, J. M., Rhodes, S. D., Ayala, G. X., Eng, E., Arceo, R., & Phipps, S. (2004). Realidad Latina: Latino adolescents, their school, and a university use photovoice to examine and address the influence of immigration. *Journal of Interprofessional Care, 18*(4), 403–415.

Sun, C. J., Stowers, J., Miller, C., Bachmann, L. H., & Rhodes, S. D. (2015). Acceptability and feasibility of using established geosocial and sexual networking mobile applications to promote HIV and STD testing among men who have sex with men. *AIDS and Behavior, 19*(3), 543–552.

Tanner, A. E., Mann, L., Song, E., Alonzo, J., K., S., Arellano, E., . . . Rhodes, S. D. (2016). weCare: A social media-based intervention designed to increase HIV care linkage, retention, and health outcomes for racially and ethnically diverse young MSM. *AIDS Education and Prevention, 28*(3), 216–230.

Wallerstein, N. (1994). Empowerment education applied to youth. In A. C. Matiella (Ed.), *The multicultural challenge in health education* (pp. 153–176). Santa Cruz, CA: ETR Associates.

Wallerstein, N., & Duran, B. (2010). Community-based participatory research contributions to intervention research: The intersection of science and practice to improve health equity. *American Journal of Public Health, 100*(Suppl 1), S40–S46.

Yardley, L., Morrison, L., Bradbury, K., & Muller, I. (2015). The person-based approach to intervention development: Application to digital health-related behavior change interventions. *Journal Medical Internet Research, 17*(1), e30. doi:10.2196/jmir.4055

PART 5

PROMISING PRACTICES: ETHICAL ISSUES

Ethics of health research traditionally focuses on the protection of human participants as carried out by institutional review boards (IRBs) (e.g., university IRBs or Indian Health Service IRBs). These protections primarily emphasize the Belmont principles of respect for persons (voluntary participation), beneficence (maximizing benefits), and justice (balancing risks and benefits) (see Chapter 15). Such focus can be categorized as research regulation. These legal protections are certainly an important part of any research project, and yet the ethical focus in CBPR expands beyond the rights of individual research participants.

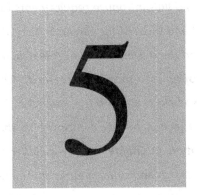

A number of scholars in the past decade have sought to expand the discussion of CBPR ethics beyond simply IRB regulations (Banks & Brydon-Miller, 2018; see also Chapters 14 to 16). For example, the stewardship of CBPR through governance can be an ethical stance (see Chapter 16). Stewardship includes the protection of community (and individual) interests, enhances the

development of equitable partnerships and effective collaboration, provides legitimacy for the research by ensuring appropriate approvals are obtained, builds capacity in the community, and ensures the community and cultural perspective is provided throughout the research process to increase the quality of the research and the effectiveness of interventions.

Stewardship can be provided by a number of sources. In Native communities, the use of tribal research review boards and IRBs introduce requirements for community protections and benefits along with cultural fit and focus of the research. They also require collaboration in all phases of the research including the dissemination of research. In Native and non-Native communities, advisory boards are often used to steward research. Further, partnership agreements and evaluation frameworks also help to steward the research.

The three chapters in this section further contribute to this expansion of ethical issues beyond simple research regulation. In Chapter 14, Myra Parker describes how the application of CBPR principles enhances research and cultural ethics in American Indian and Alaska Native (AI/AN) communities. She argues that cultural issues are critical for AI/AN communities and that CBPR principles and practices enable researchers and community members to integrate culture into the research and intervention process. This integration enables partnerships to improve the quality and impact of the research and intervention and hence meet an ethical obligation of community benefit. Further, she suggests that CBPR principles and practices throughout the research and dissemination process ensure ethical research protocols are used and help to avoid research violations and unintended consequences such as stigma for the community.

In Chapter 15, Rachel Morello-Frosch, Phil Brown, and Julia Green Brody discuss how CBPR (re)shapes the ethical oversight of human subjects protection in research. They argue that strict and traditional IRB review of CBPR can result in unintended violations of the very ethical principles review committees are charged to uphold. They argue this is in part because of the seeking of IRBs to protect research participants as individuals, whereas CBPR seeks to protect individuals and communities. This ethical tension has profound implications for the viability and logistics of CBPR projects. The authors suggest ways to manage these tensions to ensure that CBPR projects are supported, which is especially important given the increased uptake of community-engaged methods in biomedical and social science research.

In Chapter 16, Sarah Flicker, Adrian Guta, and Robb Travers broaden the focus of ethics beyond IRBs to examine "everyday ethics" of CBPR. Specifically, they note that many of the ethical issues faced by CBPR practitioners fall outside the traditional purview of IRBs. It is in the everyday choices about how to engage communities (with myriad "right" and "wrong" answers) that morals, ethics, values, and principles may conflict. The authors identify and discuss four key points in the life cycle of a typical CBPR project: (1) laying the groundwork; (2) getting "permission," governance as stewardship, and honoring community protocols; (3) project implementation and working with peer researchers; and (4) sharing work and ending the cycle. They illuminate each challenge and offer a brief case study for consideration and reflection to explore the idea of researchers "as active moral agents."

REFERENCE

Banks, S. and Brydon-Miller, M. (Eds.). (2018). Ethics in participatory research for health and social well-being, London, Routledge.

CHAPTER

14

CBPR PRINCIPLES AND RESEARCH ETHICS IN INDIAN COUNTRY

MYRA PARKER

AMERICAN INDIAN/ALASKA NATIVE (AI/AN) communities and individuals have experienced harm from research, medical practitioners, and health systems, leading to distrust of research and medicine. Over three thousand AI/AN women were sterilized without their knowledge or consent during the 1960s and through the 1970s, some as young as sixteen years old (Lawrence, 2000). Indian Health Service physicians recommended sterilizations based on discriminatory views of AI/AN people. In research, Arizona State University researcher Therese Ann Markow obtained DNA samples from Havasupai tribal members to use in a diabetes study in the early 1990s (Garrison, 2013). She gave samples to researchers at ASU and other labs across the country. Study participants and the tribe assert they were not informed these samples would be given to other researchers or that they would be used to study mental health problems, consanguinity, and tribal migrations. They further stated in court documents that these practices resulted in individual and community harm from stigma, as well as from a lack of informed consent, and went against important cultural beliefs.

These cases raise issues about the ethics of research processes, particularly the informed consent process required of research participants. Beyond research ethics specified in the Common Rule, it is also important to consider the cultural elements of research that may not fit neatly into an ethics discussions. The Common Rule refers to the federal regulations governing human subjects research. These cultural elements shape the nature of health problems and interventions and the rights of people to define those problems and interventions. Research ethics discussions limited to the Common Rule focus exclusively on individual informed consent and other Belmont principles rather than considering culture and community benefits, two critical aspects of research with AI/AN communities and individuals.

Community-based participatory research (CBPR) principles (see Chapter 3) reinforce Indigenous research ethics and help to bring Western and Indigenous research ethics into an integrated perspective (Pearson, Parker, Fisher, & Moreno, 2014). CBPR ensures inclusion of AI/AN cultures and social and environmental considerations unique to Indian Country through every stage of the research process. Adhering to CBPR principles helps researchers and AI/AN communities to accurately assess potential harms and benefits from research methods, participation, and dissemination; improves research knowledge for AI/AN in general; and can help improve external validity of research findings. For example, using CBPR principles can ensure inclusion of subgroups within the community, such as elders, who may not be part of a non-CBPR approach. Inclusion of these subgroups helps research teams gather comprehensive perspectives of public health needs and possible contributing factors, enhancing generalizability across the entire AI/AN population of interest (Wallerstein & Duran, 2010). Thus, CBPR can provide an important approach for addressing cultural issues throughout the research process in a meaningful and appropriate way.

INCORPORATING CULTURAL ELEMENTS THROUGH CBPR PRINCIPLES

One of the most important contributions of CBPR is to ensure the inclusion of culture and cultural diversity in the research process. Specifically, a culture-centered approach encourages a recognition of the importance of culture, the voice or agency of community members in defining problems and solutions, and societal transformations related to culture and agency (Dutta, 2007; Wallerstein et al., under review). Not only does a culture-centeredness approach and understanding of the culture(s) of participating communities support improved research ethics, but also it improves the overall fit and quality of the research. Kagawa-Singer, Dressler, George, and Elwood (2016) recognize culture as follows: (1) is a schema created by humans, (2) helps to support community members' survival and well-being, and (3) helps group members interpret the world through social norms of beliefs, attitudes, spiritual and emotional explanations, and practices. These authors further argue that our cultural frameworks operate through multiple dimensions. Not only do they integrate biological, psychological, and sociological aspects of our communities but also they rely on our relationships with the world around us, including the natural world. Cultures are complex and necessarily incorporate aspects of surrounding geography, historical realities, social norms and trends, and the political realm (Kagawa-Singer et al., 2016).

Research translation, application, and dissemination benefit from culture-centeredness in the research process. Ignoring culture when conducting research in diverse communities can result in a poor fit for health interventions and lower uptake of intervention content (Vaeth, Wang-Schweig, & Caetano, 2017), let alone ethical violations of informed consent and related issues such as in the Havasupai Diabetes Study. The principal investigator in the Havasupai Diabetes Study failed to obtain informed consent from individual tribal participants for research on their DNA samples for health conditions and tribal characteristics outside the scope of diabetes research originally specified. In fact, paying attention to key cultural elements can have positive health impacts. This section explores several components of Kagawa-Singer et al.'s (2016) definition of culture to illustrate how cultural elements can work with CBPR principles to shape health outcomes.

Kagawa-Singer et al. (2016) describe how culture is related to several key domains that in turn affect health behaviors including (but not limited to) spiritual and emotional explanations of health and well-being and health knowledge and practices. Spiritual and emotional explanations of health and well-being can influence health behaviors. For example, use of traditional healers is a spiritual and emotional approach to addressing health issues and varies across tribes. In a study of two large tribes, Southwest tribal members experiencing lifetime substance abuse disorder and lifetime comorbid depression or anxiety and substance disorders turned to traditional healers more frequently than members of a Northern Plains tribe (Beals et al., 2005). Using CBPR to understand these differences by involving community members early in the process and building from community strengths could help improve access to traditional healers, improve partnerships between traditional healers and mental health and medical professionals, and perhaps destigmatize mental health services and substance disorder treatment. AI/AN spiritual leaders involved through an advisory board or other meaningful roles may provide the cultural context relevant to AI/AN help-seeking behaviors, specifically for mental health or substance use issues. Such an approach helps to avoid an erroneous assumption that different tribal groups use traditional healers at the same rate, thus ensuring the CBPR principle of "fit to the local cultural context." Involving spiritual leaders and other stakeholders from both tribal communities could support hypothesis development of the circumstances under which tribal members would be likely to seek care.

A second key cultural element is health understanding and knowledge as it relates to health practices. For example, a recent study examined AI/AN parents, youth, and health providers' understanding of human papillomavirus (HPV) screening. Teens, the most at-risk group in the study, were less likely to endorse the statement that HPV can cause cervical cancer. By contrast, young adults were most likely to indicate HPV can cause cervical cancer, even compared to Indian Health Service (IHS) providers. No teens indicated that they believed HPV to be a rare infection, whereas about 40 percent of parents, young adults, and IHS providers indicated they believed it to be rare (Schmidt-Grimminger et al., 2013). Given the disparity of health knowledge across high-risk groups, parents, and providers, community partnerships supported through CBPR processes could represent an important step to improve HPV knowledge in this community. In non-Native communities, addressing these knowledge differences might include having open dialogue to enhance comprehension. However, in some AI/AN communities, discussing sexual practices may be considered taboo. Relying on a non-Native approach might dissuade participants from learning important information. Facilitating collaborative processes in all phases of the research, one of the CBPR principles, could support understanding of key cultural beliefs and norms, resulting in improved interventions and education and avoiding any unintended consequences to enhance the knowledge of HPV.

A final illustration of Kagawa-Singer et al.'s (2016) notion of culture includes structural and ecological elements. CBPR supports research partnerships in the process of integrating broader social, economic, and other environmental factors that affect population health into research plans. For example, an AI/AN family of five living ten miles outside of downtown

Seattle and without a car may need to travel two hours by bus, one way, for their children to see the doctor at the only medical facility that offers IHS-subsidized care in Seattle. Thus, the structural limitations of the Seattle urban transportation system disproportionately affect families living in poverty, resulting in barriers to health care for these families. By combining this perspective with cultural humility, researchers can gain a more comprehensive understanding of the challenges communities face, resulting in improvements in research planning, implementation, and community fit. Cultural humility (see Appendix 4) includes committing to an ongoing relationship with communities, acknowledging the fluidity and subjectivity of culture, and thereby challenging individuals and institutions to address inequalities (Fisher-Borne, Cain, & Martin, 2015). Cultural humility represents an important competency to achieve adherence to the spirit of CBPR and also ensures a strong fit with community ethics perspectives.

ENSURING ETHICS THROUGH THE APPLICATION OF CBPR PRINCIPLES

Although the previous section illustrates how application of CBPR principles can address ethical issues related to cultural elements, this section highlights how CBPR principles and practices can ensure broader ethical adherence throughout stages in the research. The CBPR principle of using a cyclical and iterative process presents opportunities to revisit study fit and the ethics of study decisions throughout the research process. From the conceptualization stage through dissemination, communities have important insight in the research that affects their communities (James et al., 2014).

Recognizing the community as a unit of identity constitutes an important first step. For AI/AN communities, some may be defined by reservation boundaries, and others, such as urban Indian communities, may be defined by community members. Defining community informs how IRBs or other research-approval entities may review human subject involvement on behalf of the community partner. Such a recognition helps to avoid unintended ethical violations and also ensures the cultural perspective of community boards are included in the research ethics processes.

Discussing research ideas constitutes a critical next step in working with AI/AN communities. All too often researchers have made decisions about research questions or selected their own priorities for health research in AI/AN communities (Walters & Simoni, 2009). Incorporating community input in the problem-definition phase could include feedback on the initial literature reviews to describe the public health issues, identifying appropriate scientific resources, and recognizing that "gray literature," non-peer-reviewed materials such as government reports, tribal reports, and Indigenous or other community resources, may provide critical information.

Scientific methodology and research design may also benefit from reliance on the CBPR framework. Communities have preferences in choosing the research design, identifying the sample, providing input on recruitment strategies, and identifying or giving feedback on the measures used for health outcomes and cofactors (Corbyn, 2011). Discussing human subjects' protections with community stakeholders fits in with CBPR practices (Harding et al., 2012; Quigley, 2015). Establishing informed consent requirements, ensuring cultural norms and expectations are met, and understanding the unique vulnerabilities without stigmatizing communities all contribute to a clear, mutual understanding of how research ethics will be upheld. CBPR approaches can support development of the plan for analysis to ensure community input.

Many diverse communities, including AI/AN communities, are ambivalent about randomized controlled trials (RCT) (Massey & Kirk, 2015). Although communities understand that the RCT is the "gold standard" for ensuring unbiased results, they also recognize that the requirements for an RCT may be challenging for community members. Discussing the methodology and analysis offers all partners opportunities to discuss potential risks and benefits, build trust, and to clarify everyone's expectations of the research process, and concerns about individual- and community-level risks.

Including community input in the study dissemination plan supports trust building (Lucero, 2013; Chapter 5), which is an important CBPR principle. Many AI/AN communities require community review and approval of publications and presentations prior to dissemination (Brugge & Missaghian, 2006; Foster et al., 1999; Navajo Nation IRB, 2003; Tribal IRBs, 2008). In addition to supporting human subjects and community protections, community contributions can assist and support meaningful dissemination (Chen, Diaz, Lucas, & Rosenthal, 2010). Academic publications may be useful for researchers or physicians, but most communities require research results in a different format for decision making, program development, and community capacity building. This may necessitate translation of research results into materials, building on community strengths, with content easily used by community stakeholders. These efforts guard against stigmatization and other community-level harms as well as ensure an equitable role in decision making for AI/AN communities.

Culture-centeredness, as a CBPR principle, represents CBPR praxis and, in research projects involving AI/AN communities, a key CBPR outcome. As CBPR praxis (or the cycle of reflection, action, reflection practice), it means developing, relying on, and incorporating a meaningful process in the research to ensure community decision making and cultural knowledge in formulating interventions and research designs. As a key CBPR outcome, culture-centeredness, brought about by the amalgamation of culture, community agency, and voice, can lead to community benefits such as cultural revitalization and community transformations. Community voice and decision making about the use of data in general, and not just about specific cultural practices, embody an important CBPR principle that recognizes the importance of cultural and community worldviews for decision making. One example is establishing a clear, multidirectional process for summarizing study results aimed to inform tribal partners. This process ensures knowledge democracy across partners and supports community action for improved health outcomes.

Incorporating community voice in decision making operationalizes another CBPR principle of supporting community empowerment. Community voice can facilitate agreement across the research partnership as to the best steps and deliverables for community use. Tribal decision making may vary by stakeholder, given the results of a research study. As an example, for a study involving elementary school children, tribal program managers may have a different need and focus for the data as compared to tribal leaders. Data at the level of the school district may reflect a high degree of school absenteeism, which may support a conclusion that improved school engagement is needed to incentivize school attendance and make the content more relevant for students. Thus, a tribal program manager would work to integrate tribal culture(s) into the educational materials.

By contrast, tribal leaders may examine the overall population-level data and identify the public health need—for example, to reduce the risk of underage alcohol use. Tribal leadership

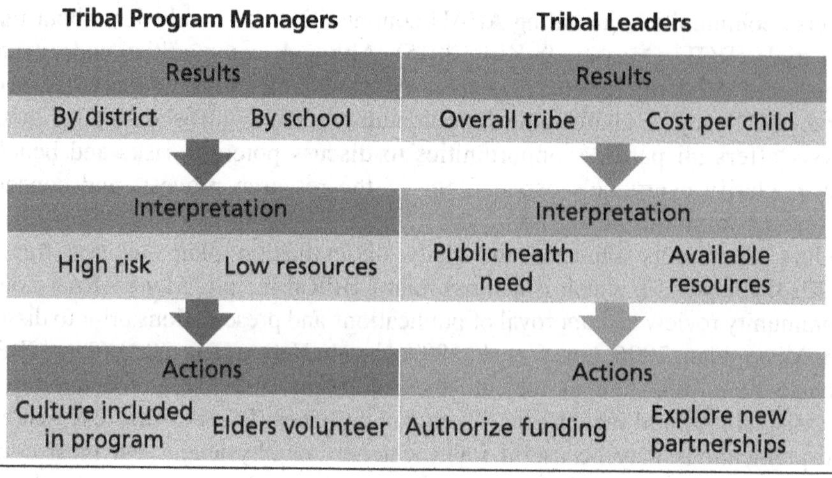

FIGURE 14.1 *Integrate Knowledge and Action for the Mutual Benefit of All Partners*

may then be able to authorize additional funding to after-school programs to ensure children have a safe alternative to settings in which alcohol use may be promoted. In this example, the research findings may focus on alcohol use and school absenteeism as major outcomes, which are then translated by tribal stakeholders into action to support improvements in overall health and well-being for elementary school students. This process supports the Indigenous research ethics principle of "doing good" across the community to ensure community benefit, which contrasts with the principle of beneficence in the Belmont Report, which espouses the notion of "do no harm" to individuals participating in research (see Figure 14.1).

CONCLUSION

Culture matters in public health research with AI/AN communities as well as in research implementation, translation, and dissemination. CBPR principles, in combination with human subject protection principles, help to include culture in public health research for improved relevance and benefit to AI/AN communities involved in the research. CBPR also reinforces adherence to ethics principles, supporting diverse communities by offering a meaningful opportunity to discuss and make decisions about what research makes sense for them and the community as a whole.

QUESTIONS FOR DISCUSSION

1. In the following scenario, how do CBPR principles inform research decisions?
2. How do ethics principles and CBPR principles relate to the community context described in the scenario?
3. How does culture play a role in understanding CBPR and ethics applications?
4. How could an understanding of structural inequities and context inform research decisions?

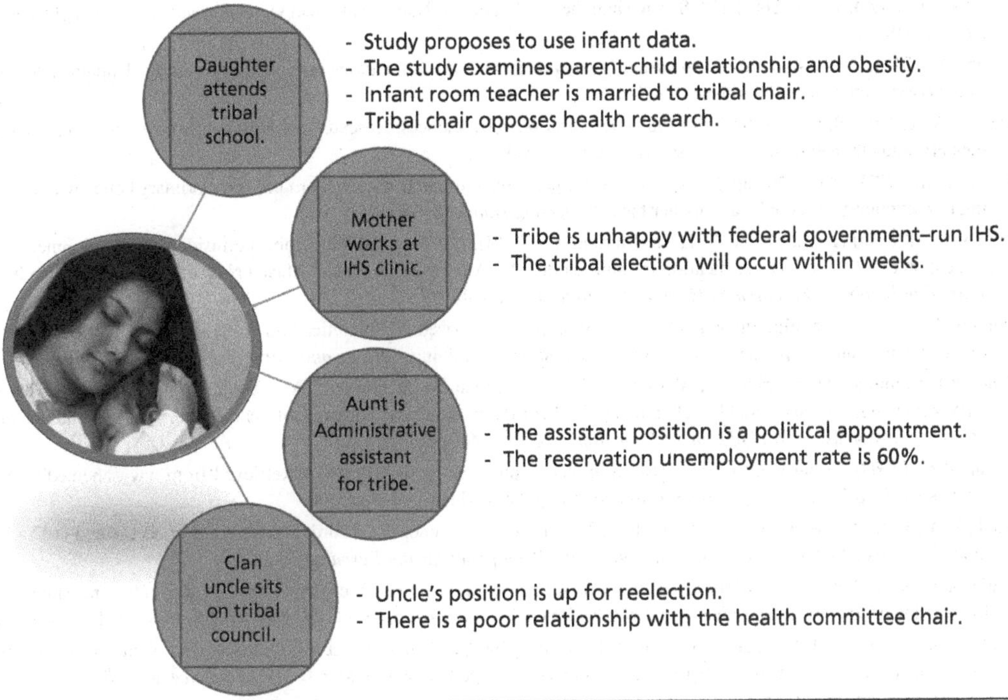
Daughter attends tribal school.
- Study proposes to use infant data.
- The study examines parent-child relationship and obesity.
- Infant room teacher is married to tribal chair.
- Tribal chair opposes health research.
Mother works at IHS clinic.
- Tribe is unhappy with federal government–run IHS.
- The tribal election will occur within weeks.
Aunt is Administrative assistant for tribe.
- The assistant position is a political appointment.
- The reservation unemployment rate is 60%.
Clan uncle sits on tribal council.
- Uncle's position is up for reelection.
- There is a poor relationship with the health committee chair.

Research Scenario: Applying CBPR in a Tribal Setting

REFERENCES

Beals, J., Manson, S. M., Whitesell, N. R., Spicer, P., Novins, D. K., & Mitchell, C. M. (2005). Prevalence of DSM-IV disorders and attendant help-seeking in two American Indian reservation populations. *Archives of General Psychiatry, 62,* 99–108.

Brugge, D., & Missaghian, M. (2006). Protecting the Navajo people through tribal regulation of research. *Science and Engineering Ethics, 12,* 491–507.

Chen, P. G., Diaz, N., Lucas, G., & Rosenthal, M. S. (2010). Dissemination of results in community-based participatory research. *American Journal of Preventive Medicine, 39,* 372–378.

Corbyn, Z. (2011). Science education: Research on the reservation. *Nature, 471,* 25–26.

Dutta, M. J. (2007). Communicating about culture and health: Theorizing culture-centered and cultural sensitivity approaches. *Communication Theory, 17,* 304–328.

Fisher-Borne, M., Cain, J. M., & Martin, S. L. (2015). From mastery to accountability: Cultural humility as an alternative to cultural competence. *Social Work Education, 34,* 165–181.

Foster, M. W., Sharp, R. R., Freeman, W. L., Chino, M., Bernsten, D., & Carter, T. H. (1999). The role of community review in evaluating the risks of human genetic variation research. *The American Journal of Human Genetics, 64,* 1719–1727.

Garrison, N. A. (2013). Genomic justice for Native Americans. *Science, Technology, & Human Values, 38,* 201–223.

Harding, A., Harper, B., Stone, D., O'Neill, C., Berger, P., Harris, S., & Donatuto, J. (2012). Conducting research with tribal communities: Sovereignty, ethics, and data-sharing issues. *Environmental Health Perspectives, 120,* 6–10.

James, R., Tsosie, R., Sahota, P., Parker, M., Dillard, D., Sylvester, I., . . . Kiana, G. (2014). Exploring pathways to trust: A tribal perspective on data sharing. *Genetics in Medicine, 16,* 820–826.

Kagawa-Singer, M., Dressler, W. W., George, S. M., & Elwood, W. N. (2016). *The cultural framework for health: An integrative approach for research and program design and evaluation.* National Institutes of Health. Retrieved from https://obssr.od.nih.gov/about-us/publications/

Lawrence, J. (2000). The Indian Health Service and the sterilization of Native American women. *American Indian Quarterly, 24,* 400–419.

Lucero, J. (2013). *Trust as an ethical construct in community-based participatory research partnerships*. Unpublished doctoral dissertation. University of New Mexico.

Massey, A., & Kirk, R. (2015). Bridging Indigenous and western sciences: Research methodologies for traditional, complementary, and alternative medicine systems. *SAGE Open, 5.*

Navajo Nation IRB. (2003). Navajo Nation IRB: A unique human research review board has three primary concerns: Protecting its community, its people, and its heritage. *Protecting Human Subjects, pp.* 1–2.

Pearson, C. R., Parker, M., Fisher, C. B., & Moreno, C. (2014). Capacity building from the inside out: Development and evaluation of a CITI ethics certification training module for American Indian and Alaska Native community researchers. *Journal of Empirical Research on Human Research Ethics, 9,* 46–57.

Quigley, D. (2015). Promoting human subjects training for place-based communities and cultural groups in environmental research: Curriculum approaches for graduate student/faculty training. *Science and Engineering Ethics, 21,* 209–226.

Schmidt-Grimminger, D., Frerichs, L., Black Bird, A. E., Workman, K., Dobberpuhl, M., & Watanabe-Galloway, S. (2013). HPV knowledge, attitudes, and beliefs among Northern Plains American Indian adolescents, parents, young adults, and health professionals. *Journal of Cancer Education, 28,* 357–366.

Tribal IRBs. (2008). Tribal IRBs shape research in Native populations. *IRB Advisor*. Retrieved from www.ahcmedia.com/articles/15543-tribal-irbs-shape-research-in-native-populations?trendmd-shared=0

Vaeth, P. A., Wang-Schweig, M., & Caetano, R. (2017). Drinking, alcohol use disorder, and treatment access and utilization among U.S. racial/ethnic groups. *Alcoholism: Clinical and Experimental Research, 41,* 6–19.

Wallerstein, N., & Duran, B. (2010). Community-based participatory research contributions to intervention research: The intersection of science and practice to improve health equity. *American Journal of Public Health, 100*(Suppl 1), S40–S46.

Wallerstein, N., Oetzel, J. G., Duran, B., Magarati, M., Pearson, C., Belone, L., et al. (under review). Conceptualizing and measuring the culture-centered approach in community based participatory research. *Social Science & Medicine.*

Walters, K. L., & Simoni, J. M. (2009). Decolonizing strategies for mentoring American Indians and Alaska Natives in HIV and mental health research. *American Journal of Public Health, 99*(Suppl 1), S71–S76.

CHAPTER 15

DEMOCRATIZING ETHICAL OVERSIGHT OF RESEARCH THROUGH CBPR

RACHEL MORELLO-FROSCH, PHIL BROWN, AND JULIA GREEN BRODY

Sections of the chapter have been adapted from the following articles with permission: Morello-Frosch, R., Varshavsky, J., Liboiron, M., Brown, P., & Brody, J. G. (2015). Communicating results in post-Belmont era biomonitoring studies: Lessons from genetics and neuroimaging research. *Environmental Research, 136,* 363–372. https://doi.org/10.1016/j.envres.2014.10.001; and Brown, P., Morello-Frosch, R., Brody, J. G., Altman, R. G., Rudel, R. A., Senier, L., . . . Simpson, R. (2010). Institutional review board challenges related to community-based participatory research on human exposure to environmental toxins: A case study. *Environmental Health: A Global Access Science Source, 9,* 39. https://doi.org/10.1186/1476-069X-9-39.

THE BENEFITS OF CBPR for community partners have been well documented and include enhanced co-learning between community members and scientists, informing organizing efforts, and linking research to policy action. Less, however, has been written on how CBPR (re)shapes the scientific enterprise itself by improving its *rigor*, *relevance,* and *reach* (Balazs & Morello-Frosch, 2013). *Rigor* refers to the practice and promotion of good science—in the study design, data collection, and interpretation phases of research. *Relevance* refers to whether science is asking the right questions and how it elucidates opportunities for individual action or collective change. *Reach* encapsulates the degree to which knowledge is disseminated to diverse audiences and translated into useful tools for the scientific, regulatory, policy, and lay arenas. Moreover, by advancing the three Rs, CBPR not only facilitates *translational* research (i.e., application of research findings to community stakeholders and policy makers) but also, more important, *transformational* research, which changes the nature of and approach to scientific inquiry itself. Figure 15.1 displays a continuum from translational to transformational research. On the left side, traditional scientific methods collect community data or conduct research translation but treat community members as passive study participants. Toward the right, community engagement increases, as members move from being mere study participants to being active research partners.

This transformative potential of CBPR also extends to the realm of research ethics and oversight of human subject protections. In general, institutional review board (IRB) review of human subjects research encourages investigators to systematically assess the ethical implications of their proposed projects. This process involves feedback and revisions of study protocols to ensure that ethical concerns are thoroughly vetted. In addition to encouraging researchers to reflect on the ethics of their work, IRB members themselves often learn about novel methodological approaches to research, such as CBPR, and their unique ethical nuances.

Increasing uptake of community-engaged methods in biomedical and social science research makes it particularly important that scientists, funders, community members, and university administrators work toward defining human subjects' protection procedures that support CBPR projects instead of inadvertently hindering them.

OVERSIGHT OF PROTECTION OF STUDY PARTICIPANTS IN RESEARCH

In 1979, the Belmont Report established principles for the use of human subjects in scientific research. Developed partly in response to the notorious Tuskegee syphilis study on poor African American men, Belmont identified three basic principles governing the ethical use of human

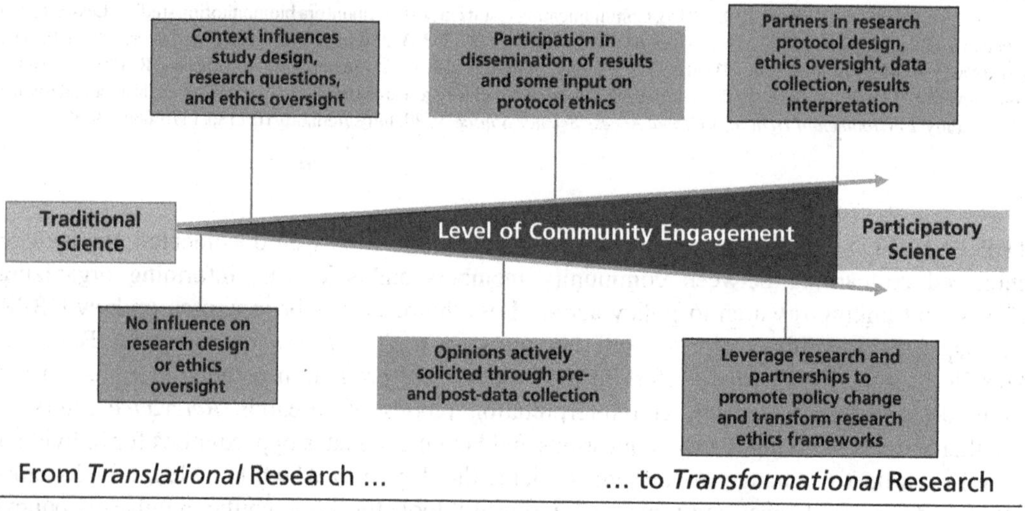

FIGURE 15.1 *The Three Rs of CBPR: Rigor, Relevance, and Reach*
Source: Adapted from Balazs and Morello-Frosch (2013).

research subjects: (1) “respect for persons,” or voluntary participation and special protection for those who lack the capacity to make their own decisions; (2) “beneficence,” or maximizing benefits and reducing risk to participants; and (3) “justice,” or balancing risk and benefits and selecting study participants only “for reasons directly related to the problem being studied” (US Department of Health and Human Services, 1979).

Implementation of the Belmont Report principles falls to IRBs that protect individual research participants through confidentiality, informed consent, and oversight of research design and communications with participants. But although IRBs have been the traditional enforcers of the Belmont principles, they are not the only place where those principles have found expression. Those same principles form the basis of CBPR, with affected communities engaging more directly in research design and the collection and analysis of individual-level human data. CBPR explicitly focuses on problems that affect whole communities—environmental toxics, for example—and thus is different from most biomedical research, which takes the individual as its primary subject. In CBPR, researchers work closely with community members and community-based organizations to develop research agendas, conduct analyses, and disseminate results and information. This merging of community interests and community action reflects another distinct quality of CBPR: its commitment to advocacy for the public good and creating open access to information (Morello-Frosch et al., 2015).

CBPR takes “respect for persons” to a new level: not only do study participants voluntarily participate in research but also they *actively* collaborate to carry it out. This inclusion reflects CBPR’s commitment to the principles of “beneficence” and “justice,” because the active involvement and scrutiny of study participants encourages the fair assessment and distribution of the research’s risks and benefits. Further, the CBPR concept of data as co-owned and the practice of giving research participants the right to decide whether to have full access to research results helps ensure they have sufficient information to make informed choices during and after the study and is thus consistent with Belmont’s emphasis on informed consent. In the process, research “subjects” are transformed into research “participants.” CBPR thus enters a “post-Belmont era,” blurring the traditional roles of researcher and subject and taking seriously the insight, energy, and objectives that members of the affected community bring (Morello-Frosch et al., 2015).

CBPR further embodies the “respect for persons” principle by protecting research participants from being objectified and dehumanized. By encouraging the active involvement of study participants in the research process, CBPR greatly reduces the chances that they will be objectified in the first place. As participants in the design and implementation of the research plan, members of the affected community have a level of “informed consent” far deeper than typically occurs in conventional research. Thus CBPR achieves “respect for persons” by democratizing the research process and encouraging scientist experts to work alongside communities, rather than treating them as objects of study.

Despite these characteristics, however, IRB review of CBPR projects can result in unintended violations of the very principles they seek to uphold. This is in part because of implicit assumptions embedded in the Belmont Report that were adopted by IRBs but that contradict other CBPR principles. For example, IRBs, following Belmont, assume that the research participant is an *individual,* whereas CBPR sees research participants as individuals and as a *community* of individuals (Deeds et al., 2008). This difference has profound implications for confidentiality, the dissemination of information, and the assessment of risks and benefits.

The differing assumptions and discord that CBPR researchers and IRBs bring to the research process come into sharpest relief in the context of two particular CBPR practices: (1) direct community participation in research and (2) the reporting back of individual results to study participants who want them. With regard to the first issue, some clinical researchers form community or patient advisory boards to promote more communication with study participants and broader community benefits of research. Still, CBPR represents a much deeper form of engagement with study communities that makes it qualitatively different. CBPR's inclusion of laypersons and others traditionally outside the research process means university IRBs must consider collaborators who are outside their conventional jurisdiction. As a result, IRBs may be reluctant to oversee human subjects' protection compliance for such outside partner organizations. This can lead to misunderstandings and unnecessary delays as IRBs deliberate about whether and how to extend their jurisdiction into new territory, and, if accommodation is not reached, it can restrict the roles that community members can play or force partner organizations to pay for independent IRB coverage. In terms of the second issue, IRBs may object when a community-based organization challenges traditional academic norms by engaging in research and advocacy. Moreover, the CBPR practice of reporting back, and the philosophy of openness that informs it, challenges IRB assumptions about who controls the flow of data produced in human subjects research, when and whether those data should be made available to members of an affected community, and what the nature and duration of the researcher–study participant relationship should be.

These differences and the unfamiliarity of many IRBs with CBPR can create undue obstacles and extensive delays to conducting research, diminish the benefit of research for study participants, and potentially cause them harm as they anxiously await unnecessarily long periods of time to receive results that could inform strategies for protecting their future health and that of their families and communities. Not surprisingly, some researchers have criticized the rigidity of IRB reviews, particularly for low-risk, non-intrusive research (Bosk & DeVries, 2004; Brown et al., 2010).

UNCERTAINTY OF STUDY RESULTS AND PARTICIPANTS' RIGHT TO KNOW

A great tension in the ethical oversight of CBPR entails reporting back individual-level results with scientific uncertainty regarding implications for health. This is particularly the case in the realm of environmental health research, specifically in studies that characterize human exposures to a diverse array of environmental chemicals, through biomonitoring, for example. Since World War II, more than eighty-three thousand chemicals have been registered for commercial use in the United States, three thousand of which are produced or imported at 1 million pounds or more per year (Environmental Protection Agency, 2010, 2011). Most of these chemicals have little to no toxicity testing data, and information on exposure sources, mitigation strategies, and health implications remains elusive in many cases. Although we increasingly know more about the effects of chemicals on health, significant data gaps remain and raise ethical and scientific challenges for whether and how to report biomonitoring results to study participants. As our analytic capacity to detect chemicals in humans surpasses our ability to interpret results, scientists and IRB members have raised the question of whether it may be detrimental to share individual biomonitoring results with study participants. Hypothetically, a participant might be psychologically harmed by receiving results if their clinical significance is unknown or if no valid options exist to address the potential health risks they reveal (Shalowitz & Miller, 2005). Indeed, the National Bioethics Advisory Committee issued guidelines directing researchers to report biomarkers only when health implications are significant and recourse is available (National Bioethics Advisory Committee, 1999). These discussions may not, however, have adequately considered the distinction between communications related to genetic biomarkers, which are not modifiable, and chemical exposures, many of which are modifiable. When these clinical guidelines are applied to chemical exposure research, people are left unaware of the presence in their own bodies of environmental chemicals, often known to be harmful in animal studies and sometimes in in vitro and human studies.

From the perspective of CBPR, such rigid reporting-back guidelines are an affront to individuals' and communities' right to know, and by extension they tarnish the scientific process. More recently, several guidance documents, including the National Academy of Sciences biomonitoring report, now support participants' right to know their personal chemical biomonitoring results (Brody et al., 2014). Nevertheless, tensions between participants' right to know their exposure results and their capacity or right to act to reduce those exposures can raise ethical challenges when developing results communication protocols. For example, in some occupations (e.g., farm workers or custodians) study participants may not be able to take action to reduce their chemical exposures, either through the use of personal protective equipment or the substitution, reformulation, and purchasing of less-toxic products used at the workplace (Holmes, 2013; Senier, Mayer, Brown, & Morello-Frosch, 2007).

Research on reporting back in personal exposure studies and genetics research has also explored study participant perspectives and expectations, and evidence indicates that although some participants might opt out of learning their results, the vast majority believe they have a right to know. One study reported that 97 percent of participants wanted their personal exposure results even if the health implications of the data were not clear (Brody et al., 2007), mirroring the strong desire of study participants in other environmental health studies to receive results (Quandt et al., 2004). As in chemical biomonitoring studies, public attitudes about genetic research also support the return of individual results. A poll concluded that for many study participants, learning their results was a large motivating factor for enrolling in such studies, with 75 percent of 4,500 respondents in one study indicating they would be less likely to volunteer if individual results were not provided (Kaufman, Murphy, Scott, & Hudson, 2008). Despite this evidence, individualized reporting back remains controversial because many IRBs question whether scientific uncertainty regarding health implications of genetic or chemical biomonitoring results can cause undue stress among study participants. This concern may not be warranted. A randomized study investigating the psychological effects of disclosure of an apolipoprotein E (APOE) allele associated with Alzheimer's disease revealed that participants who were informed that they had a genetic predisposition did not show more symptoms of anxiety or depression compared to participants who did not get their screening results (Green et al., 2009). Similarly, evaluation of reporting back in community-engaged chemical biomonitoring studies indicates that participants who learn about their chemical exposures gain valuable knowledge about environmental health, which results in behavioral changes (e.g., in purchasing decisions) and engagement in the policy process (e.g., public testimony to influence industrial permitting decisions) (Adams et al., 2011; Altman et al., 2008).

Although the biomedical-driven research approach may recommend only reporting back when health implications are clear, a CBPR right-to-know approach empowers study participants with knowledge, addresses community-level concerns such as stigmatization, and promotes policy change. Moreover, biomedical ethics are evolving to promote more open communication between patients and health care providers, which has begun to influence communication strategies in environmental health science. For example, through the Open Notes project, patients who were given electronic access to their doctors' notes reported feeling more informed and in control of their health care, which in turn fostered more productive communication and shared decision making with their health care providers (Delbanco et al., 2012). Digital communication interfaces used in the clinical setting can be adapted for applications to report back individual results in CBPR projects by providing options for receiving results, including views using text or graphs, in different languages, and aimed at diverse literacy levels (Boronow et al., 2017). Key to this reporting-back process is a collective consensus about who represents the interests of study communities and how their priorities can be effectively incorporated into protocol development.

IRB CHALLENGES RELATED TO INDIGENOUS RESEARCH

Scientific research has a sordid history in the colonization of Indigenous peoples within the United States and internationally through the devaluation, appropriation, and desecration of their beliefs, cultural practices, knowledge, environments, and bodies (Smith, 2012; Tallbear, 2013). Yet because tribes and other Indigenous peoples insist on their status as sovereigns, they also resist, regulate, initiate, collaborate in, and govern ethics in research in ways that support self-governance, cultural-centeredness, and sovereignty. (See Chapter 14.) For example, CBPR has been used to carry out innovative environmental health research projects with Native Americans and Alaska Natives in the United States (Hoover et al., 2012). US law requires extensive review by multiple IRBs; the Indian Health Service tasks area IRBs and tribal epidemiology centers with evaluating research projects involving American Indians and Alaska Natives. These committees generally include Native and non-Native members, researchers, clinicians, and community leaders (Saxton et al., 2015). In addition, tribes often have their own internal IRBs or tribal government approval processes to vet research projects to ensure that they align with their own priorities as well as legal and cultural standards (Becenti-Pigman et al., 2008; Macaulay et al., 1998; Sharp & Foster, 2002).

Although tribal IRBs seek to protect the sovereignty and interests of Indigenous communities, some external IRBs universalize ethical frameworks in ways that "homogenize" Indigenous communities as inherently vulnerable without regard to their interests, relationships to researchers, and leadership roles on research projects. These cases have been characterized as a form of "ethical imperialism" that undercuts the research priorities and methods advanced by Indigenous communities (Saxton et al., 2015). For example, a tribal collaboration with university researchers and a nongovernmental organization to conduct a CBPR breast milk biomonitoring study among Alaska Native communities was thwarted by the Alaska area IRB, despite clear support from tribal leadership, on the grounds that the study might discourage breastfeeding. For nearly five years, tribal and university researchers sought to alleviate these ethical concerns by demonstrating to the area IRB that their biomonitoring study protocol would report results to participants while actively encouraging the continuation of breastfeeding. After several rounds of protocol review, the study was effectively thwarted by the Alaska area IRB. The rigidity of the IRB review in effect undermined key Belmont tenets, including autonomy, beneficence, and justice, by hindering the project, which sought to address Alaska Native communities' concerns about exposures to environmental chemicals in the Arctic region (Saxton et al., 2015).

Most tribal research rules of conduct and reviews strongly encourage reporting back of findings to individual research participants and the tribe (American Indian Law Center, 1999; Freeman, 2004). Reporting back is viewed as a continuous process rather than something that occurs only at the conclusion of a research project (American Indian Law Center, 1999). The Indigenous Rights Protection Act (Indigenous Peoples Council on Biocolonialism, 2000) stipulates that researchers must provide a detailed plan on how they will communicate aggregate study results to diverse audiences and personal results to individual participants and how the community at large will be educated or empowered by their proposed study. A description of the frequency and manner by which the aggregate data and progress reports will be shared with research review committees along with a communication plan for presenting aggregate results to the community at large must be included in study protocols. These requirements affirm the notion of community engagement in the development of results communication protocols and the reporting back of results as a reflexive and iterative process.

DEMOCRATIZING ETHICAL OVERSIGHT OF RESEARCH

The problems that arise in IRB reviews of CBPR projects stem from the different assumptions and objectives of diverse parties and institutions. Therefore, effective solutions require engagement by all research stakeholders to successfully navigate ethical review of multi-partner CBPR projects: IRBs, CBPR researchers, community and CBO partners, study participants, and funding agencies. Researchers need to educate those IRB members who may be unfamiliar with CBPR in its basic principles, its scientific and community benefits, and the unique ethical considerations it raises. CBPR scientists can connect community partners with IRB staff members to demonstrate the community's involvement in the research process and how their perspective on human subjects' protection is key to the project's success. This might include inviting community partners to meetings with the IRB. Research partners can include this "community consent" in their IRB application. If the IRB lacks the familiarity, experience, or the skill set necessary for assessing the ethical issues posed by a research project, an outside expert should be brought in to educate the board.

Funding institutions, including National Institutes of Health and National Science Foundation, should offer human subjects guidance specific to CBPR research and should sensitize universities to the importance of supporting community groups. (See Appendix 8 for community CITI trainings.) University IRBs should be aware that community organizations may operate on different time lines and that the intense and lengthy university IRB-reporting process can create conflicts for them. Even when giving this guidance to IRBs, researchers doing grant-funded community-based research should include ample time for IRB review in their grant proposals. Similarly, funding agencies should encourage academic institutions to provide IRB oversight to academic and community partners to avoid unnecessary delays and expenses in protocol reviews. They may want to promote consortium-based approval whereby one institution's IRB is accepted by others in the consortium; indemnification may be necessary so that universities do not bear responsibility for the actions of community partners.

IRBs need to better regulate potential conflicts of interest their members may bring to the review process, particularly when an institution might have a vested interest in the outcome of a proposed study (because of its implications for a state public health agency action, for example). A survey of 893 IRB members at one hundred academic institutions found that 36 percent had at least one relationship with industry in the previous year, of which only two-thirds had been disclosed to the IRB. Of those reporting conflicts, nearly one-third had participated in the reviews anyway (Campbell et al., 2006).

Finally, IRBs must reexamine how they address situations in which participants want access to and disclosure of their own study results. In some cases, this necessitates continued interaction between researchers and participants, a process that IRBs have traditionally been reluctant to allow and are poorly designed to manage. In the case of environmental health research, iterative rounds of approval for ongoing communication with study participants can create delays that undermine researchers' relationships with participants and harm participants' capacity to take timely action to reduce their exposures. To address this challenge, IRBs can review prototypes of such communication protocols without having to repeat reviews with every iteration. Participants may also want to share their personal results with other study participants and have the collective power to disseminate their results through their own networks and broader public forums. Putting the brakes on individual reporting back could push confidentiality protections to collide with the principle of beneficence. Thus, CBPR challenges IRBs to reassess the seemingly contradictory elements of the Belmont principles and develop alternatives that do not require choosing one principle over another.

WORKING WITH COMMUNITY AND TRIBAL IRBS

University IRBs are not the only forums in which community benefits and risks of research may be assessed. Some tribes convene their own review boards to evaluate collectively whether proposed research is justified and benefits the community (Quigley, 2006). Although tribal IRBs have the power of regular IRBs, other community review boards do not meet the requirements for oversight of federally funded research, requiring an additional IRB to provide formal guarantees. Academic IRBs reviewing research proposals on behalf of such communities need to understand their form and organization, their needs and vulnerabilities, and their governance and communication structures for disseminating research (Weijer, 1998).

Community representation in the review process would be helpful not only to those explicitly engaged in CBPR but also to those engaged in individual research who may not have considered the effects of their research on communities. NIH rules were clarified in 1998 to ensure that IRBs have "knowledge of the local research context," but although one member of the IRB must be from outside the institution, direct community representation is not required (National Institutes of Health, 1998). Community representation on academic IRBs usually takes the form of large, well-established organizations rather than grassroots groups and does not usually reflect the demographic composition of the communities under study. We recommend that IRBs recruit not just any community members but those who have experience in either CBPR or other community-engaged research. This can provide benefits to many IRB reviews because of the creativity, flexibility, and respect for human subjects' protection that comes with CBPR experience.

CONCLUSION

The very CBPR practices that concern many IRBs are exactly those that make community-engaged work so valuable for communities and the scientific enterprise and that enhance ethical oversight of research. Yet, ethical tensions emerge when communities that seek to conduct research with scientific collaborators face roadblocks by IRBs, which delay or deny approval of study protocols and hinder investigations of potentially significant public questions that affect them. Efforts to overcome these IRB challenges require a holistic understanding of how CBPR researchers and study communities (whether defined by geography, class, ethnicity, or other socially salient distinctions) collaborate in ways that empower the latter to play a central role in the scientific enterprise, which includes ethical oversight of research. Ultimately, IRBs will need to go beyond simply modifying traditional review procedures to fundamentally incorporate how CBPR ethics redefines the scientific enterprise itself, including researcher-participant relationships, academic-community interactions, and the right to know the significance of study results for individual and collective action to improve public health.

QUESTIONS FOR DISCUSSION

1. What are the elements of CBPR that can advance ethical oversight of public health and medical research?
2. How can IRBs do more to integrate ethical protections for study communities and individual study participants?

REFERENCES

Adams, C., Brown, P., Morello-Frosch, R., Brody, J. G., Rudel, R., Zota, A., . . . Patton, S. (2011). Disentangling the exposure experience: The roles of community context and report-back of environmental exposure data. *Journal of Health and Social Behavior, 52*(2), 180–196. https://doi.org/10.1177/0022146510395593

Altman, R. G., Morello-Frosch, R., Brody, J. G., Rudel, R., Brown, P., & Averick, M. (2008). Pollution comes home and gets personal: Women's experience of household chemical exposure. *Journal of Health and Social Behavior, 49*(4), 417–435.

American Indian Law Center. (1999). *Model tribal research code: With materials for tribal regulation for research and checklist for Indian health boards* (3rd ed.). Albuquerque, NM: Author.

Balazs, C. L., & Morello-Frosch, R. (2013). The three R's: How community-based participatory research strengthens the rigor, relevance and reach of science. *Environmental Justice, 6*(1). https://doi.org/10.1089/env.2012.0017

Becenti-Pigman, B., White, K., Bowman, B., Palmenteer-Holder, N. L., & Duran, B. (2008). Research policies, processes and protocol: The Navajo Nation Human Research Review Board. In M. Minkler & N. Wallerstein, *Community-based participatory research for health: Processes and outcomes* (2nd ed., pp. 441–446). San Francisco, CA: Jossey-Bass.

Boronow, K. E., Sussman, H. P., Gajos, K. Z., Rudel, R. A., Arnold, K. C., Brown, P., Morello-Frosch, R., Havas, L., & Brody, J. G. (2017). DERBI: A digital method to help researchers offer "right-to-know" personal exposure results. *Environmental Health Perspectives, 125*(2), A27–A33.

Bosk, C., & DeVries R. (2004). Bureaucracies of mass deception: Institutional review boards and the ethics of ethnographic research. *Annals of the American Academy of Political and Social Science, 595*, 249–263.

Brody, J. G., Dunagan, S. C., Morello-Frosch, R., Brown, P., Patton, S., & Rudel, R. A. (2014). Reporting individual results for biomonitoring and environmental exposures: Lessons learned from environmental communication case studies. *Environmental Health: A Global Access Science Source, 13,* 40. https://doi.org/10.1186/1476-069X-13-40

Brody, J. G., Morello-Frosch, R., Brown, P., Rudel, R. A., Altman, R. G., Frye, M., . . . Seryak, L. M. (2007). Improving disclosure and consent. *American Journal of Public Health, 97*(9), 1547–1554. https://doi.org/10.2105/AJPH.2006.094813

Brown, P., Morello-Frosch, R., Brody, J. G., Altman, R. G., Rudel, R. A., Senier, L., . . . Simpson, R. (2010). Institutional review board challenges related to community-based participatory research on human exposure to environmental toxins: A case study. *Environmental Health: A Global Access Science Source, 9,* 39. https://doi.org/10.1186/1476-069X-9-39

Campbell, E. G., Weissman, J. S., Vogeli, C., Clarridge, B. R., Abraham, M., Marder, J. E., & Koski, G. (2006). Financial relationships between institutional review board members and industry. *New England Journal of Medicine, 355*(22), 2321–2329. https://doi.org/10.1056/NEJMsa061457

Deeds, B. G., Castillo, M., Beason, Z., Cunningham, S. D., Ellen, J. M., Peralta, L., & Adolescent Trials Network for HIV/AIDS interventions. (2008). An HIV prevention protocol reviewed at 15 national sites: How do ethics committees protect communities? *Journal of Empirical Research on Human Research Ethics, 3*(2), 77–86. https://doi.org/10.1525/jer.2008.3.2.77

Delbanco, T., Walker, J., Bell, S. K., Darer, J. D., Elmore, J. G., Farag, N., . . . Leveille, S. G. (2012). Inviting patients to read their doctors' notes: A quasi-experimental study and a look ahead. *Annals of Internal Medicine, 157*(7), 461. https://doi.org/10.7326/0003-4819-157-7-201210020-00002

Environmental Protection Agency. (2010). *HPV chemical hazard data availability study.* Retrieved October 15, 2011, from www.epa.gov/HPV/pubs/general/hazchem.htm

Environmental Protection Agency. (2011). *TSCA chemical substance inventory.* Retrieved December 17, 2012, from www.epa.gov/oppt/existingchemicals/pubs/tscainventory/index.html

Freeman, W. L. (2004). *The protection of potential individual volunteers and tribal communities in research involving the Indian Health Service (IHS) (IRB appendix).* Portland, OR: Northwest Portland Area Indian Health Service Institutional Review Board.

Green, R. C., Roberts, J. S., Cupples, L. A., Relkin, N. R., Whitehouse, P. J., Brown, T., . . . Farrer, L. A. (2009). Disclosure of APOE genotype for risk of Alzheimer's disease. *New England Journal of Medicine, 361*(3), 245–254. https://doi.org/10.1056/NEJMoa0809578

Holmes, S. (2013). *Fresh fruit, broken bodies.* Berkeley CA: University of California Press.

Hoover, E., Cook, K., Plain, R., Sanchez, K., Waghiyi, V., Miller, P., . . . Carpenter, D. O. (2012). Indigenous peoples of North America: Environmental exposures and reproductive justice. *Environmental Health Perspectives, 120*(12), 1645–1649. https://doi.org/10.1289/ehp.1205422

Indigenous Peoples Council on Biocolonialism. (2000). Indigenous Research Protection Act. Retrieved January 15, 2017 from www.ipcb.org/

Kaufman, D., Murphy, J., Scott, J., & Hudson, K. (2008). Subjects matter: A survey of public opinions about a large genetic cohort study. *Genetics in Medicine: Official Journal of the American College of Medical Genetics, 10*(11), 831–839. https://doi.org/10.1097/GIM.0b013e31818bb3ab

Macaulay, A. C., Delormier, T., McComber, A. M., Cross, E. J., Potvin, L. P., Paradis, G., Kirby, R. L., Saad-Haddad, C., & Desrosiers, S. (1998). Participatory research with native community of Kahnawake creates innovative code of research ethics. *Canadian Journal of Public Health, 89,* 105–108.

Morello-Frosch, R., Varshavsky, J., Liboiron, M., Brown, P., & Brody, J. G. (2015). Communicating results in post-Belmont era biomonitoring studies: Lessons from genetics and neuroimaging research. *Environmental Research, 136,* 363–372. https://doi.org/10.1016/j.envres.2014.10.001

National Bioethics Advisory Committee. (1999). *Research involving human biological materials: Ethical issues and policy guidance.* Rockville, MD: National Institutes of Health.

National Institutes of Health. (1998). *IRB knowledge of local research context.* Bethesda, MD: Division of Human Subjects Protection OPPR.

Quandt, S. A., Doran, A. M., Rao, P., Hoppin, J. A., Snively, B. M., & Arcury, T. A. (2004). Reporting pesticide assessment results to farmworker families: Development, implementation, and evaluation of a risk communication strategy. *Environmental Health Perspectives, 112*(5), 636–642.

Quigley, D. (2006). A review of improved ethical practices in environmental and public health research: Case examples from native communities. *Health Education and Behavior, 33,* 130–147.

Saxton, D. I., Brown, P., Seguinot-Medina, S., Eckstein, L., Carpenter, D. O., Miller, P., & Waghiyi, V. (2015). Environmental health and justice and the right to research: Institutional review board denials of community-based chemical biomonitoring of breast milk. *Environmental Health, 14,* 90. https://doi.org/10.1186/s12940-015-0076-x

Senier, L., Mayer, B., Brown, P., & Morello-Frosch, R. (2007). School custodians and green cleaners new approaches to labor-environment coalitions. *Organization and Environment 20,* 304–324.

Shalowitz, D. I., & Miller, F. G. (2005). Disclosing individual results of clinical research: Implications of respect for participants. *Journal of American Medical Association, 294*(6), 737–740.

Sharp, R. R., & Foster, M. W. (2002). Community involvement in the ethical review of genetic research: Lessons from American Indian and Alaska Native populations. *Environmental Health Perspectives, 110,* 145–148.

Smith, L. T. (2012). *Decolonizing methodologies: Research and indigenous peoples*. London, UK: Zed Books.

Tallbear, K. (2013). *Native American DNA: Tribal belonging and the false promise of genetic science*. Minneapolis, MN: The University of Minnesota Press.

US Department of Health and Human Services. (1979). *The Belmont report: Ethical principles and guidelines for the protection of human subjects of research*. Bethesda, MD: The National Commission for the Protection of Human Subjects of Biomedical and Behavioral Research.

Weijer, C. (1998). Protecting communities in research: Philosophical and pragmatic challenges. *Cambridge Quarterly of Healthcare Ethics, 8,* 501–513.

CHAPTER

16

EVERYDAY CHALLENGES IN THE LIFE CYCLE OF CBPR

BROADENING OUR BANDWIDTH ON ETHICS

SARAH FLICKER, ADRIAN GUTA, AND ROBB TRAVERS

IN 2007 WE began to reflect on the mismatch between traditional research ethics and institutional review board (IRB) guidelines and the kinds of issues that are encountered in community-based participatory research (CBPR) (Flicker et al., 2007). Although we recognized the importance of ethics review and the need for researchers to be accountable for their practices, we were able to show that the dominant biomedical orientation of review processes was creating challenges given the flexible, collaborative, and relational approaches found in CBPR. After assessing the applicability of institutional research ethics review to CBPR principles, we proposed suggestions for improving their relevance. Since then, Canadian research ethics board practices are demonstrating slow but promising paradigmatic and policy shifts (Guta, Wilson, et al., 2010). Many US IRBs are also improving their procedures for more effective and relevant reviews of CBPR research.

In continuing to study ethics in the context of CBPR, we have become increasingly convinced that IRB institutional changes are only one piece of the ethics puzzle. Many ethical challenges and daily dilemmas faced by CBPR practitioners fall outside the purview of review boards (Mikesell, Bromley, & Khodyakov, 2013). It is in the everyday choices about how to engage community, with myriad "right" and "wrong" answers, that ethics, morals, values, and principles may conflict.

In response to the ways in which conventional research has historically been conducted *on* community (rather than *with* or *alongside*), CBPR has been positioned as an ethical alternative, based on core principles (see Chapter 3), that seeks to engage those most affected by health inequities in the research process as full and engaged partners. These principles codified a "new" way of operating that privileged relationality, multiple voices, and different ways of knowing. IRBs were never in a position to monitor these sets of ethical commitments, nor should they be. And yet, these ethical commitments have become for many CBPR practitioners a moral compass that guides our work. In choosing to describe our work as CBPR, community and academic practitioners actively align themselves with this principled promise that boasts the potential for transformational outcomes.

However, these principles do not always work congruently and sometimes may be in tension with each other (Travers et al., 2013). It is in these moments of tension, and in the quest to honor these values, that new ethical dilemmas emerge. Work in, and with, community is often messy, complicated, and hard. In contrast to romanticized notions of empowered citizens engaging in transformational social justice work, we often become mired in the slow, tedious work of making hard quotidian decisions ranging from resource allocation to data analysis. However, the ways we go about making decisions on these matters is not trivial. As Eikeland (2006) so eloquently writes,

> the ethical questions that concern action research often seem to operate on a smaller scale, such as: who is to be involved; how and why; who makes decisions and how; whose interpretations are to prevail and why; how do we write about and publish on people involved; who owns the ideas developed; etc. . . . The consequences of letting such questions pass unattended may be—intended or not—the spontaneous, habitual emergence of subtle power structures on a micro-level, not clearly visible in the beginning, but accumulating and "petrifying" over time into larger unwanted patterns. (pp. 38–39)

Thus, in this chapter, we pay attention to what Banks and her colleagues (2013) call the "everyday ethics" of CBPR. The small and everyday decisions that represent choices about power, equity, and justice often operate at the microlevel of weighing these moment-to-moment alternatives. Together, these everyday decisions inform how CBPR practitioners understand themselves as moral agents and engage community in ethical ways.

LAYING THE GROUNDWORK

The first step in beginning a CBPR project, of gathering and establishing your team, can be one of the most ethically fraught. It brings up many questions about "who represents a community?" (Jewkes & Murcott, 1998) and who has the authority to speak or make decisions on behalf of his or her peers. These questions are particularly challenging to answer in contexts in which there is no elected or official leadership body. For many stigmatized and marginalized communities, there may be few entities that purport to represent them, and they are unlikely to reflect the diversity of community experience. In such cases, the "community" may be represented by elected officials, government bureaucrats, staff members, volunteers, board members of community-based organizations, or those with lived experience of the issue under study. If research foci are controversial, there may be strong differences of opinion and political histories between communities that are fractured and divided by the issues under study. Decisions about representation and governance will have powerful implications for the kinds of questions that get asked and the ways they get answered. For researchers who may be "outsiders" the complications multiply: they may not immediately realize the complexities of the landscape (D'Alonzo, 2010). For example, a group of CBPR practitioners were surprised to discover the range of perspectives about substance use within a small health care facility and inadvertently created conflict between clients (Strike et al., 2016). They ultimately had to redesign their project and implemented new steps to ensure participants felt supported.

Sorting out representation, governance, and human resource policies can be a fraught matter. Projects may decide to include community members as coinvestigators, create community advisory boards, hire community members as core staff, or all three. There is a wide range of the degree to which each project takes up participatory principles and is successful in democratizing power. In "Case Example 16.1: Trans PULSE," the research team intentionally developed a governance structure that ensured that trans community members' voices would always be in the majority.

CASE EXAMPLE 16.1 Trans PULSE

The Trans PULSE Project is a CBPR project that investigates the impact of social exclusion and discrimination on the health of trans people in Ontario, Canada. The project was initiated by trans community members with support from an ally who worked at a local health center. Together, these community partners sought out academic partners and built a governance model in which key decisions had to be approved in contexts when 50 percent +1 of the vote came from trans members of the investigator's team.

Source: Travers et al. (2013).

GETTING "PERMISSION": GOVERNANCE AS STEWARDSHIP AND HONORING COMMUNITY PROTOCOLS

As a result of the ongoing colonial violence done in the name of research, many Indigenous communities are now demanding that research done in, and with, their communities formally seek tribal permission and adopt more participatory practices. CBPR's decolonizing potential (Darroch & Giles, 2014) has excited many scholars who are actively trying to adapt methodologies to local contexts (Castleden, Garvin, & First Nation, 2008; Simonds & Christopher, 2013). In addition to the original principles laid out by Israel et al. (1998), CBPR projects operating in Indigenous contexts must also acknowledge history, context, tribal sovereignty, and Indigenous ways of knowing (LaVeaux & Christopher, 2009).

Furthermore, the idea of CBPR governance as stewardship has gained popularity. "Governance as stewardship enhances protection of the community, helps foster research partnerships and appropriate . . . approval of research by community bodies, ensures benefit for the community, provides legitimacy and shares responsibility for the research, provides community control, and builds research capacity in communities" (Oetzel et al., 2015, p. 1161).

Tribal and community review boards have sprung up to offer additional community relevant protections beyond traditional ethics review, attending to such issues as cultural safety, community consent, and important process concerns (Shore et al., 2011). Moreover, in Canada, research policy now requires researchers seeking to do research with Indigenous communities to first obtain formal permission from those communities (Tri-Council of Canada, 2010). Although recognizing Indigenous sovereignty, this has been complicated to put into practice. Many reserve communities have formal leadership structures or research councils, yet those seeking to do research with urban Aboriginal people may find figuring out "whom to ask" difficult. Nevertheless, this model of showing clear respect for communal rights to self-determination may be an important one to pursue when working with other groups that have also suffered colonial (and other forms) of oppression. In "Case Example 16.2: Taking Action! Building Aboriginal Youth Leadership for HIV Prevention," the research team sought informed communal consent from several formal bodies and informal stakeholders to ensure that their protocol was ethical, culturally safe, and respectful in specific local contexts.

CASE EXAMPLE 16.2 Taking Action! Building Aboriginal Youth Leadership for HIV Prevention

This CBPR project worked with six Indigenous communities across Canada. The project was governed by a national Indigenous youth council and the Canadian Aboriginal AIDS Network's National Research Advisory Committee, made up of diverse community stakeholders. In addition to formally getting approval through multiple university-based research ethics boards, the project also sought formal permission from various local entities. In urban centers, project leads met with local community-based organizations and sought permission. In a northern Inuit community, they received approval from the mayor and elected officials. In multiple First Nations communities, Taking Action approached local and regional research councils (if constituted) and band councils.

Source: Flicker et al. (2014).

PROJECT IMPLEMENTATION

Gathering data in marginalized communities can be extremely challenging. Sometimes those with lived experience of the issue under study are in the best position to navigate hidden networks. Peer researchers (PRs) are members of a research project's target population who are trained to participate as coresearchers (Flicker, Roche, & Guta, 2010; Greene et al., 2009). Recruiting, hiring, and managing peer researcher involvement can present unique ethical challenges (Guta, Flicker, & Roche, 2010).

Similar to all new staff members in a research project, peer researchers require extensive training. For some PRs, it may be the first time that they are working in professional environments, and additional supports may be necessary. This is particularly true for peer researchers who may be unintentionally triggered by the nature of their work duties (e.g., drug users collecting drug-related data). Because PRs may be navigating their own personal networks or operating in very small, tight-knit communities, special attention to helping PRs manage boundaries (e.g., maintaining confidentiality) may be challenging.

Despite the fact that PR positions may be seen as a step toward inclusion and increasing participation, care needs to be taken to think through the possibilities for real and meaningful power sharing (particularly when PRs are operating in a traditional, bureaucratic employee structure). As we have noted elsewhere, "Care should be taken to avoid research practices that benefit extensively from the labor and expertise of peer researchers, but offers little in return in the way of recognition, remuneration, or a sense of ownership of the work" (Flicker et al., 2010, p. 3). In "Case Study 16.3: Women's CBR Study," the research team had to change their original plans to accommodate the unique inclusion needs of their peer researchers.

Finding creative strategies for engaging PRs, and community partners in general, in data analysis has the potential to enrich analyses and interpretation and dissemination strategies (Cashman et al., 2008; Flicker, 2008). Evaluations reveal that this tends to be an area in which many projects fall short of their participatory promise (Flicker, Savan, Mildenberger, & Kolenda, 2008; Flicker et al., 2008); leaving PRs out of analysis can be unintentionally disempowering to those who are excluded (Travers et al., 2013).

CASE STUDY 16.3 **Women's CBR Study**

Women living with HIV were hired to conduct and facilitate focus groups with other HIV+ women. However, because of HIV-related stigma and complicated community relationships, the peer researchers did not want their names associated with project recruitment or dissemination materials. They were also reluctant to take leadership roles in focus group facilitation because many of them felt uncomfortable about the power dynamics this might set up with their peers. Peer researchers needed a number of additional (social, psychological, physical, and monetary) supports in place in order to succeed at their jobs.

Source: Logie, James, Tharao, and Loutfy (2012).

SHARING YOUR WORK AND ENDING THE CYCLE

The end of a project phase presents new ethical issues when thinking about how to share research findings in respectful and accessible formats, how to credit participation, and how to close a project. Some partners, particularly those from marginalized communities, may not see the utility of investing precious project time and resources into academic publications. Many may want to publicize results in more accessible ways (e.g., newsletters, press releases, blog posts, social media) to get the word out. Developing a comprehensive knowledge translation and exchange plan (Nixon, Casale, Flicker, & Rogan, 2012) that specifies data sharing and ownership protocols (Schnarch, 2004), often through memoranda of understanding—in advance—can be a useful strategy for figuring out *who* needs to be reached *how* and with *what* messages. Then, difficult conversations need to be had about how project resources will be allocated to realize these ambitions.

Another end-of-project issue is how people will get recognized and credited for their work. Academics and staff members from community-based organizations are often happy to have their job titles acknowledged. However, this may be more complicated when team members belong to stigmatized communities (e.g., drug using, sex working, HIV+). They may have invested substantial time and intellectual capital but have very mixed feelings about attaching their names to documents that may live on in the public record. For instance, a youth who is currently street involved and an activist on the project may not want to be affiliated as "the homeless youth" on a report or conference presentation years later when he or she may no longer identify with that experience. The traumas of disclosure may also have real legal implications for some. Care needs to be taken to carefully negotiate a plan for acknowledgment that takes into account present and potential future conditions. For instance, in "Case Study 16.4: Healing Home," the research team took extra precautions to ensure the long-term confidentiality and anonymity of previously homeless participants when a book about their project was being published.

Last, although academics and service providers often move from one project to another (following funding cycles), these research projects often become meaningful interventions for community members involved. They can provide structure, purpose, employment, and social support and referrals for health care, housing, and social services. Some community members invoke "family" when describing CBPR projects; these research projects can become a lifeline for more marginalized members of the team. Carefully planning for the end-of-project funding and creating a transition plan for all members of a team is a necessary ethical requirement.

CASE STUDY 16.4 **Healing Home**

Homeless young women were involved in a project that looked at social and structural barriers and facilitators to their health and well-being. At the time of their participation, the youth were all very excited about the project and proud of their role in it. However, a few years later, when the project was being turned into a book, some of the participants who had subsequently found housing and stability were very worried about the possible implications of being identified by current friends, partners, or employers. Extra caution was taken to ensure their anonymity.

Source: Oliver (2013).

CONCLUSION

The issues we have discussed are complex, and there are no "absolute" right ways of approaching them; careful ethical reflection throughout the research process can lead to creative and equitable responses. Reflection on the ways power operates in these micro moments can lead to strategies for opportunities to share control. For example, when a CBPR project is submitted for institutional ethics review, community partners may feel a sudden shift in power toward the university. Sharing full control in such moments is very likely not possible, but providing the space to discuss people's feelings in relation to the shift *is* possible (and necessary). Paying attention to such "relational" challenges in the life of a CBPR project is crucial.

As Banks and colleagues (2013) write, "This way of constructing the 'ethical' is to see the moral agent not just as an impartial deliberator, but also as an embedded participant with situated and partial relationships, responsibilities, values and commitments that frame and constrain ways of seeing, judging and acting in particular situations. Thus the 'ethical' is present in ways of being as well as acting, and in relationships and emotions, as well as conduct" (p. 266). In order for CBPR to truly be about reparative justice, we need to be "actuating a new type of ethical practice through mutuality, equity, and shared responsibility" (Bromley, Mikesell, Jones, & Khodyakov, 2015, p. 902).

QUESTIONS FOR DISCUSSION

Imagine you are building a new CBPR team and don't want to be caught off guard with unforeseen ethical challenges.

1. What governance, decision-making, and conflict resolution models will your team adopt to transform traditional power structures in ways that are reasonable and feasible? What could a partnership agreement cover to be helpful? What ethical principles are important for your team to uphold?
2. What kinds of training and supports will you put in place for peer researchers and other community members? How will you ensure that your research approach does not further stigmatize communities?
3. How will you plan for the end life of a project? What strategies can you build in to ensure a smooth transition for all team members?

REFERENCES

Banks, S., Armstrong, A., Carter, K., Graham, H., Hayward, P., Henry, A., . . . McNulty, A. (2013). Everyday ethics in community-based participatory research. *Contemporary Social Science, 8*(3), 263–277.

Bromley, E., Mikesell, L., Jones, F., & Khodyakov, D. (2015). From subject to participant: Ethics and the evolving role of community in health research. *American Journal of Public Health, 105*(5), 900–908.

Cashman, S., B., Adeky, S., Allen, A., J., Corburn, J., Israel, B. A., Montaño, J., . . . Wallerstein, N. (2008). The power and the promise: Working with communities to analyze data, interpret findings, and get to outcomes. *American Journal of Public Health, 98*(8), 1407–1417.

Castleden, H., Garvin, T., & First Nation, H.-a.-a. (2008). Modifying photovoice for community-based participatory Indigenous research. *Social Science & Medicine, 66*(6), 1393–1405. doi:https://dx.doi.org/10.1016/j.socscimed.2007.11.030

D'Alonzo, K. T. (2010). Getting started in CBPR: Lessons in building community partnerships for new researchers. *Nursing Inquiry, 17*(4), 282–288.

Darroch, F., & Giles, A. (2014). Decolonizing health research: Community-based participatory research and postcolonial feminist theory. *The Canadian Journal of Action Research, 15*(3), 22–36.

Eikeland, O. (2006). Condescending ethics and action research. *Action Research, 4*(1), 37–47. doi:10.1177/1476750306060054

Flicker, S. (2008). Who benefits from community-based participatory research? *Health Education & Behavior, 35*(1), 70–86.

Flicker, S., Danforth, J., Oliver, V., Konsmo, E., Wilson, C., Jackson, R., . . . Mitchell, C. (2014). "Because we have really unique art": Decolonizing research with Indigenous youth using the arts. *International Journal of Indigenous Health, 10*(1), 16–34.

Flicker, S., Roche, B., & Guta, A. (2010). *Peer research in action III: Ethical issues*. Toronto, Canada: Wellesley Institute.

Flicker, S., Savan, B., McGrath, M., Kolenda, B., & Mildenberger, M. (2008). If you could change one thing . . . What community-based researchers wish they could have done differently. *Journal of Community Development, 43*(2), 239–253.

Flicker, S., Savan, B., Mildenberger, M., & Kolenda, B. (2008). A snapshot of community-based research in Canada: Who? What? Why? How? *Health Education Research, 23*(1), 106–114.

Flicker, S., Travers, R., Guta, A., Macdonald, S., & Meagher, A. (2007). Ethical dilemmas in community-based participatory research: Recommendations for institutional review boards. *Journal of Urban Health, 84*(4), 478–493. doi:10.1007/s11524-007-9165-7

Greene, S., Ahluwalia, A., Watson, J., Tucker, R., Rourke, S. B., Koornstra, J., . . . Byers, S. (2009). Between skepticism and empowerment: The experiences of peer research assistants in HIV/AIDS, housing and homelessness community-based research. *International Journal of Social Research Methodology, 12*(4), 361–373.

Guta, A., Flicker, S., & Roche, B. (2010). *Peer research in action II: Management, support and supervision.* Toronto, Canada: Wellesley Institute.

Guta, A., Wilson, M., Flicker, S., Travers, R., Mason, C., Wenyeve, G., & O'Campo, P. (2010). Are we asking the right questions? A review of Canadian REB practices in relation to community-based participatory research. *Journal of Empirical Research on Human Research Ethics, 5*(2), 35–46.

Israel, B., Schulz, A., Parker, E., & Becker, A. (1998). Review of community-based research: Assessing partnership approaches to improve public health. *Annual Reviews Public Health, 19*(1), 173–194.

Jewkes, R., & Murcott, A. (1998). Community representatives: Representing the "community"? *Social Science and Medicine, 46*(7), 843–858.

LaVeaux, D., & Christopher, S. (2009). Contextualizing CBPR: Key principles of CBPR meet the Indigenous research context. *Pimatisiwin, 7*(1), 1.

Logie, C., James, L., Tharao, W., & Loutfy, M. R. (2012). Opportunities, ethical challenges, and lessons learned from working with peer research assistants in a multi-method HIV community-based research study in Ontario, Canada. *Journal of Empirical Research on Human Research Ethics, 7*(4), 10–19.

Mikesell, L., Bromley, E., & Khodyakov, D. (2013). Ethical community-engaged research: A literature review. *American Journal of Public Health, 103*(12), e7–e14.

Nixon, S. A., Casale, M., Flicker, S., & Rogan, M. (2012). Applying the principles of knowledge translation and exchange to inform dissemination of HIV survey results to adolescent participants in South Africa. *Health Promotion International, 28*(2), 233–243.

Oetzel, J. G., Villegas, M., Zenone, H., White Hat, E. R., Wallerstein, N., & Duran, B. (2015). Enhancing stewardship of community-engaged research through governance. *American Journal of Public Health, 105*(6), 1161–1167.

Oliver, V. (2013). *Healing home: Health and homelessness in the life stories of young women.* Toronto, Canada: University of Toronto Press.

Schnarch, B. (2004). Ownership, control, access, and possession (OCAP) or self-determination applied to research: A critical analysis of contemporary First Nations research and some options for First Nations communities. *Journal of Aboriginal Health, 1*(1), 80–95.

Shore, N., Brazauskas, R., Drew, E., Wong, K. A., Moy, L., Baden, A. C., . . . Seifer, S. D. (2011). Understanding community-based processes for research ethics review: A national study. *American Journal of Public Health, 101*(S1), S359–S364.

Simonds, V. W., & Christopher, S. (2013). Adapting Western research methods to Indigenous ways of knowing. *American Journal of Public Health, 103*(12), 2185–2192.

Strike, C., Guta, A., de Prinse, K., Switzer, S., & Carusone, S. C. (2016). Opportunities, challenges and ethical issues associated with conducting community-based participatory research in a hospital setting. *Research Ethics*, pp. 1–9. doi:10.1177/1747016115626496

Travers, R., Pyne, J., Bauer, G., Munro, L., Giambrone, B., Hammond, R., & Scanlon, K. (2013). "Community control" in CBPR: Challenges experienced and questions raised from the trans PULSE project. *Action Research, 11*(4), 403–422.

Tri-Council of Canada. (2010). Tri-Council policy statement 2: Ethical conduct for research involving humans. Retrieved May 11, 2017, from www.pre.ethics.gc.ca/pdf/eng/tcps2/TCPS_2_FINAL_Web.pdf

PART 6

PROMISING PRACTICES TO OUTCOMES: CBPR CAPACITY AND HEALTH

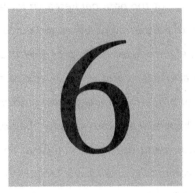

The importance of evaluation and assessment of the added value of equitable participatory practices among community, agency, other social actors and academic researchers has grown in this last decade of the consolidation of CBPR and community-engaged research approaches. An increased number of systematic reviews have identified multilevel outcomes and effective partnership practices (see Chapter 1). Although many of us are part of these national evaluation efforts, including identifying mixed-methods instruments and measures or metrics of engagement and partnering (see Appendix 10), the caution still exists to recognize the importance of contexts under which specific partnerships operate. Key questions to consider remain: (1) under what conditions and contexts do partnerships choose which practices are "best" or promising

in their experience, and (2) how will their chosen practices affect research designs and interventions to produce their desired (and also possibly unintended) outcomes within communities and the academy?

This section of the book provides three chapters on research and evaluation methodologies, measures, and outcomes as a result of using CBPR approaches. Chapter 17 by John G. Oetzel and colleagues presents the next stage of the national Research for Improved Health (RIH) study to identify measures and analyses of partnering practices and outcomes, using constructs from the four domains of the CBPR model introduced in Chapter 6. With a mixed methodology of Internet surveys of two hundred partnerships and seven diverse case studies, the authors present empirical data of associations of promising practices with outcomes, as well as options for how other partnerships can adapt the model and measures for their own evaluations.

Chapter 18 by Noelle Wiggins and colleagues compares and contrasts participatory evaluation with CBPR using two community health worker (CHW) initiatives, one in the United States and one in Nicaragua. The authors present a transformational participatory evaluation approach, as closest to CBPR's philosophy, which also incorporates decolonizing approaches to evaluation. They offer a cycle of participatory evaluation steps that enables all stakeholders, including the CHWs, to participate in all stages of the evaluation, including interpreting and dissemination of data for health improvements in their communities, and they end with lessons learned to ensure authentic participation of community.

Chapter 19 by Lorenda Belone, Derek M. Griffith, and Barbara Baquero takes a personal approach to outcomes by describing the role of CBPR training and research opportunities as pipelines to their own academic success as faculty members of color. These opportunities enabled their success in integrating their academic careers with a life calling of service to communities. Personal outcomes for participants in the research process, whether from the academy or community, are important human development outcomes, and, in this case, they served to strengthen the sustainability of CBPR within the larger research enterprise at the same time as diversifying the academy.

CHAPTER 17

EVALUATION OF CBPR PARTNERSHIPS AND OUTCOMES

LESSONS AND TOOLS FROM THE RESEARCH FOR IMPROVED HEALTH STUDY

JOHN G. OETZEL, BONNIE DURAN, ANDREW SUSSMAN, CYNTHIA PEARSON, MAYA MAGARATI, DMITRY KHODYAKOV, AND NINA WALLERSTEIN

AS NOTED IN previous chapters, community-based participatory research (CBPR) is a popular approach that uses equitable research partnerships to engage in community health improvement and reduce health inequities when working with underserved communities, Indigenous communities, communities of color, and other communities facing inequities in health or experiencing mistrust for past research issues (Atalay, 2010; Lorway et al., 2013). Despite the popularity of CBPR in practice, the science of CBPR has lagged behind. Although CBPR can and should be implemented based on social justice values (rather than simply utilitarian values) (Trickett, 2011), there is also a need to establish the conceptual and empirical rationale for its use. The development of several frameworks, the CBPR conceptual model (Chapter 6), a logic model emphasizing partnership synergy (Khodyakov et al., 2011) and a realist review of CBPR research (Jagosh et al., 2012), have advanced the theorizing and conceptual explanation of CBPR.

The empirical rationale for CBPR is starting to grow as well. As noted in Chapter 1, recent reviews demonstrate the positive impacts of community-engaged research (CEnR) in general and CBPR in particular for health outcomes (Cyril, Smith, Possamai-Inesedy, & Andre, 2015; O'Mara-Eves et al., 2015). These reviews provide strong justification for the benefit of CBPR and some evidence of its impact. At the same time, these reviews do not provide sufficient information about why CBPRs lead to health outcomes or how to evaluate the various elements of CBPR to improve partnership capacity and partnering. Further, effective evaluation requires a range of quantitative and qualitative tools. There are a number of evaluation frameworks in the literature, and yet some of the tools in these frameworks lack evidence of reliability and validity (Sandoval et al., 2012). (See Appendix 10 for further tools.)

The purpose of this chapter is twofold. First, we share the methods and measures that we developed in the Research for Improved Health (RIH) study. The quantitative and qualitative measures are valid and reliable evaluation tools that partnerships and outside evaluators can use to assess partnering process and outcomes. Second, we present evidence from the RIH study linking CBPR processes and contexts with outcomes, including CBPR capacity and system outcomes, community transformation, and health improvement. The chapter begins with a discussion of a previous different project that served as foundational for the evaluation tools and outcome data presented in the RIH study. We then discuss specific evaluations tools and outcomes of the RIH study and conclude by discussing how these tools can be used for evaluation purposes.

STUDY OF PARTNERSHIP SYNERGY

As part of the NIMH Partnered Research Center for Quality Care (PRC) in Los Angeles, a team of academic and community partners conducted the Partnership Evaluation Study (PES), which explored the process and outcomes of community engagement (CE) in research (Khodyakov et al., 2011, 2013). PES was conducted in 2010, and at that time, there was no rigorous empirical research that measured the extent to which community partners were engaged in the process of conducting research or evaluated the impact CE has on outcomes of partnered research projects. Grounded in the early conceptual model of community-academic partnerships (Wallerstein & Duran, 2010; Wallerstein et al., 2008), an existing measure of partnership synergy (Lasker, Weiss, & Miller, 2001; Weiss, Anderson, & Lasker, 2002) was supplemented with newly developed measures of CE in research and outcomes of partnered research projects.

Partnership synergy is an outcome of partnership functioning that facilitates the accomplishment of more than what can be done by individual partners on their own (Lasker et al., 2001; Weiss et al., 2002). On partnered research projects, academics contribute their research expertise and knowledge of evidence-based interventions, whereas community partners bring their understanding of community needs, local sociocultural contexts, and knowledge of community- and practice-based evidence. By benefiting from complementary strengths and areas of expertise, community-academic collaborations develop partnership synergy, which ultimately results in more comprehensive and sustainable programs as well as stronger relationships with the community at large. In a realist review of twenty-three partnerships, Jagosh et al. (2012) also found the importance of partnership synergy as a middle-range theory to explain the contribution of partnering processes to outcomes of culturally appropriate research, sustainability, capacity, and system changes. (See Appendix 6 for discussion of realist review methodology.)

The first step in the PES was the development of a logic model to link partnership characteristics (e.g., the extent of CE in research, partnership size, and duration); partnership functioning (e.g., leadership, decision making, efficiency, management, resources, and challenges encountered); partnership synergy; and partnership outcomes at a community and policy level (e.g., improved access and improved health) and personal level (e.g., professional development). A series of semi-structured interviews with academic and community leaders working on thirty-nine out of seventy-two mental health and substance abuse partnered projects affiliated with the PRC were conducted (details available in Khodyakov et al., 2011, 2013).

The primary goal of the interviews was to develop measures of CE in research and outcomes of partnered research projects to be used in the survey, which led to two approaches to measuring CE in research: (1) the community engagement in research index (CERI), which offers a multidimensional view of community participation in the research process, and (2) a three-model approach that differentiates among the levels of community participation (Khodyakov et al., 2013). The CERI included research steps from grant proposal writing and conducting background research; to developing sampling procedures and recruitment; to implementing the intervention and designing interview and survey questions, collecting, analyzing, and interpreting study findings; to dissemination. Then, three partnership models were created (Baker, Homan, Schonhoff, & Kreuter, 1999): (1) community partners only provide access to study participants and are not engaged in the research aspects of the project, (2) community partners are consulted and act as advisors but do not make any research-related decisions, and (3) community partners engage in the research activities. These three models became the response set for the activities in the CERI (1 = "Community partners did not participate in this activity"; 2 = "Community partners consulted on this activity"; 3 = "Community partners were actively engaged in this activity."). The CERI results in an index by summing the scores across the twelve research activities and dividing by three (4 = low engagement to 12 = high engagement).

The study findings suggested that more active engagement of community partners in research is positively associated with a number of perceived community- and policy-level outcomes, including more sustained partnerships among agencies, policy changes, and public recognition and acknowledgment from local policy makers and government officials. Moreover, partnerships with higher levels of community engagement in research are more likely to contribute to the perception of positive professional development of their members, whereas larger partnerships with higher levels of synergy may positively affect partners' perception of personal capacity. Finally, larger projects that actively engage community partners in research and have higher levels of synergy may yield higher levels of perceived political impact and a greater number of perceived community- and policy-level outcomes (Khodyakov et al., 2011).

Given the strength of these findings and the quality of measurement, the CERI, partnership synergy, partnership process measures, and several outcome measures were included in the RIH study. RIH researchers did change how we used the CERI by focusing on three different dimensions of what we called *community involvement in research.*

RIH STUDY METHODS

The research design for the RIH was a mixed-method, iterative integration design; we describe this as an Indigenous-transformative framework with full details found elsewhere (and more briefly in Chapter 6) (Hicks et al., 2012; Lucero et al., 2016; Oetzel, Zhou, et al., 2015; Pearson et al., 2015). The sampling frame for the study was developed in the first instance with a series of steps. A computer algorithm was used to screen 103,250 federally funded extramural projects funded in 2009 to identify projects that involved CEnR or CBPR. Staff review of abstracts provided further validation of the inclusion of projects. The projects were research-based projects from a range of health topics and funding agencies. From this search, 333 projects were identified. Among the invited projects, only 294 actually involved CBPR or CEnR (based on self-identification or rescreening of nonparticipating abstracts).

From this sample, we initiated the two key data collection elements: qualitative case study and cross-sectional survey. We selected seven partnerships for an in-depth qualitative case study. The case studies were included to account for complexity in contextual, dynamic, and temporal features and processes of the conceptual model that the cross-sectional survey could not capture. The seven cases were selected (see Chapter 6) to include successful partnerships from a range of health topics and ethnic-racial communities. The data collection involved two research team members visiting partnerships and in particular the community where the project was located. During these visits, ten to fifteen interviews and one to two focus groups were conducted with team and advisory board members. Further, observations of meetings and review of documents were completed. Three case studies were completed prior to initiating the survey, so we also used these data to inform and change the cross-sectional survey, particularly when no previous measures could be identified. The two components continued in parallel until the completion, at which time the qualitative and quantitative findings informed each other and provided triangulation of conclusions.

The cross-sectional survey involved a two-stage sample. First, two hundred (68.0 percent) of the principal investigators (PIs) or project directors (PDs) participated in a key informant survey (KIS) during the latter part of 2011. The KIS asked the PIs to identify project characteristics and also up to four partners (one academic and three community) to participate in the second survey, the community engagement survey (CES). The PIs identified 404 partners, and 312 completed the survey. Of the 200 eligible PIs, 138 completed the CES. These 450 participants represented 82 percent of the total projects in which a KIS was completed and 56 percent of the original 294 projects. In addition, the PIs and PDs were invited to complete the CES and to nominate community partners to complete the CES. All data were collected via DatStat Illume, a web-based survey platform.

All research processes and measures were developed in consultation and collaboration with two advisory groups of academic and community partners with expertise in CBPR. One group focused on the qualitative measures and research design, and the other group focused on the quantitative elements. These steps allowed for the creation of items with face and content validity consistent with the CBPR conceptual model. The specific measures and tools are described in the following three sections, and URLs for these and other tools can be found in Appendix 10 and in http://cpr.unm.edu/research-projects/cbpr-project/research-for-improved-health.html.

QUALITATIVE MEASURES AND TOOLS

We employed a multi-method data collection strategy during the case studies. The purpose of this approach was to triangulate varied sources of data from different stakeholders as well as create more visually engaging and interactive opportunities to ensure participation from partnership members who may have different preferences for sharing their views. The qualitative tools involved two primary components: interview guides and historical time lines.

The qualitative interview guides—individual and focus group—were developed following an iterative process of review and refinement with multiple study team stakeholders. The CBPR conceptual model grounded this effort because it provided a foundational base from which to create relevant questions across the domains. Given that our goal was to conduct interviews and focus groups with a diverse range of partnership participants—university as well as community members—we recognized that the interview guides needed to be flexible and adaptive to the respondents' specific role. The overarching purpose of the guides was to link stakeholder perspectives and actions to broader historical, cultural, and political contexts, partnership functioning, group dynamics, specific implementation strategies, and a range of potential outcomes (e.g., personal, health, and policy).

A common and effective strategy in the development of qualitative interview guides is to begin by eliciting narrative reflection and stories through personal engagement and experience. We recognized that interviewees across the partnership spectrum may not have engaged in a process of considering their own personal roles in these projects or how such efforts have been influenced by larger sociohistorical and interactional forces. Therefore, questions in the domains concentrated on probing descriptions of existing conditions and partnership dynamics derived from actual experience rather than focusing on more abstract associations among model components. Once final draft guides were developed, we conducted a series of pilot interviews with CBPR partnership members connected to our research team as a way to test and modify the guides. We reviewed these initial transcripts as a team to modify the content and sequencing of questions until we reached consensus on a final version. Individual interviews were conducted with a broad cross-section of partnership members, and focus group sessions were held with typically a core group of academic and community members, emphasizing group dynamic processes over individual perceptions and roles.

During a previously agreed time during the case study visit, we gathered academic and community partnership members together and guided them through a historic time line exercise. A research team moderator instructed the group to consider the most salient events that have influenced the historical development of the partnership. We informed them that there was no predetermined start or end date to this time line. Participants were free to consider past historical events as relevant ranging from broader political-economic structures that influence social conditions, receipt of grant funding, or the arrival or departures of partnership members. To enhance the experience, we typically gave people a large piece of butcher paper (or several pieces taped together) to either lay on a table or tape to a wall (3 ft × 9–12 ft) and handed out markers. There was very little direct research team facilitation for this exercise, and after some initial hesitation, participants began interacting with each other about specific events and dates while reflecting further on their partnership history. Appendix 7 displays the historical time line (also known as the River of Life tool).

We found this exercise to be a rich complement to other sources of data collection. In some case studies, participants began the time lines several decades before the present time period and a few traced the origins of their collective interests back well over a century. For example, one case study site identified slavery and the civil rights movement as foundational to partnership activities. Following the completion of the time line (which usually took about an hour), we then moderated a semi-structured focus group to explore the items and events featured on the scroll. These sessions were highly interactive because they provided an opportunity for partnership members to learn from each other and to assess where the partnership came from and what progress has been made.

KEY INFORMANT SURVEY

Guided by the CBPR conceptual model, we first identified project-level measures that included project descriptors and structural features that could be collected via self-report from the PI or abstracted from the RePORTER database. We obtained measures from a library of available CBPR measures that mapped onto constructs and domains represented in the CBPR conceptual model (Pearson et al., 2011).

Project descriptive measures were primarily gathered from RePORTER and included funding for specific areas of research, conditions, or diseases; specific organizations; specific geographical regions; application success rates; and information on the researcher (PI) and his or her organization, project details including abstracts, key words, start and end dates, and type of award (R: research, K: career development, U: center grants) mechanisms used by the National Institutes of Health, and so on.

Structural features included measures to address the nature of agreements among partners and the ways that the partners work together. They included the following elements:

- Project features (twelve items: for example, length of partnership and confidence in goal achievement)
- Resource control and power sharing (four items: for example, who hires personnel and decides how the resources are shared)
- Research integrity (three items: for example, research ethics training and guidelines on confidentiality)
- Formal agreements (seven items: for example, memoranda of understanding or written agreement and the contents of those agreements)
- Formal trainings or substantial discussions (eight items: for example, training about cultural humility, privilege, and power and conflict resolution)
- Partnership roles and involvement (thirteen items: for example, CERI items with one new item).
- Research outcomes (four items: for example, papers in press or published, additional research, or funding)

COMMUNITY ENGAGEMENT SURVEY

The CES measures academic and community partners' perceptions of partnership context, processes, research design, and outcomes as guided by the CBPR conceptual model. Overall, there were twenty-two measures with 101 items included in the CES. For the partnership context domain, the CES included (1) a measure of the capacity of the partnership to meet its aims; and (2) a measure of the degree of trust at the beginning of the partnership.

For the partnership processes domain, the CES contained (1) four measures of structural and individual features and (2) eight measures of relational dynamics. The structural and individual measures comprised the following: bridging social capital, alignment with CBPR principles-partner focus, alignment with CBPR principles-community focus, and partner values (degree of agreement with the mission of the project). Relational dynamics included the following measures: cooperation, participation, respect, trust, influence, participatory decision making, leadership effectiveness, and resource management.

For the intervention and research design domain, the CES had a measure of partnership synergy from PES and measures of community involvement in background research, community involvement in data collection, and community involvement in analysis and dissemination (the last three derived from the CERI). For the partnership outcomes, we included four measures of systems and capacity changes: individual capacity building, agency capacity building, shared power relations in research, and sustainability. We also provided two measures of long-term outcomes: community transformation and community health improvement.

We conducted a rigorous assessment of the psychometric properties of these scales (Oetzel, Zhou, et al., 2015). Confirmatory factor analysis demonstrated that the twenty-two measures have strong factorial validity, and Pearson correlation analysis established convergent and discriminant construct validity. Internal consistency was strong, with eighteen of twenty measures with multiple items achieving at least a .78 Cronbach's alpha (two measures were single items).

Finally, we also developed a measure of culture-centeredness based on the CES measures and qualitative methods (Wallerstein et al., under review). Ensuring cultural fit of research methods, design, and co-development of interventions is necessary for meaningful research outcomes, research integrity, ethical conduct, external validity, and effectiveness to enhance health equity. The culture-centered approach identifies communication processes that marginalize certain communities and suggests three core constructs that challenge this marginalization by validating communication knowledge: community voice and agency (inclusion of community perspective in defining problems and identify solutions), reflexivity (awareness of unstated power and privilege), and structural transformation (changing rules and resources) (Dutta, 2007). The measure includes seven subscales related to these three core constructs.

KEY OUTCOMES

The quantitative and qualitative analyses have been conducted in an integrative manner and aligned with the CBPR conceptual model. We organize the findings on four key areas: (1) conceptualizing outcomes, (2) promising practices, (3) context and culture, and (4) structure and governance. A fifth key evaluation area was the testing of the conceptual model itself, using structural equation modeling, which is presented in Chapter 6.

Conceptualizing Outcomes

Our qualitative and quantitative analyses identified a series of outcomes, reflecting different levels of change and values. The initial desired outcome for a partnership might be the health or research outcome as identified in the specific objectives of a project or grant. Yet, CBPR projects have a potentially much greater breadth of outcomes, including advances toward social justice goals of reduced inequities and knowledge democracy. Qualitative analyses from the case studies showcased this range. Case study participants noted the importance of community and system transformation as core desired intermediate and long-term outcomes of their partnership. These outcomes related to changes in the policy environment, that is, greater recognition of the community partners' strengths as sources of data and as advocates with influence, specific policy changes (e.g., local ordinance enacted by policy makers based on partnership data and advocacy), or improved services and programs. At an intermediate level, case studies identified outcomes in the university environment through changes in IRB processes, for example, as well as community capacity outcomes, such as increased skills in partner agencies related to research. On a personal level, we found that involvement in partnership activities led to positive changes for community members, such as new motivations for pursuing further education or new skills to enhance personal and professional goals. Through the historical time line, we also found greater interest in evaluating the partnership itself in terms of which practices led to greater partnership synergy and effectiveness.

These findings relate closely with our conceptualization of quantitative outcomes at three different levels: (1) short term, (2) intermediate, and (3) long term (Oetzel, Zhou, et al., 2015). Short-term outcomes are the immediate output of partnership dynamics and include partnership synergy. Intermediate outcomes consist of system and capacity outcomes of individual and agency capacity building, shared power relations in research, and sustainability. The long-term outcomes are the community transformations, such as improved programs, policies, and services, and improving the status of the community health issue being addressed.

Promising Practices

One of our specific aims of the RIH study was to identify a set of promising practices for CBPR. These promising practices are contextual and process variables for partnering that are associated with the three different types of outcomes. Building on community consultations (Belone et al., 2016), we categorize these promising practices in congruence with our model: *context* (partnership has capacity to meet aims); *partnership structures* (which ensure bridging social capital, value alignment, and power sharing through written agreements and control of resources); *relationships* (mutual dialogue, influence, ethical management, and trust); and *research-intervention* (ensuring community involvement in all research phases).

We completed a multilevel multiple regression analysis of the KIS and CES data to identify which of these promising practices is associated with each of the specific outcomes including a composite outcome (a combination of the seven outcomes). These practices accounted for 21 to 67 percent of the variance in the specific outcomes. For example, the following specific constructs were associated with the composite outcome: (1) having a formal written agreement, (2) having shared academic and community control of resources, (3) a partnership with strong capacity, (4) following CBPR principles, (5) community involvement in multiple stages of the research, (6) partners having influence on the project, (7) effective leadership, and (8) effective resource management (Duran et al., under review).

The qualitative analysis also explored promising practices, particularly related to partner dynamics. We specifically sought examples of how partnerships built and nurtured relationships of trust and used a trust typology to categorize varying stages of this process (see Chapter 5). Trust is an essential component of partnership synergy yet remains a fragile and ongoing dynamic that requires nurturing in even experienced partnerships. Other aspects of group dynamics included strategies for collaborative decision making and how partnerships managed and distributed relationships of power. Finally, we identified the importance of "bridging characteristics" of certain partnership members (often academic staff members who come from similar communities that the partnership works with). Bridging social capital was seen as an essential quality given the importance of effective communication and "translation" across the academic-community boundary and across ongoing structural barriers of institutional racism and privileged academic knowledge (see Chapter 4).

Context and Culture

Perhaps the most overarching finding in the qualitative analysis related to the social and historical context in which partnerships developed and ultimately drove priorities and goals (Muhammad et al., 2015). Community members cited a deep historical awareness of the processes leading to disparities and current needs. Indeed, without exception, all of the intervention and policy projects we encountered were directly linked to these dynamics and were rooted in cultural knowledge. Although the case studies varied across a range of sociopolitical climates, we found that there was a high degree of recognition regarding how contextual factors influenced project and partnership decisions. The quantitative analysis included limited contextual elements because context is hard to measure across partnerships (quantitative exceptions were partnership capacity and trust at beginning of partnership).

We also identified culture-centeredness as a central feature of partnership project development and adhering to core CBPR principles (Muhammad et al., 2015; Wallerstein et al., under review). Themes of cultural revitalization and identity were consistently reported across the case studies. In some cases, the importance of culture-centeredness related to grounding program and research materials within linguistic and social norms of communities, whereas in other settings, recognition of historical and structural racism served as a common basis to function as a social movement aimed at achieving forms of justice (Devia et al., 2017). The lack of culture-centeredness would be a significant deterrent to positive group dynamics and mutuality in academic-community member relationships. Our measure of culture-centeredness validates this conclusion because it was moderately correlated with group dynamics constructs. Further, the measure was also moderately correlated with intermediate and long-term outcomes.

Structure and Governance

Another major thematic focus included processes of structure and governance. We were interested in understanding how projects were conceptualized and approved as well as in identifying the relevant advisory structures for decision making and reporting. The issue of governance was particularly salient in Native (American Indian, Alaska Native, or Native Hawaiian) partnerships given the central role of such processes as a fundamental basis for engaging in partnership efforts and respecting Native sovereignty. In non-Native partnerships, we observed other oversight processes, though these were typically less formal and based on the context of the partnership itself.

Our quantitative findings showed that Native-serving projects receive less funding compared to other communities of color and multiple race–unspecified groups (Pearson et al., 2015). However, the research outputs in Native communities were no different than those in other communities. This may be explained by the fact that Native communities were more likely to have a written agreement, and perhaps these protected the resources and time of the community partners.

A key aspect of governance is the stewardship of projects (Oetzel, Villegas et al., 2015). Much of governance of research projects focused on research ethics. However, this is insufficient oversight of the research project. Stewardship means ensuring that the research project is administered appropriately to meet specific aims and is accountable to community values and priorities. Our research explored the approval of a project as a form of stewardship. We found that projects approved by a tribal government or health board were more likely to have control of resources, written agreements, and agreements about publishing compared to other types of approval, such as advisory boards, agencies, or individuals. These steps help to ensure that the project is well resourced and thus benefits the community.

MEASURES AND TOOLS FOR EVALUATION

Collectively, all of these findings demonstrate a robust set of measures and tools that identify key and promising CBPR practices. The constructs we have measured have empirical evidence of relevance for the various outcomes. Further, the combined qualitative and quantitative results provide a level of triangulation and also complementarity.

We end the chapter with recommendations on how to use the model as a planning and quality improvement and reflection tool for ongoing evaluation of community-engaged partnerships in innovative and simple ways. For example, community-academic partnerships can use these valid and reliable measures, with qualitative interview guides, to self-assess their partnership practices and outcomes in order to strengthen their partnerships to achieve desired outcomes. Partners can use their own data results to choose the constructs they perceive best fit their project and partnership needs by (1) assessing where their partnership stands for a particular construct of interest compared to national community-engaged project data (e.g., based on empirical results from our cited studies) and prioritizing strategies to address that particular partnering process and (2) evaluating the quality of the measures in relation to other constructs within their own partnership (e.g., are higher levels of participation related to higher capacity building?).

To use the model as a visioning tool for planning or to create an evaluation strategy, there are inductive and deductive approaches. Inductively, partnerships can use the four domains (context, partnership processes, intervention and research, and outcomes) as the starting point to drive their planning, beginning from their own interests and contexts. For example, partners could first reflect on their "desired outcomes," reflecting on which constructs resonate and which need to be changed. They then can return to contexts and continue with partnership processes and intervention and research issues, identifying constructs that resonate or new ones. The result is an adapted model specific to their partnership. If the partnership is just starting, the same approach would lead to documenting desired outcomes, then brainstorming issues in their context, their desired strategies for creating equitable relationships, the potential impact on research design, and revisiting outcomes (see http://cpr.unm.edu/research-projects/cbpr-project/facilitation_tools.html).

A deductive approach might start with a set of outcomes the partnership is interested in (e.g., agency capacity building and shared power relations in research). Examining the identified promising practices from RIH (Duran et al., under review), there are a set of processes associated with each of these outcomes. The partnership can administer these measures to see where they currently stand and whether there are areas for growth.

In 2015, we were invited by Mayo Clinic partners to work with the ten-year-old Rochester Healthy Community Partnership, a collaboration between local community organizations and health researchers in Rochester, Minnesota to undertake such an application of our work. Through an iterative process of meetings and document review, they created their own version of the model (http://cpr.unm.edu/research-projects/cbpr-project/rhcp-cbpr-model-final-ppt.pdf) and modified existing instruments—individual and focus group guides, historical time line, and surveys—to evaluate partnership functioning and future goals. Our RIH instruments served as templates representing a range of domains that a partnership could select from and adapt to their needs and priorities. Analysis of eleven interviews and thirty-six surveys led to community voices reports of core areas of strength and challenge (comparing their response to RIH national averages) and of questions for the partnership to reflect on as they use the evaluation for their future directions. To use the model as a visioning tool for evaluating existing partnerships, also see http://cpr.unm.edu/research-projects/cbpr-project/facilitation_tools.html.

We are fortunate to have received further funding (2015–2020) for the next iteration of our project. In this new R01 funding called Engage for Equity (E^2), from the National Institute of Nursing Research, we are revising, improving, and translating into Spanish our KIS and CES measures. For the KIS, we have developed new measures of stewardship, community organizing capacity to complement community partnership capacity, academic practices, and advisory boards. For the CES, we enhanced measures of influence, culture centeredness, shortened many relational measures while also adding reflexivity, time commitment, satisfaction, and personal costs.

We are also developing a two-day workshop and web-based tools for partnerships at various stages on how to engage in self-assessment and reflection to strengthen their practice and achieve their own goals. The underlying assumption of the workshop and tools is that reflexivity (using Freirean empowerment methodologies) about one's partnership practices strengthens equitable practices, enabling partners to be more effective in reaching their goals. The tools for reflexivity, including evaluation quantitative measures, qualitative guides, and other resources, are being tested and refined and then will be made available to partnerships for use and adaptation to their own priorities and contexts (http://cpr.unm.edu/research-projects/cbpr-project/index.html). These tools are also complemented by the empowerment, social participation, and CBPR curriculum, available in English, Spanish, and Portuguese (http://cpr.unm.edu/curricula--classes/empowerment-curriculum.html).

In conclusion, this chapter, along with tools in Appendices 7, 10, and 11, identified methods, measures, and tools from RIH (the first national study of two hundred federally funded partnerships) that are useful for evaluation of community engagement, which can be started at baseline and maintained over time. We reported some of the key findings and psychometric properties to support the CBPR conceptual model as a guide for evaluation. These findings illustrate demonstrable outcomes of CBPR contexts and partnering practices that together can lead to enhanced recognition of the power of community and academic knowledge working together to reach specific grant goals as well as the broadest goal of health equity for all.

QUESTIONS FOR DISCUSSION

1. Think about your community and imagine a community-engaged intervention being done there (or think about an actual intervention you have read about or experienced). How would you suggest you evaluate that project?
2. Imagine you are a member of a participatory research project. How would you go about using the tools and methods presented here? How would you use them to engage in critical self-reflection? How would you ensure that the evaluation process is participatory?

ACKNOWLEDGMENTS

The research described in this chapter was supported by NARCH: (U261HS300293; U261IHS0036-04-00), with Indian Health Service in partnership with the National Institute of General Medical Sciences, National Institute of Minority Health and Health Disparities, National Institute on Drug Abuse, National Center for Research Resources, Office of Behavioral Social Sciences Research, National Cancer Institute, and Health Resources Services Administration. Engage for Equity (1R01NR015241-01A1) is funded by the National Institute of Nursing Research. We thank members of each research team, the think tank, and the academic and community partners who participated in the surveys and case studies.

REFERENCES

Atalay, S. (2010). "We don't talk about Catalhoyuk, we live it": Sustainable archaeological practice through community-based participatory research. *World Archaeology, 42,* 418–429.

Baker, E., Homan, S., Schonhoff, R., Sr., & Kreuter, M. (1999). Principles of practice for academic/practice/community research partnerships. *American Journal of Preventive Medicine, 16*(3), 86–93.

Belone, L., Lucero, J., Duran, B., Tafoya, G., Baker, E., Chan, D., et al. (2016). Community-based participatory research conceptual model: Community partner consultation and face validity. *Qualitative Health Research, 26,* 117–135.

Cyril, S., Smith, B. J., Possamai-Inesedy, A., & Andre, M.N.R. (2015). Exploring the role of community engagement in improving the health of disadvantaged populations: A systematic review. *Global Health Action, 8,* 1–12.

Devia, C., Baker, E., Sanchez-Youngman, S., Barnidge, E., Golub, M., Motton, F., Muhammad, M., Ruddock, C., Vicuña, B., & Wallerstein, N. (2017). CBPR to advance social and racial equity: Urban and rural partnerships in black and Latino communities. *BMC International Journal of Health Equity, 16,* 17. doi:10.1186/s12939-016-0509-3

Duran, B., Oetzel, J. G., Pearson, C., Magarati, M., Zhou, C., Villegas, M., & Wallerstein, N. (under review). Promising practices in community-based participatory research: Evidence from a national study. *Progress in Community Health Partnerships: Research, Education, and Action.*

Dutta, M. J. (2007). Communicating about culture and health: Theorizing culture-centered and cultural sensitivity approaches. *Communication Theory, 17,* 304–328.

Hicks, S., Duran, B., Wallerstein, N., Avila, M., Belone, L., Lucero, J., et al. (2012). Evaluating community-based participatory research to improve community-partnered science and community health. *Progress in Community Health Partnerships: Research, Education, and Action, 6,* 289–299.

Jagosh, J., Macaulay, A. C., Pluye, P., Salsberg, J., Bush, P. L., Henderson, J., et al. (2012). Uncovering the benefits of participatory research: Implications of a realist review for health research and practice. *The Milbank Quarterly, 90,* 311–346.

Khodyakov, D., Stockdale, S., Jones, A., Mango, J., Jones, F., & Lizaola, E. (2013). On measuring community participation in research. *Health Education & Behavior, 40,* 346–354.

Khodyakov, D., Stockdale, S., Jones, F., Ohito, E., Jones, A., Lizaola, E., et al. (2011). An exploration of the effect of community engagement in research on perceived outcomes of partnered mental health services projects. *Society and Mental Health, 1*(3), 185–199.

Lasker, R., Weiss, E., & Miller, R. (2001). Partnership synergy: A practical framework for studying and strengthening the collaborative advantage. *The Milbank Quarterly, 79,* 179–205.

Lorway, R., Thompson, L. H., Lazarus, L., du Plessis, E., Pasha, A., Fathima Mary, P., et al. (2013). Going beyond the clinic: Confronting stigma and discrimination among men who have sex with men in Mysore through community-based participatory research. *Critical Public Health, 24*(1), 1–15.

Lucero, J., Wallerstein, N., Duran, B., Alegria, M., Green-Moten, E., Israel, B. A., et al. (2016). Development of a mixed methods investigation of process and outcomes of community-based participatory research. *Journal of Mixed Methods Research.* doi:10.1177/1558689816633309

Muhammad, M., Wallerstein, M., Sussman, A. L., Avila, M., Belone, L., & Duran, B. (2015). Reflections on researcher identity and power: The impact of positionality on community-based participatory research (CBPR) processes and outcomes. *Critical Sociology, 41,* 1045–1063.

O'Mara-Eves, A., Brunton, G., Oliver, S., Kavanagh, J., Jamal, F., & Thomas, J. (2015). The effectiveness of community engagement in public health interventions for disadvantaged groups: A meta-analysis. *BMC Public Health, 15*(1), 1352.

Oetzel, J. G., Villegas, M., Zenone, H., White Hat, E. R., Wallerstein, N., & Duran, B. (2015). Enhancing stewardship of community-engaged research through governance. *American Journal of Public Health, 105*(6), 1161–1167.

Oetzel, J. G., Zhou, C., Duran, B., Pearson, C., Magarati, M., Lucero, J., Wallerstein, N., Villegas, M. (2015). Establishing the psychometric properties of constructs in a community-based participatory research conceptual model. *American Journal of Health Promotion, 29,* e188–e202.

Pearson, C., Duran, B., Lucero, J., Sandoval, J., Oetzel, J., Tafoya, G., Belone, L., Avila, M., Martin, D., Wallerstein, N., & Hicks, S. (2011). CBPR variable matrix: Research for improved health in academic/community partnerships. CES4Health.info. Retrieved from http://ces4health.info/find-products/view-product.aspx?code=FWYC2L2T

Pearson, C., Duran, B., Oetzel, J., Magarati, M., Villegas, M., Lucero, J., & Wallerstein, N. (2015). Research for improved health: Variability and impact of structural characteristics in federally-funded community engaged research. *Progress in Community Health Partnerships, 9,* 17–29.

Sandoval, J. A., Iglesias Rios, L., Wallerstein, N., Lucero, J., Oetzel, J., Avila, M., et al. (2012). Process and outcome constructs for evaluating community-based participatory research projects: A matrix of existing measures. *Health Education Research, 27,* 680–690.

Trickett, E. J. (2011). Community-based participatory research as worldview or instrumental strategy: Is it lost in translation(al) research? *American Journal of Public Health, 101,* 1353–1355.

Wallerstein, N., & Duran, B. (2010). Community-based participatory research contributions to intervention research: The intersection of science and practice to improve health equity. *American Journal of Public Health, 100,* S40–S46.

Wallerstein, N., Oetzel, J. G., Duran, B., Magarati, M., Pearson, C., Belone, L., Davis, J., Dewindt, L., Lucero, J., Ruddock, C., Sutter, E., Villegas, M., Dutta., M. (under review). Conceptualizing and measuring the culture-centered approach in community based participatory research. *Social Science and Medicine.*

Wallerstein, N., Oetzel, J. G., Duran, B., Tafoya, G., Belone, L., & Rae, R. (2008). CBPR: What predicts outcomes? In M. Minkler & N. Wallerstein (Eds.), *Community-based participatory research for health: From process to outcomes* (2nd ed., pp. 371–392). San Francisco, CA: Jossey-Bass.

Weiss, E., Anderson, R., & Lasker, R. (2002). Making the most of collaboration: Exploring the relationship between partnership synergy and partnership functioning. *Health Education & Behavior, 29,* 683–698.

CHAPTER 18

PARTICIPATORY EVALUATION AS A PROCESS OF EMPOWERMENT

EXPERIENCES WITH COMMUNITY HEALTH WORKERS IN THE UNITED STATES AND LATIN AMERICA

NOELLE WIGGINS, LAURA CHANCHIEN PARAJÓN, CHRIS M. COOMBE, AILEEN ALFONSO DULDULAO, LETICIA RODRIGUEZ GARCIA, AND PEI-RU WANG

PARTICIPATORY EVALUATION IS an approach to assessing the strengths and weaknesses of a program, intervention, or activity and making recommendations for improvements that involve those directly affected in the evaluation process. It can be considered a subfield of participatory research and a discipline in its own right. Given the proper combination of skills, relationships, conditions, and value orientations, participatory evaluation can produce more valid and actionable results than more conventional approaches to evaluation, while at the same time contributing to the empowerment of individuals and communities.

In this chapter, we will provide a solid grounding in the fundamentals of participatory evaluation as distinct from research, explore transformative participatory evaluation as most consistent with CBPR, offer a cyclical process for conducting transformative participatory evaluation, and end with two examples of how participatory evaluation is being used in two community health worker (CHW) programs, one in the United States and one in Nicaragua. Throughout, we seek to demonstrate how context, skills, and values influence how we conduct empowerment-oriented participatory evaluation and research.

WHAT IS EVALUATION?

There are many ways of thinking about the relationship between evaluation and research; the development of new paradigms for research over the last thirty years has further blurred an already hazy distinction. Nonetheless, differences remain, and it is important to understand those differences in order to conduct effective evaluations (Springett & Wallerstein, 2008).

Perhaps the key difference between evaluation and research lies within the word *evaluation*. At its heart, evaluation is a systematic process of *assigning value* or making a judgment about a program, intervention, or activity to improve effectiveness or inform decision making (Morelli & Mataira, 2010). Although most practitioners now agree that research is never value-free, assigning value is not an inherent function of research.

Because evaluation is conducted about a specific program, evaluators must constantly take *context* into account, whereas some researchers (though not those influenced by CBPR) try to exclude context. Although participatory researchers may have additional goals, a central goal of research is the *creation of new knowledge* (and ensuring the *external validity* of findings), whereas a central goal of evaluation is *program improvement* (and ensuring the *internal validity* of findings) (Levin-Rozalis, 2003).

Many of these factors—the explicit goal of assigning value, the influence of context, the orientation of service to some group—mean that evaluation is inherently political. Evaluators therefore must be prepared to understand and mitigate the effects of power, especially participatory evaluators who wish to contribute to empowerment.

WHAT IS PARTICIPATORY EVALUATION?

Cousins and Chouinard (2012) define participatory evaluation as a range of collaborative approaches to evaluation "in which trained evaluators work in partnership with [program] stakeholders to produce evaluative knowledge" (p. 10). This range includes the empowerment evaluation pioneered by Fetterman (2000). They contrast these approaches to more conventional approaches to evaluation in which the evaluator is an outsider who strives to maintain "objectivity" and distance from the program being evaluated. Based on a positivist or post-positivist worldview, conventional forms of evaluation assume that objective truth exists and can be known through hypothesis generation and testing. Participatory and collaborative approaches to evaluation are based on a worldview that "includes the ways in which the people involved with facts perceive them" and acknowledges that "concrete reality is the connection between subjectivity and objectivity, never objectivity isolated from subjectivity" (Freire, 1982, p. 30).

Cousins and Chouinard (2012) divide the range of participatory evaluation into two principal streams: practical participatory evaluation (P-PE) and transformative participatory evaluation (T-PE). P-PE is motivated primarily by a pragmatic philosophy and a desire to produce valid findings that can be used for program improvement (Brisolara, 1998). P-PE is based on a democratic pluralist theory of power, which assumes people choose to participate or not based on free will. By contrast, T-PE grows out of a desire, originally from Latin America, South Asia, and Africa, to create a just society by challenging unequal power structures. (See Chapter 2 for analogous Northern and Southern participatory research traditions.)

TRANSFORMATIVE PARTICIPATORY EVALUATION

In terms of its historical antecedents and its current uses, T-PE is the participatory evaluation stream most in line with CBPR and thus is the focus of this chapter. T-PE has two primary sources: the participatory action research (PAR) work conducted by Colombian sociologist Orlando Fals-Borda and colleagues in Latin America in the 1960s to 1990s (Fals-Borda & Rahman, 1991) and the participatory research and evaluation work conducted by Walter Fernandes and Rajesh Tandon (1981) and colleagues in South Asia during roughly the same period of time (Hall et al., 2013). These practitioner authors were working in the context of community development amid the social-political ferment occurring in many parts of the Global South. Influenced by thinkers such as Marx, Engels, Gramsci (1971), and Frankfurt School theorists, these researchers identified mechanisms that maintain inequity and developed research and evaluation strategies for empowering those most marginalized in society by ceding power to them and making them the agents, rather than the objects, of research (Brisolara,1998).

Although the historical context of the United States is different, similar disparities of wealth, power, and control produced the need for participatory research and evaluation, inspiring practitioner academics such as John Gaventa (1980, 1991), along with popular educators at the Highlander School for Research and Education, such as Myles Horton (2003), to produce participatory research that bears many similarities to the approach developed in the Global South. These approaches are closely connected to the popular education methodology that was systematized and disseminated by Brazilian educator Paulo Freire (Freire, 2003; Wallerstein & Auerbach, 2004; Wiggins, 2012; Wiggins et al., 2014). Popular education can help to create an organizational and community climate that promotes and sustains participatory evaluation and is profiled in the case studies.

Power is a central issue in participatory evaluation generally. In the context of community health programs and interventions, power takes on added significance. With lack of power understood as an overarching disease risk factor (Wallerstein, 1992), it stands to reason that the way to reverse health inequities is to shift and balance power between dominant and oppressed communities. This occurs through the process of *empowerment,* which is understood in public health not as a process that is done by the powerful *to* or *for* those lacking power but rather as a process that communities most affected by inequities do for and with themselves. Public health studies suggest that empowerment independently predicts better self-reported health and decreased depressive symptoms (Wallerstein, 2006) and that popular education is an effective way of increasing empowerment and improving community health (Wiggins, 2012).

DECOLONIZING PARTICIPATORY EVALUATION

T-PE developed in the Global South as it emerged from colonization and has always been concerned with the question of who gets to assign value and define knowledge. In 1991,

Rahman wrote of the need to "return to the people the legitimacy of the knowledge they are capable of producing through their own verification systems, as fully scientific" (p. 15). This statement prefigures the "decolonizing methodologies" of Indigenous scholar Linda Tuhiwai Smith (1999), who states that "imperialism and colonialism brought complete disorder to colonized peoples, disconnecting them from their histories, their landscapes, their languages, their social relations and their own ways of thinking, feeling and interacting with the world" (p. 29).

One of the insights of a decolonizing approach is that research and evaluation are critical and important sites of struggle where colonization and Western science can be challenged and Indigenous ways of knowing centralized (Kawakami et al., 2007; Morelli & Mataira, 2010; Tuhiwai Smith, 1999; Zavala, 2013). A decolonizing approach changes the Western paradigm of evaluation by challenging the meaning of value, what constitutes value, and whether an intervention should be improved on or cease to exist. It empowers communities to set evaluation agendas; incorporate historical, cultural, spiritual, social, environmental, and emotional "data"; and have their evaluation findings returned to their communities (Kawakami et al., 2007; Morelli & Mataira, 2010). Adopting a decolonizing approach to evaluation represents a return to the roots of transformative participatory evaluation, as well as a further step toward conducting evaluation from within the worldview of those most directly affected by the program, intervention, or activity under study.

A PROCESS FOR CARRYING OUT TRANSFORMATIVE PARTICIPATORY EVALUATION

Similar to CBPR, T-PE is not a specific methodology but rather an approach to evaluation based on a worldview and set of key principles that guide evaluation design, process, and methods (Shulha et al., 2016). A number of frameworks have been developed that lay out key steps in participatory evaluation (Coombe, 2012; Fawcett et al., 1996; Fetterman, Kaftarian, & Wandersman, 2015; Maltrud, Polacsek, & Wallerstein, 1997; Springett & Wallerstein, 2008). Represented initially as sequential steps in Coombe (2012; see Figure 18.1), T-PE is in practice a cyclical, iterative process of learning from the past, applying new understandings to the future, and cycling back through processes as needed.

Step 1: Identify Purpose and Commit to Participatory Evaluation

Together, those groups and organizations with a vested interest in the program, intervention, or activity identify the purpose and objectives of the evaluation, decide whether to commit to a participatory approach, and determine the extent and type of participation by different groups. Important considerations are the project's stage of development, past experience with evaluation and research, resources available and needed, and potential benefits of carrying out a participatory evaluation.

Community, program, and institutional contexts are essential considerations throughout the process. Contextual factors include power relationships between and among community members, funders, outside evaluators, and policy makers; the level at which the program is being conducted (e.g., local, state, national); and support or lack thereof for the participatory process from program funders and organizational leaders. In participatory evaluation there is "a role for program sponsors/funders to support the inquiry in ways that move well beyond the provision of fiscal resources" (Cousins & Chouinard, 2012, p. 130).

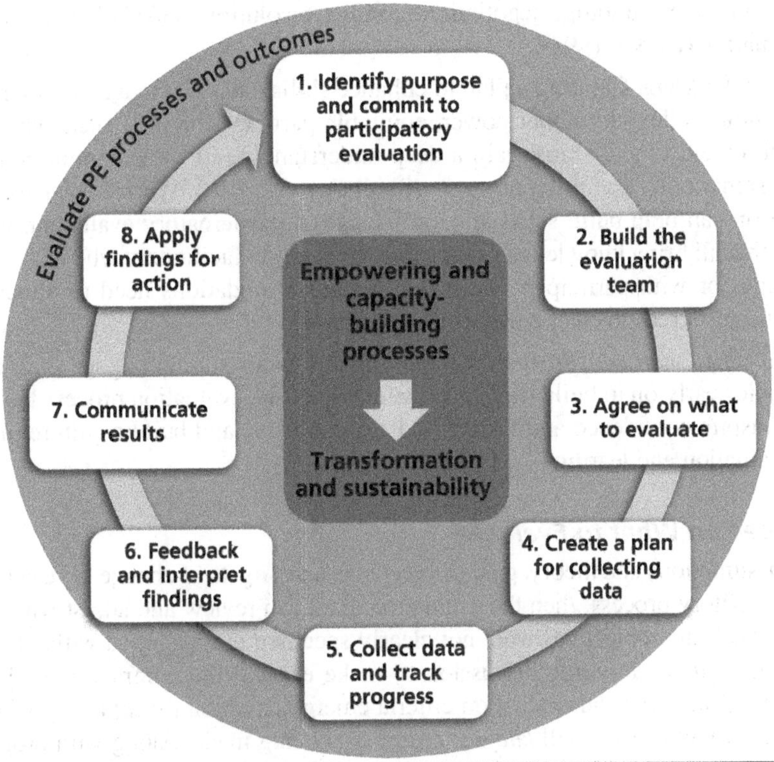

FIGURE 18.1 *Key Steps in Participatory Evaluation Process*

Step 2: Build the Participatory Evaluation Team

Collaborative partnerships require a shared commitment to equity and adequate time and skills to establish and maintain relationships, build mutual trust, understand differences, and resolve conflicts. Laying the proper groundwork is critical to success and involves four key tasks:

1. *Core team.* It is important to formally identify who will be involved, the level and nature of participation expected, and what personal and institutional resources each partner brings to the table. Although diverse stakeholder groups can generally produce more credible and valid findings, extremely unequal levels of power and privilege among stakeholders can complicate the goal of transformation. Guiding principles and operating norms can help address power differentials to foster equitable participation and make the best use of everyone's time.
2. *Roles and multiple mechanisms for participation.* Identifying the roles and strategies for substantive participation is an important early step for an equitable and high-quality evaluation. In some projects, stakeholders participate in certain stages (e.g., data collection, dissemination, etc.) and in others they are involved throughout. Also, depth of participation can vary over time. To accomplish the goals of T-PE, evaluation facilitators often work in teams and employ a constellation of skills that include facilitation, popular or liberating

education, team building, negotiation, conflict resolution, stakeholder involvement, and coordination (Burke, 1998).

3. *Capacity building*. Creating a plan to enhance skills and knowledge of all partners fosters co-learning, reflexivity about power, equitable participation, and sustainability. External evaluators and funders must gain a deep understanding of the community, the historical and current context, and the program (Shulha et al., 2016). Workshops based on popular education can help build skills and knowledge of participatory evaluation while emphasizing that all bring knowledge to the table. Evaluation facilitators who are working across languages or with participants who require accommodations need to allocate sufficient time and resources to ensure that all can participate fully.
4. *Relationships with constituencies*. Finally, participants should engage their broader constituencies early on to build trust and ownership of the evaluation process beyond the core team, inspire confidence and vision, address concerns, and build a culture of transformative evaluation and learning.

Step 3: Agree on What to Evaluate

If program assumptions and theory, goals, objectives, and targets of change have been spelled out using a participatory process, then the evaluation team can review and adjust what was initially proposed. If goals and objectives were not clearly specified or developed without participation, evaluation facilitators can guide discussion to make explicit the community's implicit theory (Weiss, 1995). Objectives and evaluation criteria emerge from jointly exploring what results are desired and how participants will *know* if progress is being made. Along with program-specific outcomes such as improved health, it is important to measure process and systems outcomes such as participation (Rifkin, 2014), collaboration (Granner & Sharpe, 2004), empowerment and community control (Cyril, Smith, & Renzaho, 2015; Wallerstein, 2006), and community competence or capacity (Eng & Parker, 1994; Goodman et al., 1998; Liberato et al., 2011).

Step 4: Create a Plan for Collecting Data

The participatory evaluation team collaboratively develops a design and methodology for the evaluation that is made up of quantitative and qualitative methods for collecting information to track progress and document change. Feuerstein (1988) recommends building confidence in participants by starting with existing methods of monitoring. The evaluation plan needs to be feasible and make the best use of community resources while ensuring that results are valid and credible. Popular education activities can be used to develop an evaluation design that values and integrates multiple ways of knowing.

Step 5: Collect Data and Track Progress

T-PE involves community members in documenting the program and its effects. Systems for recording activities and events as they unfold should be developed with those who will be using them, including partner organizations to enhance sustainability (Zukoski & Luluquisen, 2002). Use of technology and online resources, such as handheld devices for recording data in the field (Gravlee et al., 2006), expand the community's ability to create and use knowledge. See for example, the Community Tool Box Online Documentation System (see Appendix 11).

Step 6: Feedback and Interpret Findings Collectively

Making sense of the data is a collaborative effort that combines technical expertise, experiential knowledge, and deep understanding of the community. The evaluation facilitator and project staff members organize different types of data into a common body of information that participants can check for meaning and validity and then identify gaps or connections among the data. The aim is to build consensus and incorporate preliminary implications and recommendations to set the stage for moving from knowledge to action using a decolonizing lens, incorporating larger structural factors into the analysis.

Step 7: Communicate Results to Relevant Audiences

Participatory evaluation communicates findings to key insider and outsider stakeholders in multiple ways and at multiple time points. Sharing achievements as they occur and framing evaluation data in terms of strengths rather than weaknesses can energize the community and build trust and commitment to the project. Creative media, such as video, theater, art, posters, websites, and social media, using the expertise of community team members, may communicate results more effectively than reports and presentations.

Step 8: Apply Findings for Action

Using the lessons learned, the group can strengthen or expand community efforts, institutionalize changes, and plan future actions. Valuable information on program processes and outcomes may lead the project to redefine objectives, redirect scarce resources or seek out new ones, modify strategies, and strengthen leadership structures. Community efforts that aim for transformative change focus on evaluating collective power, equity, systems change, and policy advocacy (Cheezum et al., 2013; Israel et al., 2010; Minkler, Garcia, Rubin, & Wallerstein, 2012).

CASE STUDY ONE: THE OREGON COMMUNITY EDUCATION WORKER (CEW) PROGRAM

In the following, we provide two case studies of how participatory evaluation is being used to foster and facilitate empowerment in two community health worker programs. The case studies provide concrete applications of the theory and action steps previously described.

Background and Lead Partners

The Community Education Worker (CEW) Program, based in Multnomah County, Oregon, is a two-year-old partnership between culturally specific and mainstream community-based organizations (CBOs), a public agency, and several local funders. The CEW Program is the result of a community-based process that aimed to ensure that all children in Multnomah County can achieve educational success and obtain a fulfilling career that pays a living wage.

The idea for the CEW Program came from a Latina mother, who expressed a need for people from her own community who could help her prepare her children to succeed in kindergarten. In response, the "Ready for Kindergarten (R4K) Collaborative" decided to adapt the CHW model. In its first year, individuals who had participated in a CHW-certification course using popular education were hired by three culturally specific agencies: Native American Youth and Family Association (NAYA), Latino Network, and the Urban League of Portland. The Immigrant and Refugee Community Organization (IRCO) added CEWs serving the Zomi (Burmese) and Somali communities in year 2. CEWs conduct visits with families, facilitate parent-child learning groups, serve as cultural mediators between families and systems, and organize parents to address early childhood education inequities.

The Multnomah County Community Capacitation Center (CCC) was chosen by the R4K Collaborative to lead the CEW Program and conduct the evaluation. For fifteen years, the CCC has supported communities most affected by inequities to identify and address their own most pressing health issues, using popular education, the CHW model, and community-based participatory research and evaluation (CBPR/E). As the staff members and communities involved have grown and become more diverse, the theoretical framework of the CCC has expanded from its original Latin American influences to include the civil rights movement, disability rights movement, and movements to decolonize evaluation and community practice.

To date, the participatory evaluation experience of the CEW Program can be divided into two phases. In year 1, CCC developed an evaluation plan that, although it had participatory elements, was largely driven by the CCC staff members. During year 2, CCC is deepening stakeholder participation to develop a truly participatory evaluation. The experience of the CEW Program demonstrates how an evaluation can progress along a continuum from evaluator-driven to community-driven.

Context

Portland, Oregon, is the whitest major city in the United States (Badger, 2015). Although Oregon has a reputation (at least in dominant culture) for being politically progressive, this reputation obscures a history of oppression and exclusion directed at people of color and immigrants. As Portland has become a highly desirable place to live, gentrification and an acute shortage of affordable housing have led to substantial displacement and homelessness among low-income people of color. Families of color are now moving into areas where they have not traditionally lived, where they do not feel welcome, and where schools are ill-prepared to effectively serve their children.

Initial Steps in the T-PE Process

After the idea for the CEW Program had been developed, CCC staff members and a supervisor at one of the culturally specific agencies co-facilitated a workshop at an R4K meeting to develop a logic model. This resulted in a draft set of desired outcomes as well as short-, medium-, and long-term indicators for these outcomes. Social Venture Partners (SVP) Portland, one of the local funders, contributed other intermediate and long-term outcomes associated with kindergarten readiness.

The CCC proposal for year 1 evaluation funding to SVP was not yet participatory because CEWs had not yet been hired. CCC included a proviso in the proposal that a commitment to developmental and participatory evaluation would likely mean changes in the future based on CEW and community input.

Once the CEWs were hired, the next step was to begin to bring them into the evaluation process, which occurred during their initial training. Following discussions on how assessment can be used as a tool for oppression or for empowerment, the new CEWs were introduced to the logic model, which was compared to a "road to educational equity," starting at "now" and ending twenty to twenty-five years in the future. On the far right were outcomes such as "all children graduate from high school." In the middle were indicators such as "families express increased ability to advocate for their children with systems." On the left were short-term measures such as "children have a primary care home." CEWs were given placards with the outcomes and indicators. They were asked to read their outcome or indicator and then place it on the road. They started on the far right and worked backward so that they could see what the program's ultimate goals were and how their actions as CEWs would contribute to achieving the long-term goals. Finally, the group reflected on several questions: (1) How does our work now contribute to achieving outcomes twenty and twenty-five years into the future? (2) What do you think about these outcomes? and (3) In order to show that we are moving along this time line, what do we have to do?

The "road to educational equity" activity set the stage for the participatory development of tools to track outcomes and indicators. In a series of meetings conducted separately with both major language groups (Spanish and English), a draft set of tracking forms was workshopped with the CEWs. At each stage, changes made with one language group were translated into the other language and reviewed by the other language group until initial forms were developed. Forms have continued to change based on input from CEWs, such as simplifying "case management" sections to allow more flexibility for CEWs and participants to record and track their goals and activities.

Deepening Participatory Processes

In year 2, evaluation staff members expressed a desire at a steering committee meeting to make the evaluation a fully participatory process. Despite the extra time involved for frontline and supervision staff members, whose time was already limited, they supported this idea. An e-mail invitation was sent to key stakeholders, who included CEWs, supervisors, and funders. Since then, meetings of the participatory evaluation team have been held monthly. In these fully bilingual meetings, popular education has been used to build collective knowledge about topics such as (1) the meaning of evaluation and the range of evaluation paradigms; (2) how beliefs about truth, knowledge, and values influence approaches to evaluation; (3) the role of evaluation questions; (4) evaluation design; and (5) data collection methods. The year 1 evaluation plan has been used as an example of the phenomena the team is discussing. Participants have expressed excitement about learning to use terms such as *ontology* and *epistemology* (in two languages) and satisfaction that no assumptions were made about their interest in or ability to learn these concepts. The team has made changes to better reflect the collective paradigm and revised evaluation questions.

The process of developing a participatory evaluation for the CEW Program reflects many of the lessons described in the background section of this chapter. Despite their heavy workload, CBO staff members, including CEWs, have been eager to engage in the participatory process, as long as meetings are fully accessible to them and their time is well spent. They bring insights from their cultural groups that could not be accessed if they were not a part of the process, leading to better evaluation questions and stronger outcomes. Staff members and partners from SVP have not only supported the process but also have eagerly participated in it. Because many of the evaluation team members, including CEWs, have extensive experience with popular education, there is a shared, preexisting commitment to popular education values including solidarity, compassion, humility, and love for the cause of the people. This commitment provides solid grounding for the participatory evaluation process.

CASE STUDY TWO: AMOS HEALTH AND HOPE, NICARAGUA

This case study describes the T-PE approach of a community-based nonprofit public health organization in Nicaragua called AMOS Health and Hope (www.amoshealth.org). Despite being in a low-resourced global health setting, AMOS has prioritized T-PE as an integral part of the CBPR conceptual model (see Chapter 6) to improve program impact and facilitate community empowerment.

Context

Nicaragua is the second poorest country in Latin America and has a long history of man-made and natural disasters. Starting with the death of the majority of the Indigenous populations during Spanish colonization, followed by years of dictatorship under the Somozas, a revolution in the 1980s, and earthquakes, hurricanes, and International Monetary Funds (IMF) structural adjustment policies in the 1990s, the country is characterized by extreme disparities in wealth and health.

Passionate about reducing health inequities and informed by the work of global health, popular education, and public health practitioners, AMOS cofounder, the late Dr. Gustavo Parajón, pioneered the first Nicaraguan CHW program and later gave the best advice possible: "A doctor in Nicaragua should not be a doctor but a teacher to share our knowledge and empower others to serve." In this spirit, AMOS was founded as a place to learn alongside communities to continuously evaluate, reflect, and improve the practice of CBPR, community empowerment, and participatory evaluation. AMOS currently works in twenty-six communities and four departments throughout Nicaragua, serving a population of thirteen thousand people.

CHW and Staff Training for CBPR and Participatory Evaluation

When the current codirectors cofounded AMOS in 2006, an emphasis was placed on designing the program using CBPR principles, including participatory evaluation. Not having funds for an evaluator, AMOS integrated participatory evaluation into every aspect of the program. CHWs are trained using popular education methodologies and often refer to themselves as "agents of change" who work to transform root causes of inequities in their own communities. The CHWs in each of the communities comprise a community health promoter, community leaders, and volunteer mothers who form a community health committee. The current evaluation staff members at AMOS mentor and annually train field staff members and CHWs to ensure that the principles of T-PE occur throughout the organization.

AMOS's multidisciplinary staff members comprise CHWs, nurses, doctors, and nutritionists from a range of social classes, ethnicities, and countries and are conscious of colonization, the bidirectionality of relationships between communities and themselves, and the continuous need to inspire and be inspired using transformative educational methods.

Participatory Evaluation Processes

AMOS's approach is to start by developing trust with the communities, understanding the geographic boundaries of the community (which often may not be the same as governmental boundaries), as well as developing an inventory to identify community strengths. The approach is assets-based and seeks to bring together multi-sectoral collaboration for increased impact through a three-way partnership: the *community* identifying their key community priorities and issues, the *government* providing top-down policy guidance and epidemiological priority guidance, and *nongovernmental partners* such as nonprofits and churches offering the support and facilitation for participatory processes and evaluation.

Once the three-way partnership is established, a health committee (HC) is formed by community leaders representing diverse geographic, political, and cultural groups and who receive training by AMOS staff members using popular education methods. The cornerstone of the community's participatory evaluation process is the census, which is based on the motto "Every person is counted, and every person counts." Conducted by community members, the census is analyzed in coordination with AMOS staff members, who do the initial tabulation of data. Once data are interpreted with the community, the HC develops a community plan of action. Communities have developed priority projects, such as installation of clean water filters, clean-up campaigns for vector control, and community advocacy to close down bars.

A balance of community-driven priorities (such as clean water projects) and the governmental epidemiological priorities (such as ensuring systematic home visitation of pregnant women and newborns to prevent high neonatal mortality rates) is facilitated by AMOS support staff members, who visit communities monthly. Community data are analyzed by the health promoter and HC on a quarterly and annual basis. Popular education methodologies such as the River of Life (see Appendix 7) are used to support participatory evaluation. The process is iterative with several steps done annually to prioritize issues, implement a community health plan, and evaluate impact together.

Many lessons have been learned over the years:

1. *"Staff not stuff" approach.* Participatory evaluation requires staff time and resources to organize and integrate real-time data into an understandable form to allow for deeper discussion at the community level. This is a challenge in low-resource international health settings where donors tend to give money for "stuff"—commodities such as vitamins, vaccines, educational flipcharts, deworming pills—but not for trained and committed staff members needed for CBPR and participatory evaluation. With many competing needs for funding, strong organizational leadership and a commitment to CBPR is necessary to ensure adequate staff and resources for T-PE.
2. *Continuing education for T-PE.* Despite Latin America being the birthplace of many transformative education methodologies, most education still uses "banking" methodology (Freire, 2003). Intensive CBPR training for new staff members followed by ongoing training and mentoring is key to ensuring T-PE becomes part of the organizational culture. Having a T-PE-oriented evaluator on staff to facilitate this process is key!
3. *Balancing epidemiological and community priorities.* In the framework of transformational community development work, epidemiological priorities often must be balanced with community priorities. For example, patients who have walked three hours carrying their child to the clinic expect curative services, such as antibiotics for a common cold, even though international protocols prohibit this use. Communities don't clamor for preventive care even though it is more cost-effective. Through the T-PE process, AMOS has ensured

that data collected on the use of antibiotics is shared with the community. This practice, combined with educational messages using popular education methodologies, has resulted in significant improvement on the rational use of antibiotics in communities. Balancing these two priorities is a long-term process that includes the use of T-PE to help establish priorities based on real data that can be used to change social and cultural norms.

4. *Real-time data use by communities*. For T-PE to create momentum for change in communities, there is a need for constant feedback of data to communities, which can be very time-consuming when a paper-based system is used. Future plans at AMOS include seeking funding to design and implement robust mobile data collection and evaluation systems that can provide real-time data for CHWs and training CHWs to use these mobile data systems with their community evaluation teams in order to enhance the impact of T-PE processes.

AMOS provides lessons for practitioners and researchers in the development of participatory evaluation tools for low-resource settings. Participatory evaluation as practiced by AMOS is not a separate project or intervention, but a way of life. In the words of one CHW: "We are investigators because we collect information on what is going on in our own communities. And because we know, we can take that knowledge and make a difference in our own communities."

CONCLUSION

Transformative participatory evaluation is a process of skill building and power sharing that, when conducted with intention and integrity, can promote the empowerment of individuals and communities, as well as contribute to a range of other desirable outcomes. Facilitation of a successful participatory evaluation process requires careful attention to composition of the stakeholder group, relationship building across a range of stakeholders, deep awareness of one's own cultural worldviews, open acknowledgment and constant renegotiation of power and control, use of liberatory educational philosophies and methods, selection of appropriate data collection methods, and prevention of stakeholder burnout through optimal use of their time. It carefully balances education, investigation, and action, and in so doing, it provides a crucial opportunity to challenge assumptions of value and shift and balance power.

QUESTIONS FOR DISCUSSION

1. What are the key differences between transformative participatory evaluation and more conventional approaches to evaluation? How does T-PE challenge dominant Western assumptions about value and the meaning of knowledge?
2. Based on your experience as well as what you read, why is it important to constantly attend to power relationships when working on diverse teams? What strategies can we use to do this?
3. How do you reconcile balancing epidemiological priorities with community priorities in a participatory evaluation process?

REFERENCES

Badger, E. (2015, March 24). *How the whitest city in American appears through the eyes of its black residents.* Washington Post. Available at: https://www.washingtonpost.com/news/wonk/wp/2015/03/24/how-the-whitest-city-in-america-appears-through-the-eyes-of-its-black-residents/?utm_term=.0c2665705ec2

Brisolara, S. (1998). The history of participatory evaluation and current debates in the field. In E. Whitmore (Ed.), *New directions for evaluation: Understanding and practicing participatory evaluation, 80,* 25–37.

Burke, B. (1998). Evaluating for a change: Reflections on participatory methodology. In E. Whitmore (Ed.), *New directions for evaluation: Understanding and practicing participatory evaluation, 80,* 43–55.

Cheezum, R. R., Coombe, C. M., Israel, B. A., McGranaghan, R. J., Burris, A. N., Grant-White, S., … Anderson, M. (2013). Building community capacity to advocate for policy change: An impact evaluation of the Neighborhoods Working in Partnership Project in Detroit. *Journal of Community Practice, 21*(3), 228–247.

Coombe, C. M. (2012). Participatory approaches to evaluating community organizing and coalition building. In M. Minkler (Ed.), *Community organizing and community building for health and welfare* (pp. 346–365). New Brunswick, NJ: Rutgers University Press.

Cousins, J. B., & Chouinard, J. A. (2012). *Participatory evaluation up close: An integration of research-based knowledge.* Charlotte, NC: Information-Age Publishing.

Cyril, S., Smith, B. J., & Renzaho, A. M. (2015). Systematic review of empowerment measures in health promotion. *Health Promotion International (2015*), 1–18.

Eng, E., & Parker, E. (1994). Measuring community competence in the Mississippi Delta: The interface between program evaluation and empowerment. *Health Education & Behavior, 21*(2), 199–220.

Fals-Borda, O., & Rahman, M. A. (1991). *Action and knowledge: Breaking the monopoly with participatory action research.* New York, NY: The Apex Press.

Fawcett, S. B., Paine-Andrews, A., Francisco, V. T., Schultz, J. A., Richter, K. P., Lewis, R. K., … Fisher, J. L. (1996). Empowering community health initiatives through evaluation. In D. M. Fetterman, S. J. Kaftarian, & A. Wandersman (Eds.), *Empowerment evaluation: Knowledge and tools for self-assessment and accountability* (pp. 161–187). Thousand Oaks, CA: Sage

Fernandes, W., & Tandon, R. (1981). *Participatory research and evaluation: Experiments in research as a process of liberation.* New Delhi, India: Indian Social Institute.

Fetterman, D. M. (2000). *Foundations of empowerment evaluation.* Thousand Oaks, CA: Sage.

Fetterman, D. M., Kaftarian, S. J., & Wandersman, A. (2015). *Empowerment evaluation: Knowledge and tools for self-assessment and accountability* (2nd ed.). Thousand Oaks, CA: Sage.

Feuerstein, M. T. (1988). Finding the methods to fit the people: Training for participatory evaluation. *Community Development Journal, 23*(1), 16–25.

Freire, P. (1982). Creating alternative research methods: Learning to do it by doing it. In B. Hall, A. Gillette, & R. Tandon (Eds.), *Creating knowledge: A monopoly? Participatory research in development* (pp. 29–37). New Delhi, India: Society for Participatory Research in Asia.

Freire, P. (2003). *Pedagogy of the oppressed.* New York, NY: Continuum.

Gaventa, J. (1980). *Power and powerlessness: Quiescence and rebellion in an Appalachian valley.* Chicago: University of Illinois Press.

Gaventa, J. (1991). Toward a knowledge democracy: Viewpoints on participatory research in North America. In O. Fals-Borda & M. A. Rahman (Eds.), *Action and knowledge: Breaking the monopoly with participatory action-research* (pp. 121–131). New York, NY: The Apex Press.

Goodman, R. M., Speers, M. A., McLeroy, K., Fawcett, S., Kegler, M., Parker, E., Sterling, T., & Wallerstein, N. (1998). Identifying and defining the dimensions of community capacity to provide a basis for measurement. *Health Education & Behavior, 25*(3), 258–278.

Gramsci, A. (1971). *Selections from the prison notebook of Antonio Gramsci.* Q. Hoare & G. N. Smith (Eds.). London, UK: The Electric Book Company.

Granner, M. L., & Sharpe, P. A. (2004). Evaluating community coalition characteristics and functioning: A summary of measurement tools. *Health Education Research, 19*(5), 514–532.

Gravlee, C. C., Zenk, S. N., Woods, S., Rowe, Z., & Schulz, A. J. (2006). Handheld computers for direct observation of the social and physical environment. *Field Methods, 18*(4), 382–397.

Hall, B., Jackson, E., Tandon, R., Fontan, J. M., & Lall, N. (2013). *Knowledge, democracy, and action: Community-university partnerships in global perspectives*. Manchester, UK: Manchester University Press.

Horton, M. (2003). *The Miles Horton reader: Education for social change*. D. Jacobs (Ed.). Knoxville, TN: The University of Tennessee Press.

Israel, B. A., Coombe, C. M., Cheezum, R. R., Schulz, A. J., McGranaghan, R. J., Lichtenstein, R., ... Burris A. (2010). Community-based participatory research: A capacity building approach for policy advocacy aimed at eliminating health disparities. *American Journal of Public Health, 100*(11), 2094–2102.

Kawakami, A. J., Aton, K., Cram, F., Lai, M. K., & Porima, L. (2007). Improving the practice of evaluation through Indigenous values and methods: Decolonizing evaluation practice returning the gaze from Hawai'i and Aotearoa. *Hülili: Multidisciplinary Research on Hawaiian Well-Being, 4*(1), 319–348.

Levin-Rozalis, M. (2003). Evaluation and research: Differences and similarities. *The Canadian Journal of Program Evaluation, 18*(2), 1–31.

Liberato, S. C., Brimblecombe, J., Ritchie, J., Ferguson, M., & Coveney, J. (2011). Measuring capacity building in communities: A review of the literature. *BMC Public Health, 11*(1), 1–10.

Maltrud, K., Polacsek, M., & Wallerstein, N. (1997). *Participatory evaluation workbook for community initiatives: A toolkit for healthy communities in New Mexico*. Albuquerque, NM: University of New Mexico, MPH Program.

Minkler, M., Garcia, A. P., Rubin, V., & Wallerstein, N. (2012). Community-based participatory research: A strategy for building healthy communities and promoting health through policy change. Retrieved from www.policylink.org/sites/default/files/CBPR.pdf

Morelli, P. T., & Mataira, P. J. (2010). Indigenizing evaluation research: A long-awaited paradigm shift. *Journal of Indigenous Voices in Social Work, 1*(2010), 1–12.

Rahman, M. A. (1991). The theoretical standpoint of PAR. In O. Fals-Borda & M. A. Rahman, *Action and knowledge: Breaking the monopoly with participatory action-research* (pp. 13–23). New York, NY: The Apex Press.

Rifkin, S. B. (2014). Examining the links between community participation and health outcomes: A review of the literature. *Health Policy and Planning, 29*(2014), ii98–ii106.

Shulha, L. M., Whitmore, E., Cousins, J. B., Gilbert, N., & Al Hadib, H. (2016). Introducing evidence-based principles to guide collaborative approaches to evaluation results of an empirical process. *American Journal of Evaluation, 37*(2), 193–215.

Springett, J., & Wallerstein, N. (2008). Issues in participatory evaluation. In M. Minkler & N. Wallerstein (Eds.), *Community-based participatory research for health: From process to outcomes* (pp. 199–220). San Francisco, CA: Jossey-Bass.

Tuhiwai Smith, L. (1999). *Decolonizing methodologies: Research and Indigenous peoples*. New York, NY: St. Martin's Press.

Wallerstein, N. (1992). Powerlessness, empowerment, and health: Implications for health promotion programs. *American Journal of Health Promotion, 6*(3), 197–205.

Wallerstein, N. (2006). *What is the evidence on effectiveness of empowerment to improve health?* Retrieved from www.euro.who.int/__data/assets/pdf_file/0010/74656/E88086.pdf

Wallerstein, N., & Auerbach, E. (2004). *Problem-posing at work: Popular educator's guide*. Edmonton, Alberta: Grass Roots Press.

Weiss, C. H. (1995). Nothing as practical as good theory: Exploring theory-based evaluation for comprehensive community initiatives for children and families. *New Approaches to Evaluating Community Initiatives: Concepts, Methods, and Contexts, 1*(1995), 65–92.

Wiggins, N. (2012). Popular education for health promotion and community empowerment: A review of the literature. *Health Promotion International, 27*(3), 356–371.

Wiggins, N., Hughes, A., Rodriguez, A., Potter, C., & Rios-Campos, T. (2014). *La Palabra es Salud* (The word is health): Combining mixed methods and CBPR to understand the comparative effectiveness of popular and conventional education. *Journal of Mixed Methods Research, 8*(3), 278–298.

Zavala, M. (2013). What do we mean by decolonizing research strategies? Lessons from decolonizing; Indigenous research projects in New Zealand and Latin America. *Decolonization: Indigeneity, Education & Society, 2*(1), 55–71.

Zukoski, A., & Luluquisen, M. (2002). Participatory evaluation: What is it? What are the challenges? *Community-Based Public Health, 5*(2002), 1–6.

CHAPTER 19

ACADEMIC POSITIONS FOR FACULTY OF COLOR

COMBINING LIFE CALLING, COMMUNITY SERVICE, AND RESEARCH

LORENDA BELONE, DEREK M. GRIFFITH, AND BARBARA BAQUERO

Since 2003, the Institute of Medicine (IOM) (Gebbie, Rosenstock, & Hernandez, 2003), the W.K. Kellogg Foundation and others have declared community-based participatory research (CBPR) to be an essential area of education for public health professionals. One of the core outcomes of CBPR partnerships is in fact the development of personal skills and capacities among all stakeholders, leading often to more formal education for community partners, students, or junior researchers. For academics, training researchers to use a CBPR approach, however, is complex, and it is particularly complex for faculty members of color. Few formal programs have sought to train doctoral-level researchers, especially scholars of color, to achieve the metrics necessary for success in university or other academic research settings through a CBPR approach. This chapter will introduce three formal training programs as experienced by three faculty members of color while using a CBPR approach.

Fortunately, there has been the Native American Research Centers for Health (NARCH) initiative funded by the National Institutes of Health (NIH) in partnership with the Indian Health Service (IHS), and two W.K. Kellogg Foundation–funded postdoctoral training programs focused on the use of CBPR: the Community Health Scholars Program and the Kellogg Health Scholars Program. In this chapter, as faculty of color, we discuss some of the unique challenges and benefits of employing a CBPR approach. We begin by briefly describing each program and the scholar representing the program. We discuss our own history and culture and how that has led each of us to see CBPR research as not only a job but as a life calling and a service to communities of color. We conclude by offering some collective reflections on how CBPR makes research more meaningful in our ability to simultaneously serve our own communities as well as the scientific community.

THE NATIVE AMERICAN RESEARCH CENTERS FOR HEALTH (NARCH)

Since 2000, the purpose of NARCH has been to fund American Indian/Alaska Native (AI/AN) research, reduce AI/AN health disparities, address the distrust of research, and support a pipeline for Native researchers. To date, there have been nine NARCH funding cycles (www.nigms.nih.gov/Research/CRCB/NARCH/Pages/default.aspx). Unlike any other NIH-funding mechanism, NARCH funding requires tribes or inter-tribal organizations to be the principal investigator of a NARCH Center, which can have multiple research and training components.

Lorenda: An Indigenous Scholar and the Contribution of NARCH

I am a Navajo woman, raised in a matriarchal society that focuses on the importance of clan relationships and the roles of daughters, mothers, grandmothers, etc., which are central to one's identity. As a child I had very loving grandparents who raised me, which is not uncommon in Navajo childrearing. Navajo grandparents often take on a very active role in raising grandchildren, something I proudly do as a grandmother of a four-year-old granddaughter. I grew up in a home where education was highly valued. I was fortunate, due to the fact that in other Navajo homes education was viewed as traumatic due to prior abusive boarding school experiences. My grandfather was a life-long learner who instilled this passion in me, along with the values of respect and the importance of service to my community.

As a Native researcher who instills the importance of service to Native communities, I utilize a community-based participatory research approach with an Indigenous paradigm. For the past seventeen years, I have been engaged in health disparities research with Native communities of the Southwest. For twelve of the seventeen years I have collaborated in the creation, piloting, and now rigorous testing of an intergenerational family prevention program with three tribal sovereign nations. In addition, for eleven years I have coinvestigated the examination of the partnering processes of CBPR across the country in the hopes of improving health equity.

As a Native scholar I obtained research experience, skills, and mentoring while a master's and then doctoral student on federally funded Centers for Disease Control and NARCH studies, each study involving a New Mexico Native community, although none of these communities were my own. Though I did not officially participate in a NARCH training component, the training I received from mentorship from faculty members at UNM's Center for Participatory Research, and on-the-job research field experiences were invaluable. When I was a pre- and postdoctoral fellow, this training led to me becoming a principal investigator on a NARCH V study with an Apache community, and I then began to participate in the national NARCH investigator network.

My dissertation examined the communicative dialectical tensions and paradoxical situations faced by other Native scholars across the county and found that they experienced multiple communicative struggles while conducting research with Native communities (Belone, 2010). A major struggle included the tension of being both insider-outsider on research involving tribal communities and serving these communities yet being held to academic requirements of publishing. Native scholars also stated they struggled with the paradox of wanting to walk the talk in the academy (for those who used a CBPR approach), which was appropriate in community settings, but not fully rewarded in the academy, and the challenges of navigating when to have (or not have) open and honest communication within academic departments about the additional accountability to the community.

As an Indigenous disparities researcher, I incorporate the centering of culture in the design and dissemination of research and when possible utilize a decolonizing methodological process with a public health socioecological holistic framework. For the past twelve years, I have been actively engaged with three New Mexico Native communities. Being responsive to these communities' voices have spurred the creation of culturally specific Navajo, Pueblo, and Apache intergenerational family curricula called the *Family Listening/Circle Program (FL/CP)* that was built upon the empirically supported and culturally embedded intervention work of Whitbeck and the Anishinabe Tribe of Minnesota. The CBPR development and piloting of the culturally specific FL/CP intervention was funded by NARCH III and V (Belone et al., 2016). The findings from these pilots included the importance of acknowledging and overcoming historical negative research experiences; using community resources; listening to the voices of the young and old in guiding the family prevention program; maintaining a continuing presence in the community, even during periods without funding; and transforming each tribe's community advisory board to an effective tribal research team.

This collaborative work resulted in a continued commitment to the tribal-university partnership and the collective decision to submit and successfully obtain an NIH R01 study to test the effectiveness of FL/CP with the tribal communities. Our intention has been to establish an empirically tested program, co-developed using CBPR processes with tribal research teams, that could eventually be offered as a nationally acknowledged evidence-based program. Historically, tribes do not have options to choose Indigenous-centered programs when using federal funds for prevention-intervention programs. The rigorous testing, therefore, of FL/CP would have huge implications for tribes across the country to adopt and then adapt their own version of the culture-centered prevention-intervention program. This result not only holds the promise of improved health outcomes for tribal communities but also makes a strong contribution to health disparities research with AI/AN populations. As a Native scholar I am a proud product of the NARCH initiative.

W.K. KELLOGG COMMUNITY HEALTH SCHOLARS (CHSP) AND KELLOGG HEALTH SCHOLARS PROGRAMS (KHSP)

From 1998 to 2007, the W.K. Kellogg Community Health Scholars Program (CHSP) provided postdoctoral training fellowships to develop and enhance their CBPR research skills in working with communities while concurrently following the core principles of CBPR by contributing to the health of communities where scholars were trained (Baquero et al., 2014; Griffith et al., 2009). The CHSP grew out of the experience of an earlier Kellogg-funded program, the community-based public health initiative (CBPHI). The initial aim of the program was to enhance community understanding of social determinants of health, identify and map Indigenous leadership, build coalitions, and increase competency in working in cross-cultural settings (www.kellogghealthscholars.org).

As the CHSP program was ending, the W.K. Kellogg Foundation decided to create the Kellogg Health Scholars program, beginning in 2007. Building on the success of CHSP, the KHSP helped scholars build skills in working with communities and in translating the findings of CBPR into policy. The KHSP also sought to strengthen the capacity of community-based organizations working in communities experiencing health disparities to initiate and participate in health disparities research, to apply this research in addressing their own health challenges, and to advocate effectively for policy changes that address these disparities. As part of the agenda of the annual networking meeting in Washington, DC, KHSP scholars and their academic and community mentors participated in a "hill walk," visiting with members of Congress, staffers, and advocacy organizations to share their work and establish relationships with these policy makers and advocates. At each of these visits, scholars and their accompanying mentors shared one-page summaries of their work and its application to policy. The program ended in 2012 after training a number of scholars in CBPR who also understood how to influence policy.

Barbara: A Latina Scholar and the Contribution of KHSP

I emigrated from Venezuela with a degree in clinical psychology to pursue my graduate education in 1998, receiving my MPH and doctoral degree from the University of California, San Diego and San Diego State University.

Living in Southern California as a Latina, I now realize I had many privileges and was shielded from racial-ethnic discrimination that occurs in other parts of the country. I am the daughter of immigrants; my parents and nuclear family immigrated from Colombia to Venezuela in the early 1970s to look for better opportunities; twenty years later I did it myself. These experiences have shaped and influenced my pre- and postdoctoral research training and career. My research focuses on addressing health disparities in obesity and cancer prevention and control through the design, implementation, and evaluation of community-based interventions to promote healthy eating and active lifestyles for Latinos and rural communities in the United States.

As an immigrant, training with mentors committed to Latino health and working in a diverse and Latino majority community, I was able to leverage my cultural background, immigrant experience, language skills, and passion for research toward learning about and addressing Latino public health issues. As a complement, my predoctoral training consisted of health behavior intervention design and implementation, with an emphasis on CBPR. Mentors, professors, and supervisors shared their power with me and used their power and privilege to offer me opportunities and connection to their networks. They took the time to polish my talents, trained me as a scientist, and supported me to continue in academia. This environment proved to be important in my development as a Latina scholar. Training in that environment made it possible for me to see myself as a researcher and allowed me to believe I could achieve that goal.

From that foundation, I was able to secure a spot in the W.K. Kellogg Health Scholar Program (KHSP) in CBPR. I would describe my experience as a scholar as empowering, eye opening, and challenging. Coming from an academic community where I was part of the dominant group, then moving to UNC, Chapel Hill was a culture shock not only because the academic experience was different but also because it was a different state with different cultural politics and history. This challenged me to think about the experiences of Latinos who do not live in California and my own power and privilege as being a highly educated Latina who shared cultural and immigrant experiences but at the same time was an outsider to the same Latino community. Realizing my outsider-insider roles as Latina and a researcher has helped me to stay grounded and connected to my Latino and academic communities. From these roles, I have drawn strength to continue my work and advocate for issues I consider important without assuming that I can represent the Latino community as a whole. But also having these roles and understanding my experience have been taxing as I am never an insider nor an outsider in either community.

Professionally, the KHSP provided me the opportunity to train and practice CBPR and to find an identity as an independent researcher. The combination of having academic and community mentors taught me how to navigate and integrate both worlds into my research and to negotiate the demands and resources of each.

Personally, I have benefited from the networks I have created, the new prestigious mentors I gained, and the reputation I acquired from being in the KHSP. As a scholar of color, I have borrowed power from academic and community mentors who have provided the currency to gain entry and acceptance into the academic community. I realize now that when I introduce myself to a new group I include my postdoctoral training as a Kellogg scholar to validate my CBPR expertise and presence in the room. In addition, the training and networks allowed for the growth of my professional and peer network of like-minded and racial-ethnic diverse researchers and scholars. I am now a part of a far-reaching network of CBPR researchers who work all across the country with whom I can collaborate and obtain support and mentorship that I would not have if I had not participated in the program. Among this diverse and rich network, I know people like me, who share similar professional experiences and work toward the same goals.

Derek: An African American Man and the Contribution of CHSP and KHSP

I am an African American man who is second-generation American. My parents immigrated here from Jamaica and Guyana and both have had careers in the health field. My interest in racial and gender disparities in health grew out of a desire to understand the relationship between racism and health and how we could reduce and eliminate racial disparities in health. I earned a PhD in clinical-community psychology from DePaul University, where my research explored people's capacity to envision and act to change political and social systems.

From this work on activism and social change, I successfully competed for a position in the CHSP, where I trained at the UNC School of Public Health. During this time, I began to study institutional racism in public health systems, and I started exploring social determinants of African American men's health. This work led to me developing an academic career studying social determinants of health, strategies to achieve health equity, and men's health disparities, first at the University of Michigan School of Public Health then at Vanderbilt University. During my time on the faculty at Michigan, I also had the honor of becoming an academic mentor at Michigan in the CHSP and KHSP programs. I mentored three postdoctoral fellows, alongside my community co-mentor, Mrs. Bettina Campbell, the executive director of YOUR Center.

In my experience, being a faculty person of color presents three unique challenges and opportunities. First, while many of us bring strong political and philosophical beliefs about fairness, justice, and equity to the work, the role of a professor is not that of a philosopher or activist who operates solely on opinion. Our jobs are to use science and scholarship to inform and make change, and we have to prioritize publishing and funding this science if we want the opportunity to use our platform to make social change. Thus, it is critical to recognize that what allows you to keep your job is meeting and exceeding the expectations of promotion and tenure in the form of peer-reviewed publications and grants. Second, while recognizing this context and its constraints, it is critical to be present in the community, all the while being transparent about who we are and what we are doing. Trust is difficult to earn, easy to lose, and hard to regain once broken. Being true to CBPR principles and successful in academia may seem at odds, but they are more complicated if you try to solve these problems without sharing them with your community partners. Good community members are willing to work with you to balance their needs and your professional needs, and part of doing this work is having enough faith in them to be honest about what you need and willing to find ways that both of you can achieve goals that are mutually beneficial. There may be some potential partners who reject this notion, but perhaps that person should not be your primary partner in this work.

Third and finally, CBPR approaches to public health research and health promotion are personal. When we do this work, we are affecting the lives of real people and their friends and loved ones who eventually should become people whom you love and care about, too. It is incumbent upon us to utilize the best of our skills and the best of ourselves, along with the resources we can marshal, to not only do the best work we can but to help others in the process. There will be community members whom you may be able to help learn about educational opportunities, jobs, and careers, not to mention junior colleagues who would benefit from your ear, support, and opinions, which are hopefully reflecting wisdom. Doing this work, as I have learned from my mentors, is not just about the job but recognizing the awesome opportunity and responsibility that we have to be successful in our careers and also to make tangible change where possible, leaving the communities better than when we arrived. We also should recognize that if you leave this work or the communities of interest without relationships that extend beyond the professional, you are likely doing something wrong.

CONCLUSION

Faculty of color who use a CBPR approach face even greater challenges than colleagues who use more traditional approaches (Belone, 2010; Walters & Simoni, 2002). As we illustrate in this chapter, one tool that has been instrumental in the professional success of faculty of color who are committed to using a CBPR approach in academia has been their participation in formal funding programs that have a pipeline orientation, such as the NARCH initiative, and more formal training programs, such as the CHSP and the KHSP. These programs provided the opportunities, supports, networks, and mentoring—during and after the formal training—that have propelled us and other scholars into successful academic careers. CBPR reflects the embodiment of specific goals, values, and beliefs, and the motivation to employ this approach as a way to realize how generations of sacrifice and struggle can be honored through not only what work we do but also how we do it. In this way, scholarship created using a CBPR approach takes on more substance and meaning by the scholars and the communities they serve or represent by creating the space for bidirectional learning for new levels of critical thinking and action (Muhammad et al., 2014).

QUESTIONS FOR DISCUSSION

1. This chapter shared training opportunities that supported the authors to be trained in CBPR and to be able to conduct CBPR research. Can you identify additional training opportunities in CBPR that were not mentioned?
2. From your experience as a scholar or community member, how can you support advancing scholars of color to engage in CBPR?

REFERENCES

Baquero, B., Goldman, S. N., Siman, F., Muqueeth, S., Eng, E., & Rhodes, S. D. (2014). Mi Cuerpo Nuestro Responsabilidad: Using photovoice to describe the assets and barriers to sexual reproductive health among Latinos. *Journal of Health Disparities Research and Practice, 7*(1 Special Issue).

Belone, L. (2010). *An examination of communicative dialectical tensions and paradoxes encountered by Native American researchers in the field and in the academy.* Dissertation, Communication and Journalism, University of New Mexico, Albuquerque, NM.

Belone, L., Tosa, J., Shendo, K., Toya, A., Straits, K., Tafoya, G., Rebecca, Rae, Noyes, E., Bird, D., & Wallerstein, N. (2016). Community-based participatory research for co-creating interventions with Native communities: A partnership between the University of New Mexico and the Pueblo of Jemez. In N. Zane, G. Bernal, & F. T. L. Leong (Eds.), *Evidence-based psychological practice with ethnic minorities: Culturally informed research and clinical strategies* (pp. 199–220). Baltimore, MD: United Book Press.

Gebbie, K., Rosenstock, L., & Hernandez, L. M. (2003). *Who will keep the public healthy? Educating public health professionals for the 21st century.* Washington, DC: The National Academies Press.

Griffith, D. M., Citrin, T., Jerome, N. W., Bayer, I., & Mebane, E. (2009). The origins and overview of the W.K. Kellogg community health scholars program. *Progress in Community Health Partnerships: Research, Education, and Action, 3*(Winter), 335–348. doi:10.1353/cpr.0.0098

Muhammad, M., Wallerstein, N., Sussman, A. L., Avila, M., Belone, L., & Duran, B. (2014). Reflections on researcher identity and power: The impact of positionality on community-based participatory research (CBPR) processes and outcomes. *Critical Sociology, 41*(7—8), 1045–1063.

Walters, K. L., & Simoni, J. M. (2002). Reconceptualizing native women's health: An "Indigenist" stress-coping model. *American Journal of Public Health, 92*(4), 520–524.

PART 7

PROMISING PRACTICES TO OUTCOMES: HEALTHY PUBLIC POLICY

As illustrated throughout this book, a distinguishing feature of community-based participatory research (CBPR) is its commitment to action as part of the research process itself and not something simply left for others to do once the study is complete. By understanding policy change as a potent "action component," CBPR has the potential for improving the lives and the health of large numbers of people, beyond the partners involved or the particular communities and populations they serve.

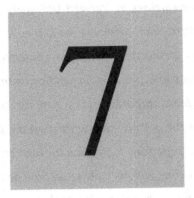

One of the most celebrated examples of the potency of community-driven and policy-focused CBPR in the United States began almost forty years ago, when residents of Woburn, Massachusetts, worried about the high rates of childhood leukemia in their neighborhood. They gathered data that led them to suspect a link to the community's water supply and tried, unsuccessfully, to convince local government authorities to test the water. Undeterred, community members then approached researchers at Harvard University's School of Public Health, and a partnership was born. Harvard team members worked collaboratively with the community in data gathering while also conducting their own epidemiological analyses to document what the community had long suspected. Not only did community members in Woburn win a multimillion-dollar civil suit against corporations that had, for years, dumped harmful chemicals in the local water supply, but the partnership's work played a key role in the federal government's decision to reauthorize Superfund legislation for toxic cleanups around the country.

In Chapter 20, Lisa Cacari-Stone and her colleagues provide an overview of CBPR and policy making, with particular attention to health equity. As they point out, although a "fundamental disconnect" often exists between researchers and policy makers, CBPR's engagement of a diversity of stakeholders including constituents most affected by a problem can build bridges among research, policy, and practice to help bring about needed change. After viewing CBPR within the context of the social ecology of research use, Chapter 20 offers and illustrates Cacari-Stone et al.'s conceptual model for CBPR in policy making. Building in part on earlier "steps and stages" frameworks, the new model moves from the contexts in which CBPR is embedded, to partnership dynamics and the roles of scientific evidence and civic engagement, to the roles partnerships may play in different phases of the policy-making process, and finally, to multi-level outcomes. An environmental justice case study illustrates the model's utility in practice, and principles of CBPR are revisited through the lens of equity policy. The chapter ends with policy competencies for CBPR partnerships interested in helping effect change on this critical macro level.

Chapter 21 by Meredith Minkler and colleagues again puts CBPR policy theory into action, analyzing a case study of food insecurity and tobacco saturation in neighborhoods that depend on small corner stores for food access. A healthy retail coalition in San Francisco's low-income Tenderloin neighborhood is examined with a focus on the roles of community, academic, health department, and other coalition partners in collecting data critical to building the local evidence base, engaging residents and merchants, and helping craft, pass, and implement a healthy retail policy enabling store conversions in such neighborhoods. The pathways model of CBPR and policy making introduced in Chapter 20 is used together with Kingdon's three streams in the policy-making process, to explore the contexts, dynamics, and diverse policy roles played by partnership members and their allies. Diverse outcomes, including successful policy passage on the municipal level, the conversion of nine initial stores to healthy retail, enhanced community and partnership capacity, and substantial increases in the availability of healthy produce and decreases in tobacco advertising and sales, also are presented, as are findings of a ripple effect in other neighborhood stores. The key role of the coalition "food justice leaders" in monitoring outcomes is discussed, as are challenges and implications for other municipalities interested in a healthy retail approach to food justice.

In Chapter 22 by Saneta deVuono-Powell and colleagues, we turn to an area in which health and social inequities in the United States are among the sharpest: the differential treatment of African Americans and Latinos in the criminal justice system. Following a brief review of the dimensions of this reality, the need for a broader, public health approach to criminal justice reform is emphasized. This broad approach is illustrated through participatory research studies of and by recently incarcerated people of color in Richmond, California, and by African Americans and Latinos in the South Bronx, New York. The two cases highlight policy outcomes, including Richmond's creation of one of the strongest "ban-the-box" measures in the country (stopping employers from asking about criminal convictions in the application and hiring process), and in the Bronx, ending such racial-profiling practices as police "stop-and-frisk" in private apartment buildings. Although the role of partnerships in such outcomes are best assessed in terms of contribution, rather than attribution, multiple data sources suggest the importance of each partnerships' efforts in bringing about these critical policy changes. Both case studies used the term participatory action research (PAR) *and use methods, such as surveys and interviews, "sidewalk science," and other methods to gather actionable data for change. Although a different term than used in the rest of the book, PAR shares similar values and principles to CBPR and offers similar promise for improving the processes and outcomes of equity-focused research on the policy level.*

In Chapter 23, Jason Corburn and colleagues broaden our gaze to explore two case studies of community-driven mapping in the global South, where slum or informal settlement dwellers and their outside partners have long mobilized to map their social and health conditions and use findings to advocate for policy change The first case study, in a large slum settlement in Rio de Janeiro, Brazil, illustrates how youth-led digital mapping, with the support of partners at UNICEF and CEDAPS, a local Non-Government Organization (NGO), involved mapping tools, including mobile phones for youth to photograph and upload images of risk in their communities to Google Maps and create a symbolic spatial representation of areas of environmental risk. They subsequently use key findings to graphically make the case to government policy actors for improvements in sanitation, reclaimed play spaces, and safer paths. In the second case study, we learn how the residents of the Mathare informal settlement in Nairobi, Kenya, have for years worked with partners at the University of Nairobi and the University of California, Berkeley, to spatially map communities, help design place-based physical and social improvements, and advocate for policies to increase health equity. The mapping led to tangible outcomes (e.g., beginning implementation of a community-designed water plan and road building and upgrades). Part of their success was their ability to help government decision makers recognize the role that settlement youth could play, working collaboratively with adult academic and other research partners to provide accurate and relevant data for policy deliberations.

Although each chapter discusses challenges, they also make the case for strong, often community-led research partnerships for collecting and translating policy-relevant data and using the findings to promote equity-focused policy change. Particularly in the unchartered waters that characterize the current historical epoch, civic engagement on all levels and in all sectors, including high-level engagement in research to inform and advocate for policy promoting health and social equity, cannot be overstated.

CHAPTER

20

COMMUNITY-BASED PARTICIPATORY RESEARCH FOR HEALTH EQUITY POLICY MAKING

LISA CACARI-STONE, MEREDITH MINKLER, NICHOLAS FREUDENBERG, AND MAKANI N. THEMBA

DESPITE DECADES OF evidence of the disproportionately adverse impacts of social disadvantage on the health of diverse populations in the United States, insufficient attention has been paid to how research can be leveraged with community partnerships to promote sound policies that advance health equity. Although research plays an important role in documenting racial and ethnic health inequities, there are ongoing challenges to moving evidence into a strategic policy agenda and focused political action. First, a fundamental disconnect typically exists between policy makers and researchers. A study of policy makers demonstrated the need for improving their understanding of the relative merits of different evidence and for researchers to better understand the demands on policy makers to better provide customer-sensitive products (Rigby, 2005).

Second, research competes with other political and world events, such as institutional constraints and rules, interest group pressure, and citizens' values (Campbell et al., 2007). The likelihood for evidence to be used in the policy-making process is increased if the research is perceived as useful to policy makers (Lavis Lomas, Hamid, & Sewankambo, 2006). Policy makers need real-life timely analysis, availability of financial and staff resources to meet demands, high technical quality, research tailored to different needs and users, and translation into user-friendly materials (Rigby, 2005).

Third, moving data into policy making requires more than the skills of researchers to package and disseminate their research for use. Northington-Gamble and Stone (2006) argue for the role of political action as a catalyst for research and policy:

> Thirty years of scholarship on agenda-setting and issues framing have shown that societal problems do not become policy issues just because they exist as problems or because careful scientific research has documented that they are problems. They must be converted into political issues by an array of leaders and defined in a way that government can do something about them. (p. 95)

To bridge the divide between scientific knowledge and policy actions, research must be shepherded through the policy-making process, from policy formulation to evaluation (Longest, 2006). The influence of research on evidence-based health equity policies relies on political momentum and civic engagement of minority populations experiencing disproportionate health inequities to move the disparities agenda from low to high importance. Community-based participatory research (CBPR) spans the division among research, policy, and practice by engaging diverse stakeholders, including those who are most affected by a policy problem of concern.

CBPR policy–focused efforts aimed at advancing health equity share values rooted in social justice and human rights, connecting people to social resources, power, or prestige. CBPR links to these values through policy-directed action. Many CBPR policy partnerships, especially those that focus on environmental and occupational justice, also highlight the utility of bridging "street science" with academic-based evidence and advocacy (Garcia et al., 2013; Gonzalez et al., 2011; see Chapter 23).

This chapter briefly reviews the role of CBPR in the social ecology of research use, presents a CBPR policy conceptual model for illustrating the role of CBPR in policy making, and reviews principles of CBPR within an equity policy framework. It then recommends equity policy competencies for CBPR partnerships that are critical for taking action. As this chapter demonstrates, although not all CBPR lends itself to policy change, CBPR partnerships with explicit goals of working within the policy arena and incorporating political action hold promise for advancing structural and systemic changes for health equity.

THE SOCIAL ECOLOGY OF RESEARCH USE

Tseng (2012, p. 7) describes the social ecology of research use as the process by which "research unfolds through linkages of relationships, organizational settings, and political and policy contexts in which policy decisions are made." In a landmark report, Prewitt, Schwandt, and Straf (2012) highlight the uncertain connection between scientific knowledge and how it is used in public policy and how it can be more effectively used. Shonkoff (2000) describes the transmission of knowledge to policy making as a complex process characterized as a daunting challenge because of the three different cultures involved (human services practice, research, and policy). Each embodies distinct cultures that it needs to learn and adapt in an atmosphere of mutual respect and understanding of a common purpose (Shonkoff, 2000).

For policy making, academic research needs to be enhanced by the knowledge and voice of those communities who can speak to their real-world experience. Research evidence needs to be locally relevant with links to local cultural and political context. Empirically supported policy interventions in the western mainstream culture may not translate to Indigenous cultures, especially if culturally supported interventions, theories, and local context are excluded from the research (Nelson, Leffler, & Hansen, 2009). Our definition of evidence within a CBPR approach embraces a variety of forms of evidence including social and basic science research; expert testimony and local cultural stories; street science; practitioner knowledge; and parent, youth, and community input.

CBPR creates a pathway by which community members or practitioners, researchers, and policy makers acquire, interpret, and use research in policy making to advance health equity. CBPR partnerships have the potential to bridge the "know-do" gap illustrated in Table 20.1 by fostering integration and translation of three types of cultures that can be linked to policy making to reduce social inequalities: (1) science, (2) policy, and (3) community-practice. This involves bringing together the three types of partners to pursue a course of targeted action that transcends deeply rooted, and sometimes self-serving, interests of politicians or scientists and researchers to advance their own agendas or keep political or academic power within their respective circles. CBPR partnerships rooted in equity policy change can help facilitate the willingness of social scientists to engage in the political process with their community partners and help forge the willingness of politicians to engage with a set of ideas beyond their class interests (Cacari Stone, Wallerstein, Minkler, & Garcia, 2014).

Although CBPR has the capacity to bridge the gap between science and practice through community engagement and social action to increase health equity (Wallerstein & Duran, 2010), fewer CBPR partnerships in the nation have explicitly targeted policy change. As discussed in Appendix 5, funders investing in CBPR have traditionally come

TABLE 20.1 The "Know-Do" Gap in Advancing Health Equity

How Policy Makers Perceive Research	How Researchers Perceive Policy	How Communities and Practitioners Perceive Policy and Research
■ Lack of timeliness ■ Politically irrelevant research ■ Research for the sake of research ■ Too much focus on describing and managing the problem ■ Lack of applicability to "real-life" solutions	■ Decisions based on political preferences and money ■ Lack of scientific evidence ■ Too much partisanship ■ Manipulation of data to support a political position or agenda ■ Lack of political will or action	■ Both disconnected from real lived experiences of the persons on whom they are doing research or for whom they are making policy ■ Lack of personal contact among researchers, policy makers, and those most affected by the problem ■ Not enough action

Source: Cacari Stone (2016).

from federal agencies, which have slowly begun to support research in environmental and structural determinants of health. This investment in CBPR in turn has manifested in an increased interest in a health-in-all-policies approach, which integrates health considerations into policy making and programming to improve the health of all communities and people (ASTHO, 2016).

Two important studies have highlighted the importance of CBPR and health policy. In 2007 and 2012, the W.K. Kellogg Foundation and the California Endowment/Policylink, together with the School of Public Health, University of California, Berkeley, published reports highlighting sixteen case studies of CBPR as a strategy for promoting health through policy change. The cases, in diverse parts of the United States ($n = 10$) and California ($n = 6$), respectively (Minkler, Garcia, Rubin, & Wallerstein, 2012; Minkler et al., 2008), were selected in part for their contributions to successful policy outcomes and with input from national and statewide advisory committees. Using in-depth, multi-method case study data collection and analysis, the partnerships ranged geographically from South Central Los Angeles; to Tar Creek, Oklahoma; to East Harlem, New York. Topics included air pollution and childhood asthma, coercive institutionalization of people with disabilities, lead paint exposure in Native and rural communities, food insecurity, and an unusual partnership with homeless skid row youth for education and criminal justice reform to end punitive practices.

THE LINK BETWEEN CBPR AND POLICY MAKING

To understand the pathways and linkages between community-based participatory research and healthy public policy, new theoretical frameworks and their testing through the use of "real-time" policy-focused CBPR projects are needed.

A Conceptual Model

As one important bridge, we present a conceptual model on CBPR and policy making that has proved useful in theorizing about and in exploring the interplay among civic engagement, political participation, and evidence as it contributes to policy changes that reduce social inequalities (Cacari Stone et al., 2014) (see Figure 20.1). Initial testing of the model focused on two environmental justice CBPR partnerships in California, one of which, the Environmental Health Coalition's (EHC) Toxic Free Campaign in the heavily Latino Old Town National City (OTNC), San Diego County, is used here to briefly illustrate the model. The coalition and its partners sought to change policy at the local level, the arena most accessible to community-based participants, and particularly at the stage of building an equity-focused agenda with multiple partners and sectors.

The majority of policy strategies developed by diverse policy partners across this and other sites were instrumental in facilitating policy formulation through systematic problem identification, creating public awareness and bringing "legitimate" attention to the issues affecting the communities, constructing policy alternatives, and adopting politically feasible policy objectives. Following is a brief description of the CBPR conceptual model along with examples from the OTNC project that illustrate how CBPR engages partners who intentionally set data-informed policy goals and direct strategies toward policy-oriented outcomes (Cacari Stone et al., 2014; Minkler et al., 2010).

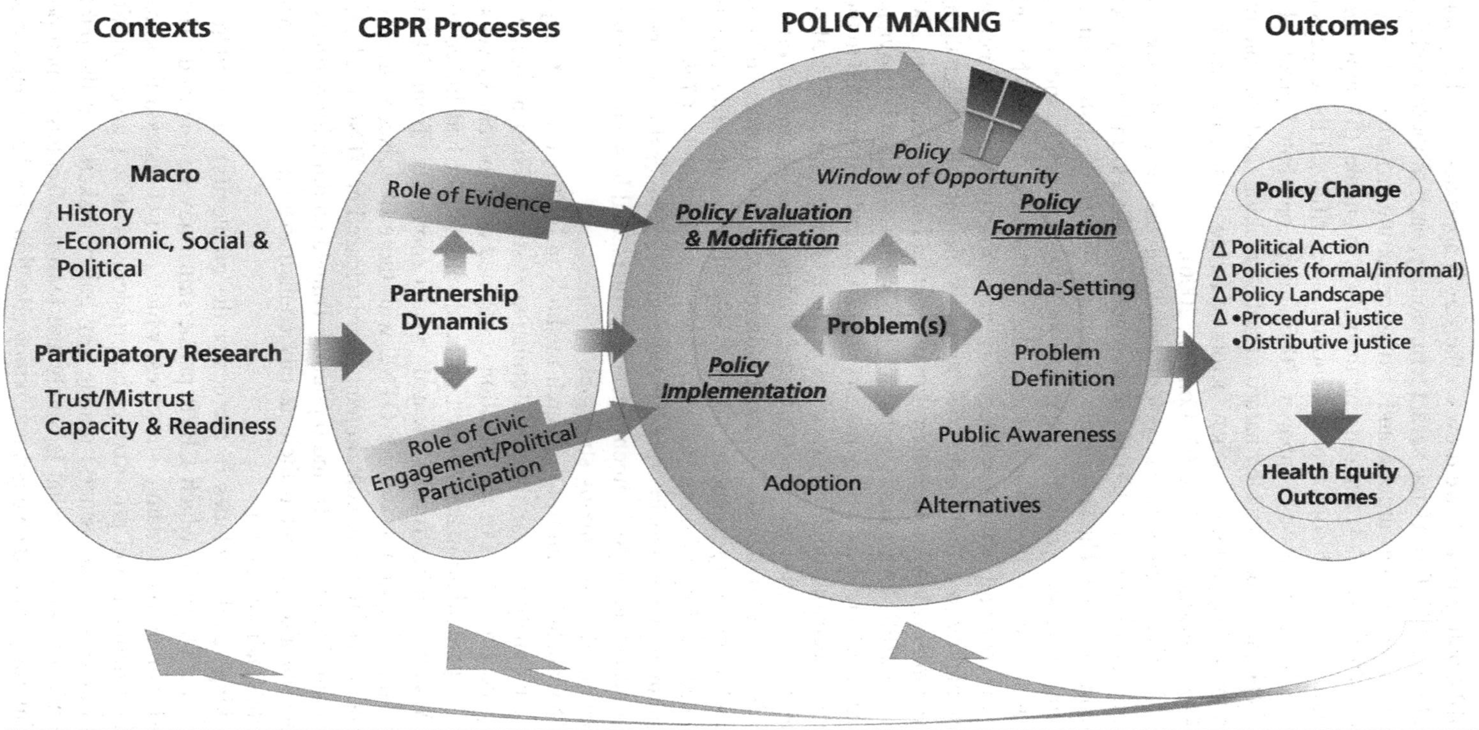

FIGURE 20.1 *CBPR Policy Model*

Source: Reprinted with permission from Cacari Stone, L., Wallerstein, N., Garcia, A., & Minkler, M. (2014). The promise of community-based participatory research for health equity: A conceptual model for bridging evidence with policy. *American Journal of Public Health, 104*(9), 1615–1623.

To create our CBPR policy model, we drew on the stages approaches of Kingdon (2003), Bardach (2000), and Longest (2006). Using varied terminology, each of these models included (1) problem definition, (2) creating awareness and setting (or getting on) policy-maker agendas, (3) constructing policy alternatives, (4) deciding on the policy to pursue, (5) implementing the policy, and (6) evaluation. Although some policy scholars have criticized these steps for oversimplifying complex political processes (Sabatier, 2007), they contributed practical insights, emphasizing the cyclical and interconnected nature of policy making, and the role of contextual factors and "windows of opportunity" when factors converge to increase the likelihood of policy change (Breckwich Vasquez et al., 2007; Longest, 2006).

The first oval, "Context," refers to *macro-contextual factors* (e.g., the socio-cultural-economic environments, political leadership and power, public attitudes, and policy trends) and the *participatory research context*. The latter includes patterns of trust (or distrust) among communities, agencies, and university partners; organizational characteristics; and their capacity for high-quality collaborative research. For instance, the macro context in OTNC included a decades' earlier decision by an all-white San Diego city council to transform the neighborhood from a residential community to a "light industrial/mixed-use neighborhood," enabling polluting industries to move into this low-income area (Environmental Health Coalition, 2005).

The second oval, "CBPR Processes," includes partnership (stakeholder) dynamics and addresses questions such as "Are there policy makers who are already committed to the issue?" and "Are there democratic decision-making processes in place among partners?" It also includes the dynamic interplay between *the role of science and evidence* and *the role of civic engagement*. Such work includes traditional outside expert–driven research studies and compelling street science, in which community members take the lead in collecting data capturing their often-sophisticated understanding of issues affecting their neighborhoods. *Civic engagement* refers to the role of community partners in organizing and advocacy, roles that may be more difficult or restricted for academic or government agency partners, and how community partners can integrate evidence into their organizing strategies.

The EHC in OTNC included multiple research methods in its Toxic Free Campaign, for example, secondary data analysis, geographic information systems (GIS) mapping, surveys, and air sampling. Resident members of the coalition conducted door-to-door surveys and collected data on ultrafine particulate matter, which an academic partner had linked to adverse lung development. A staff member further created "visual footprints" from GIS mapping, which graphically compared toxic releases for OTNC with those of adjacent areas with startling results: 23,000 pounds of toxic air contaminants were released in OTNC in 2005, whereas nearby footprints contained 6,000, 3,500, and 0 pounds. Trained community partners not only understood these data but also presented them at city council meetings and in other venues (Environmental Health Coalition, 2005).

The "Policy Making" circle includes in the center the problem(s) to be addressed and, around the periphery, the stages in which CBPR partnerships may be engaged. The policy-formation stage involves multiple dynamic strategies, which are not necessarily linear. These include agenda-setting; defining and prioritizing the problems within a given political environment, creating awareness of the issue(s) among key policy makers and the public, constructing policy alternatives based on what is timely and feasible, deciding which policies to pursue, and advocating for proposed changes and policy adoption. The last stages in particular typically involve drawing on research findings and community members' stories and experiences. Choices tend to be made when the right combination of conditions, politics (e.g., moods or leadership turnover), and policies (acceptance of ideas by policy makers) converge, creating "policy windows" of opportunity. These windows may open at any stage of the policy-making process (Kingdon, 2003).

The EHC's (2005) publication of surveys, GIS findings, and recommendations in a widely cited report was described by policy makers as having played an important role in formulating policy strategies, such as media advocacy, door-knocking, briefing public officials, and testifying at hearings. Although the academically trained research partners participated in testimony, promotoras and other residents were at the center of such efforts, including identifying policy strategies most likely to be effective (Minkler et al., 2010).

Finally, the "Outcomes" circles include policy changes, such as catalyzing political activity (i.e., new leadership, increased civic engagement), formal and informal policies (ordinances, action plans), and changes in the policy landscape. These outcomes, in turn, may increase the likelihood of future policy change and greater opportunity for two forms of justice: *distributive justice,* or equal protection and fair allocation of burdens and resources, and *procedural justice,* or fairness in how the decision-making process takes place, with marginalized communities participating in the policy-making process (Minkler, 2010; see Chapter 21).

In OTNC, policy maker and other stakeholder interviews, review of mass media, documents, and observations at hearings suggested that the EHC partnership played a key role in the unanimous passage, by the city council, of an amortization ordinance, requiring that polluting businesses be relocated outside the community within a specified period of time. The partnership's continued efforts further contributed to OTNC's becoming the first city in the state to include environmental justice in its general plan (Minkler et al., 2010). Evidence of increased *procedural justice* also was seen, including enhanced involvement of community members in city council meetings, growing youth interest in advocacy work their parents began, and one former promotora not only winning a seat on the city council but also going on to serve twice as the town's vice mayor (Minkler et al., 2010).

TAKING ACTION TO ADVANCE HEALTH EQUITY: CBPR POLICY PRINCIPLES, GOALS, STRATEGIES, TARGETS, AND TOOLS

In addition to using the CBPR policy model to identify partnership contexts, participatory strategies, and policy actions for an equity vision, CBPR partnerships may also consider several benchmarks for readiness: (1) adapting principles of equity that challenge the underlying ideologies that influence the decisions made by powerful industries, political insiders, and elites; (2) framing a policy goal from an equity lens; (3) selecting policy strategies; (4) identifying a target; and (5) using policy analysis tools.

Adapting Principles of Equity That Challenge the Underlying Ideologies That Influence the Decisions Made by Powerful Industries, Political Insiders, and Elites

In applying CBPR for policy change, we underscore the importance of a partnership's adoption of principles that span three approaches: CBPR, equity, and equity policy (see Box 20.1). CBPR

Box 20.1 Adding Principles of Equity and Equity Policy to CBPR Principles

Health Equity

- Recognizes the human right to health, defined as the right to attain the highest possible standard of health—remove obstacles to health in any sector (e.g., education, housing, or transportation) (Whitehead, 1992)
- Embraces nondiscrimination and equality—everyone has equal rights, and governments are obligated to prohibit policies that have either the intention or the effect of discriminating against particular social groups; prohibit de facto (unintentional or structural) as well as intentional discrimination
- Addresses social justice in health—striving for the highest possible standard of health for all people and giving special attention to the needs of those at greatest risk of poor health and who are economically and socially disadvantaged (Braveman et al., 2017)

Equity Policy

- Commits to distributive justice, equal protection and fair allocation of burdens and resources and procedural justice or fairness in how the decision-making process takes place with marginalized communities participating in the policy-making process (Minkler, 2010); beyond (re)allocation of resources, includes equal concerns about the nature of relationships among persons (Powers & Faden, 2006)
- Respects mutuality in relationships
- Equalizes power dynamics among diverse partners in the policy-making process
- Confronts social subordination as a threat to social justice and human rights
- Counteracts stigma of diverse populations, especially those who have been traditionally defined as "other"
- Supports capacities for self-determination
- Recognizes the role of intersectional positions of power and privilege and cultural humility in conducting community and applied research policy research
- Leverages social policies to ameliorate economic or social disadvantage, such as minimum wage laws, progressive taxation, and statutes barring discrimination in housing or employment based on race, gender, disability, or sexual orientation

partnerships often have principles that value the rich diversity and contributions of partners. Yet, this may not necessarily carry over into work for more distal structural changes that tackle the unfair distribution of resources or systemic issues related to power and privilege.

The complementarities of CBPR and policy-focused change are well captured in social justice concerns with *distributive justice* and *procedural justice*. Freudenberg expands on the principle of equity in policy by calling for identifying intersectional positions of power and privilege (see Chapter 4) and cultural humility (see Appendix 4) in modifying the social determinants of health (Freudenberg & Tsui, 2014). To best realize this potential, however, a deeper understanding of key factors is needed. These include the roles of scientific evidence and political power in bringing about policy change; the appropriate scales for policy change, from community to global; and the participatory processes that best acknowledge the interplay between power and evidence. Themba (1999) argues that community-academic partnerships should address power and help move accountability, pushing the public debate to the next level by growing and moving the parameters of research into the political realm.

To complement the principles of CBPR discussed in this book (see Chapter 3), principles of equity and equity policy may help further strengthen policy-focused CBPR practice.

Framing a Policy Goal from an Equity Lens

The first step in a CBPR partnership is to establish processes for the community to identify and frame the goal from an equity lens. In the National Academy of Sciences publication "Get Ready for Equity," Burke (2016) lists several central "equity competencies": common language, historical context, privilege and oppression, and policy and commitment to ongoing learning. In agreeing on a common language, partners should find a shared meaning in ways that support the intent of the collaboration. Going beyond the use of the term *disparities,* as the noting of *differences,* for example, the term *equity* connotes unfair and avoidable conditions, with deep understanding of the historical context of oppression, power suppression, and their intergenerational impacts on communities. To build collective wisdom and insights on systemic patterns in inequitable relationships, Jones (2016) underscores the importance of recognizing and rectifying historical injustices as a fundamental action step toward achieving health equity. In a comparison of an urban and rural CBPR case study, Devia and colleagues (2017) report how partners shaped social justice strategies for policy change based on analyses of local histories and root causes of inequities.

Setting a goal to address privilege and oppression is another avenue for developing an equity lens. It is important to name racism, sexism, homophobia, ableism, xenophobia, and Islamophobia as forces in determining how these social determinants are distributed within a given geography or community. Collective insights as to how power and oppression interplay at the personal, community, and systemic levels are core to evaluating, developing, or implementing policy. It is important to embrace ongoing learning and a commitment to humility in seeking growth in knowledge and skills among partners. Talking about privilege, oppression, and historical injustices such as racism and genocide can be challenging for diverse audiences, yet they are core to creating a policy goal from an equity lens.

Selecting Policy Strategies

After adapting principles of equity policy and selecting a policy goal, CBPR partners will need to determine who has the power to make the change, whether that be an elected official, a planning commission, or a business. Although the focus of this chapter is primarily on efforts to influence local public policy, efforts to bring about similar policy changes at higher levels or in relevant private sector arenas should also be considered, especially in partnership with other CBPR or advocacy groups in other jurisdictions. Let us now look at a range of possible policy-related strategies.

Voluntary Agreements Voluntary agreements are "pacts between a community and one or more institutions that outline conditions, expectations, or obligations without the force of law" (Themba, 1999, p. 91). Such agreements provide a useful alternative to more formal regulations when there is not sufficient support for enacting such regulations. A voluntary agreement may be an interim step toward more meaningful changes in policy, either because the voluntary agreements do not solve the problem or because some large organizations prefer public policy change to negotiating many agreements with many communities. Ideally, a written memorandum of understanding (MOU) should be developed that clearly spells out the conditions of each agreement, with appropriate oversight of implementation.

Prior to working for a healthy retail measure in San Francisco, incentivizing merchants in low-income "food swamps" to offer less alcohol and tobacco and more fresh produce (see Chapter 21), a CBPR partnership in one low-income neighborhood campaigned to get local merchants to sign voluntary agreements to stock healthier foods. These agreements led to improvements in nutritional choices for local residents and helped provide some of the evidence base for later efforts to pass legislation supporting a more formalized program citywide (Breckwich Vasquez et al., 2007; Chapter 21).

Legal Actions Well-framed legal actions, such as lawsuits and other court actions, can also accomplish significant long- and short-term goals, even if they simply result in getting the other party to the table. Yet such actions can be tedious and expensive as well as a major distraction if not integrated into a broader community agenda (Themba, 1999). Further, failure to identify the right defendants (for example, the parent company of a major local polluter) can lead to embarrassing and demoralizing defeats. In lieu of (or in addition to) bringing a lawsuit, simply filing complaints about bad or illegal practices with the appropriate regulatory agency can be an effective policy approach. In recent years, community and advocacy groups have used legal action against the food, pharmaceutical, and tobacco industries (Freudenberg, 2014) and against local governments. In the South Bronx, New York, the Morris Justice Project (MJP) is a participatory research partnership of residents, academics, lawyers, artists, and activists. Although legal challenges have not been central to their work, the MJP was in fact born in 2011 after local mothers, upset about the frequency of police harassment experienced by their sons under a "stop-and-frisk" policy, took part in a court case that effectively challenged such policing in private apartment buildings (see Chapter 22). More recently, the MJP worked with the law firm helping a California city successfully call for the reform of a controversial police "carding" policy, which also had been based on racial profiling.

Studies and Moratoriums Mandated studies and moratoriums pending data collection can be helpful under certain circumstances. Although CBPR can uncover valuable information about an unhealthy or unlawful institutional practice, far more extensive study may be necessary to collect the hard data needed to support a policy change. In such instances, CBPR partners may identify a policy goal of getting a mandated study or other data collection activity performed (or protecting what is currently being collected, such as data on racial or ethnic disparities in health).

Relatedly, a useful policy approach may involve calling for a moratorium on continued enactment of existing policy until more data are available. For example, during conflicts about local and state laws that would dictate the process for locating polluting facilities, environmental justice activists in West Harlem called for a moratorium on siting new facilities in their neighborhood to protect their community and to set a precedent that could guide future action. The breathing time allowed by a moratorium may also permit CBPR partners to organize neighborhood hearings or town hall meetings, with stories and numbers, for legislators in attendance (Wallack, Woodruff, Dorfman, & Diaz, 1999).

Electoral Strategies Electoral strategies, similar to legal approaches, tend to be time-consuming and labor intensive. Yet such approaches, including ballot initiatives, referendums by citizens, and even support of candidates, can have a considerable payoff over the longer term. There may be short-term payoffs as well. Electoral campaigns can raise the profile of an issue, attract volunteers, and pull an issue out of the purview of non-supportive policy makers and place it directly before a more supportive public. CBPR partners can often facilitate bringing an issue to public attention.

Each of these policy-related approaches—voluntary agreements, legal actions, mandated studies, moratoriums, and electoral strategies—has advantages and disadvantages that must be carefully weighed by CBPR partners in their efforts to select the alternative most likely to succeed.

Identifying a Target

As noted, decisions about the particular policy approach best suited to a given CBPR effort should be driven, in part, by a careful analysis of the most appropriate change target or decision-making body with the power to bring about the changes sought. Several key questions may be helpful to community members and their outside research partners as they choose an appropriate target:

- Who or what institutions have the power to solve or ameliorate the problem and grant the community's demands?
- Are there key actors who must be approached first as gatekeepers to the people with real power?
- What are the most powerful and strategic influences on the targets (for example, voters, consumers, faith-based organizations, investors, neighborhood organizations)?
- Who would have jurisdiction if you redefined the issue (for example, if you turned a tobacco advertising issue into a question of fair business practices)? Would this increase your likelihood of success? (Themba, 1999).

As these questions suggest, each decision-making body or target selected will require different organizing strategies to move it to action. A critical part of the CBPR process will, therefore, be conducting strategic analyses to narrow down potential targets and researching each target's self-interests, strengths, and vulnerabilities (Appendix 12). Not infrequently, such research will reveal the existence of a more vulnerable primary target with whom the possibility of success is greater. In other instances, CBPR partners may need to identify additional, secondary targets to bring about the desired change.

Finally, CBPR participants need to assess the capacities of their partnership and identify the existing competencies and needed training for conducting policy analysis.

Using Policy Analysis Tools

In CBPR partnerships, tools for achieving policy-oriented outcomes include raising public awareness of the impact of socioeconomic factors in health; engaging low-resourced and racial-ethnic communities in policy-making activities; building momentum of coalitions for grassroots organizing; applying media advocacy; and strengthening leadership, research, and policy-advocacy skills of communities.

CBPR partnerships need to invest in their ability to conduct policy analysis using various forms of evidence to make the case for change. Our CBPR policy model overemphasizes the role of CBPR in policy making and underemphasizes other factors that usually dominate the agendas and decision-making process. These include economic pressures, the role of the media, and other social and political forces that have independent and direct paths to the policy-making process. CBPR partners may wish to conduct a strategic *power analysis* to determine who has the power to make the change at the local or larger jurisdiction. Power mapping (see Appendix 12) and other tools are useful in enabling partners to become well versed in determining and analyzing the key set of players in the policy-making process.

It is also important for CBPR partnerships to diversify their focus of analysis beyond programmatic, clinical, or community-based interventions to a focus on the "structures" that determine health (systems and policies) (WHO, 2005). The use of qualitative and quantitative data may be necessary to link the interrelationships between factors at the individual level and within the social context that increase the likelihood of achieving and maintaining good health. Tools such as health equity impact assessments, digital storytelling, and mapping of visual data (see youth mapping environmental hazards in Brazil, Chapter 23), geocoding, and development of indices or measures of the SDoH (e.g., racial segregation indices, redlining) may be useful here. Similarly, the use of storytelling and side-by-side comparisons of promising or evidence-based policy interventions that list each of their trade-offs (human, economic) often are instrumental in equity-focused policy analyses.

Finally, through the use of social media and alternative communication strategies (e.g., radio, storytelling, infographics), CBPR expands the potential for translation and dissemination of various forms of evidence across diverse communities through strategies to redress power imbalances (Wallerstein & Duran, 2010). CBPR presents exciting opportunities for multimedia and multi-sectoral dissemination of research results and policy change, especially concerning the impact of research on health equity for underrepresented populations.

CONCLUSION

CBPR has been an important asset in bridging the gap among researchers, policy makers, and community members and practitioners. CBPR partners have identified, made visible, and legitimized issues so that they get on the public's agenda. It has also helped community advocates and their CBPR partners to attract media attention for long-standing but long-ignored issues when there are newsworthy findings. The best initiatives use research as a means of documenting and elucidating problems that are already of concern to communities, and they do so in ways that build confidence in community-based knowledge and ways of knowing (Chapter 2).

CBPR focused on policy change faces numerous obstacles, including the reluctance of some partners to participate, believing that they cannot legally do so, or that policy is too abstract to deal with effectively. Further, even powerful community data may be addressed informally yet discounted in policy considerations as not being rigorous enough to inform decision making. Despite such constraints, however, CBPR can be an agent for the democratization of information through bringing about the active involvement of communities in data gathering and by giving community-based groups equal access to the kinds of data that drive policy making. It can help communities influence the policy process in ways that can benefit the groups of which they are a part. CBPR partnerships are, of course, only one influence on policy. Yet, as examples in this and other chapters illustrate, community groups, academic researchers, and policy makers who are intentional about setting and achieving equity policy outcomes from the beginning can build CBPR projects that result in lasting, formal changes that, in turn, can promote health and help tackle structural and historical inequities.

QUESTIONS FOR DISCUSSION

1. Although its action orientation would seem to make policy work a natural for CBPR, community and academic partners may be reluctant to move into this area. What are some reasons for this reluctance? As a partner who sees potential for engaging in a policy-related action, what arguments might you make to encourage your partners to consider becoming engaged in this arena?
2. In what ways are goals different between CBPR partnerships that seek to advance population health (at individual, organizational, or community levels) and those that explicitly set an equity vision toward policy change? (Compare examples of CBPR partnerships you know or are described this book.)
3. Using the CBPR policy model, divide into groups based on common interests (for example, reproductive rights, environmental justice, or health care for the uninsured). Think of a real or hypothetical policy you would like to see enacted and identify where in the policy-making process is the leverage point of action (for example, agenda setting, modifying an existing policy to include equity-oriented provisions). Brainstorm strategies described in this chapter that your partnership could take to make policy, strengthen your allies, and help bring about the change you seek.

REFERENCES

Association of State and Territorial Health Officials (ASTHO). (2016). Triple aim: Implementing a "health in all policies" approach with health equity as the goal. Retrieved February 22, 2017, from www.astho.org/Health-Equity/2016-Challenge/Implementing-a-health-in-all-policies-approach-with-health-equity-as-the-goal/

Bardach, E. (2000). *A practical guide for policy analysis: The eightfold path to more efffective problem solving.* New York, NY: Chatham House.

Braveman, P., Arkin, E., Orleans, T., Proctor, D., & Plough, A. (2017). *What is health equity? And what difference does a definition make?* Princeton, NJ: Robert Wood Johnson Foundation.

Breckwich Vasquez, V., Lanz, D., Hennessey Lavery, S., Facente, S., Halpin, H. A., & Minkler, M. (2007). Addressing food security through public policy action in a community-based participatory research partnership. *Health Promotion Practice, 8*(4), 342–349.

Burke, N. (2016). Get ready for equity. *Framing the dialogue on race and ethnicity to advance health equity*. Proceedings of a Workshop. National Academy of Sciences.

Cacari Stone, L. (2016). *Lost in translation learning module: Health policy, politics and social justice*. PH 554. Albuquerque, NM: College of Population Health, University of New Mexico.

Cacari Stone, L., Wallerstein, N., Garcia, A., & Minkler, M. (2014). The promise of community-based participatory research for health equity: A conceptual model for bridging evidence with policy. *American Journal of Public Health, 104*(9), 1615–1623. doi:10.2105/AJPH.2014.301961

Campbell, S., Benita, S., Coates, E., Davies, P., & Penn, G. (2007). *Analysis for policy: Evidence-based policy in practice*. London, UK: Government Social Research Unit.

Devia, C., Baker, E., Sanchez-Youngman, S., Barnidge, E., Golub, M., Motton, F., Muhammad, M., Ruddock, C., Vicuña, B., & Wallerstein, N. (2017). CBPR to advance social and racial equity: Urban and rural partnerships in Black and Latino communities. *BMC International Journal of Health Equity, 16*, 17. doi:10.1186/s12939–016–0509–3

Environmental Health Coalition. (2005). *Reclaiming Old Town National City: A community survey*. National City, CA: Author.

Freudenberg, N. (2014). *Lethal but legal: Corportations, consumption, and protecting public health*. Oxford, UK: Oxford University Press.

Freudenberg, N., & Tsui, E. (2014). Evidence, power, and policy change in community-based participatory research. *American Journal of Public Health, 104*(1), 11–24.

Garcia, A. P., Wallerstein, N., Hricko, A., Marquez, J. N., Logan, A., Nasser, E. G., & Minkler, M. (2013). THE (Trade, Health, Environment) Impact Project: A community-based participatory research justice case study. *Environmental Justice, 6*(1), 17–26.

Gonzalez, P. A., Minkler, M., Garcia, A. P., Gordon, M., Garzon, C., Palaniappan, M.S.C., Prakash, S., & Beveridge, B. (2011). Community-based participatory research and policy advocacy to reduce diesel exposure in West Oakland, California. *American Journal of Public Health, 101*(S1), S166–S175.

Jones, C. (2016, November). Keynote address to the American Public Health Association, Denver, Colorado.

Kingdon, J. W. (2003). *Agendas, alternatives, and public policies* (2nd ed.). New York, NY: Longman.

Lavis, J. N., Lomas, J., Hamid, M., & Sewankambo, N. K. (2006). Assessing country-level efforts to link research to action. *Bulletin of the World Health Organization, 84*(8), 620–628.

Longest, B. B., Jr. (2006). *Health policymaking in the United States* (4th ed.). Chicago, IL: AUPH/Health Administration Press.

Minkler, M. (2010). Linking science and policy through community-based participatory research to study and address health disparities. *American Journal of Public Health, 100*(S1), S81–S87.

Minkler, M., Breckwich Vásquez, V., Chang, C., et al. (2008). *Promoting healthy public policy through community-based participatory research: Ten case studies*. Oakland, CA: PolicyLink.

Minkler, M., Garcia, A., Rubin, V., & Wallerstein, N. (2012). *Community-based participatory research: A strategy for building healthy communities and promoting health through policy change*. Oakland, CA: PolicyLink. Retrieved February 22, 2017, from www.policylink.org/sites/default/files/CBPR.pdf

Minkler, M., Garcia, A. P., Williams, J., LoPresti, T., & Lilly, J. (2010) Si Se Puede: Using participatory research to promote environmental justice in a Latino community in San Diego, California. *Journal of Urban Health, 87*(5), 796–812.

Nelson, S. R., Leffler, J. C., & Hansen, B. A. (2009). Toward a research agenda for understanding and improving the use of research evidence. Portland, OR: Northwest Regional Educational Laboratory. Retrieved from www.nwrel.org/researchuse/report.pdf

Northington-Gamble, V., & Stone, D. (2006). U.S. policy on health inequities: The interplay of politics and research. *Journal of Health Politics, Policy and Law, 31*(1), 93–126.

Powers, M., & Fadden, R. (2006). *Social justice: The moral foundations of public health and health policy*. Oxford, UK: Oxford University Press.

Prewitt, K., Schwandt, T. A., & Straf, M. L. (2012). Research on the use of science in policy: A framework. *Using science as evidence in public policy* (Chap. 4, pp. 53–63). Washington, DC: National Research Council, The National Academies Press. doi:https://doi.org/10.17226/13460

Rigby, E. (2005). Linking research and policy on Capitol Hill: Insights from research brokers. *Evidence and Policy, 1*(2), 195–213.

Sabatier, P. A. (2007). *Theories of the policy process* (2nd ed.). Boulder, CO: Westview Press.

Shonkoff, J. P. (2000). Science, policy and practice: Three cultures in search of a shared mission. *Child Development, 71*(1), 181–187.

Themba, M. N. (1999). *Making policy, making change: How communities are taking law into their own hands*. San Francisco, CA: Jossey-Bass.

Tseng, V., & the Senior Program Team. (2012). The use of research in policy and practice. *William T. Grant Foundation Social Policy Report, 26*(2).

Wallack, L., Woodruff, K., Dorfman, L., & Diaz, I. (1999). *News for a change: An advocate's guide to working with the media*. Thousand Oaks, CA: Sage Publications.

Wallerstein, N., & Duran, B. (2010). Community-based participatory research contributions to intervention research: The intersection of science and practice to improve health equity. *American Journal of Public Health, 100*(S1), S40–S46. doi:10.2105/AJPH.2009.184036

Whitehead, M. (1992). Concepts and principles of health equity. *Health Promotion International, 6*(3), 216–228.

WHO. (2005). Priorities for research to take forward the health equity policy agenda. WHO Task Force on Research Priorities for Equity in Health WHO Equity Team. *Bulletin of the World Health Organization, 83*, 948–995.

CHAPTER 21

IMPROVING FOOD SECURITY AND TOBACCO CONTROL THROUGH POLICY-FOCUSED CBPR

A CASE STUDY OF HEALTHY RETAIL IN SAN FRANCISCO

MEREDITH MINKLER, JENNIFER FALBE, SUSANA HENNESSEY LAVERY, JESSICA ESTRADA, AND RYAN THAYER

FOOD INSECURITY, OR "limited or uncertain access to adequate food" (Coleman-Jensen, Gregory, & Singh, 2014, p. 4), is a fact of life for one in seven Americans. As Farley and Sykes (2015) point out, however, "the problem in poor neighborhoods isn't a shortage of food, but a shortage of healthy food" (p. A19). Although half of high-income zip codes have at least one supermarket, just one in six low-income zip codes do. Further, although supermarkets in high-income zip codes devote an average of almost 280 feet of shelf space to fresh produce, small stores had just 9 feet, with three times as much space going to chips, sugary beverages, candy, and the like (Farley et al., 2009).

In neighborhoods such as San Francisco's low-income Tenderloin District, the problem of food insecurity intersects with an overabundance of advertising, display, and availability of alcohol and tobacco in the local retail environment. Poor diets, smoking, and heavy drinking contribute to the disproportionately high rates of morbidity and premature mortality (San Francisco Department of Public Health [SFDPH], 2012). This chapter begins with a brief overview of San Francisco's Tenderloin neighborhood and the Tenderloin Healthy Corner Store Coalition (the coalition). We then present the conceptual framework and methods used to explore the coalition's CBPR processes, findings, and contributions to neighborhood and policy-level change (e.g., through municipal legislation creating a successful healthy corner store retail program). We conclude by discussing some of the challenges and takeaway lessons from this case study.

OVERVIEW OF THE TENDERLOIN AND ITS HEALTHY CORNER STORE COALITION

The Tenderloin is one of San Francisco's poorest neighborhoods, with 35 percent of its thirty-two thousand residents living below the federal poverty line compared to a citywide average of 14 percent (City Data, 2015). With no full-service grocery store and more than seventy corner stores primarily stocking prepackaged food, sodas, tobacco, and alcohol, lack of access to healthy food is a significant problem. The Tenderloin also has by far the highest tobacco and alcohol outlet density in the city and correspondingly elevated rates of tobacco use and alcoholism (SFDPH, 2012). Together with deep health and social inequities and the chronic stressors associated with life in poor neighborhoods, these forces are key contributors to the poor health of residents, who have some of San Francisco's highest rates of heart disease, cancer, and premature death (SFDPH, 2012).

The precursor to what was to become the Tenderloin Healthy Corner Store Coalition (www.healthyTL.org) evolved in 2011 from a tobacco-free initiative in the neighborhood. When a youth-driven assessment graphically illustrated the plethora of tobacco advertising and availability and poor access to healthy foods in the neighborhood's corner stores, it resonated with several community-based organizations and agencies, which began meeting to discuss the problem. Formalized the following year, the coalition was initially co-led by two organizations—the Vietnamese Youth Development Center (VYDC) and the Tenderloin Neighborhood Development Corporation (TNDC)—and included diverse community-based organizations, staff members from the local health department (DPH), and other city agencies, local residents, and university partners from UC Berkeley and UCSF.

Central to the work of the coalition was the training and hiring of five local residents as "food justice leaders" (FJLs). Modeled in part on the food guardians active in the similarly food insecure Bayview Hunters Point neighborhood through its Southeast Food Access (SEFA) coalition (www.southeastfoodaccess.org), FJLs are local residents hired and trained for their roles as participatory researchers, community organizers, and advocates. Their detailed corner store assessments, resident surveys, merchant and resident education, organizing, and policy advocacy, together with the work of the larger coalition and its allies, played an important role in helping secure the passage and implementation of legislation in fall 2013, creating the city's Healthy Food Retailer Incentive Program (www.HealthyRetailSF.org) described in this chapter.

CONCEPTUAL FRAMEWORK

To explore the processes and outcomes of the coalition and its work, particularly in helping effect policy change and monitor and evaluate implementation outcomes, we used a theoretical framework that combined Kingdon's (2003) model of the three streams in the policy-making process with the CBPR and policy engagement model described in Chapter 20 (see also Cacari Stone, Wallerstein, Garcia, & Minkler, 2014).

Although policy making proceeds in a nonlinear fashion and is embedded within changing sociohistorical contexts (Bardach, 2005; Birkland, 2015; Cacari Stone et al., 2014), several policy steps "shape the content, course, pace, and development of policy" (Breckwich Vásquez et al., 2007, p. 358). Typically, they include problem definition or identification of an issue, creating awareness and getting on the policy makers' agenda, considering different policy options and deciding on one to pursue, negotiating for a policy win, and implementing the policy. Finally, and although not included in all policy-making models, monitoring and evaluating outcomes of policy implementation is a critical part of the process.

Kingdon (2003) combined these steps into three streams: the *problem stream,* convincing decision makers a problem exists and building awareness; the *politics stream,* proposing feasible, politically attractive solutions; and the *policy stream,* negotiating the politics to get approval of a proposed measure. Kingdon further noted that when positive developments occur in all three streams, a policy window of opportunity opens, increasing the likelihood of success.

As described in Chapter 20, Cacari Stone and her colleagues' (2014) pathways model of how CBPR can help promote policy change builds on the broader CBPR model used through much of this book, while adding an explicit focus on policy-making stages. It highlights, as well, "the interaction between evidence and civic engagement to shift political power" toward equity-focused policy outcomes (Cacari-Stone et al., 2014, p. 1621).

ROLE OF THE COALITION IN LINKING CBPR AND POLICY MAKING

Drawing on Kingdon's (2003) three streams in the policy-making process, and Cacari-Stone et al.'s (2014) pathways model of CBPR and policy making previously described, we now examine the role and functioning of the Tenderloin Healthy Corner Store Coalition and its CBPR efforts and contributions to policy and related change.

The "Problem Stream" and Creation of a Grassroots Coalition

Although substantial literature exists on the associations among tobacco marketing, lack of access to healthy foods, and poor health (Butler, Aboelata, Cohen, & Spilker, 2013; Farley et al., 2009; Feeding America, 2014), to effectively create awareness of the problem and reach the public and policy makers, local data that "hit home" are particularly useful.

In the Tenderloin, an "apple map" created by the Vietnamese Youth Development Center, with support from DPH, was exemplary. Based on data they had collected from thirty-five of the Tenderloin's then seventy-three corner stores, the youth created an apple map by using Google Maps, using the image of an apple, half an apple, and most often, a rotten apple core to help bring their findings alive. They showed that 42.4 percent of stores had no fresh produce, 85 percent lacked the required "no smoking" signs posted, and 75.8 percent had more than one-third of their storefronts covered with advertising, mostly for alcohol, tobacco, sugary drinks, and junk food. In all, just 19 percent of the stores received a "good apple" rating, with close to two-thirds (65.6 percent) rated "rotten apples" (Estrada & Mathews, 2012). Together with earlier CBPR studies on the lack of healthy food access and heavy tobacco concentration in the city's Bayview neighborhood (Breckwich Vásquez et al., 2007; Hennessey Lavery et al., 2005), this local evidence attracted attention and helped effect change. On the neighborhood level, the DPH encouraged the youth researchers to distribute the mandatory no smoking signs to all of the stores that were not in compliance, an action that boosted compliance by 82 percent (Estrada & Mathews, 2012).

Effective sharing of their data also increased policy maker attention to the problem. After seeing the apple map, a local supervisor visited the Tenderloin and commented, "A lot of stores are covered in cigarette and alcohol ads, or junk food and drink ads. . . I've really come to see food access as a civil rights issue. Many people don't have access to affordable, good-quality food at a fair price, and corner stores are a key part of this."

In CBPR, as Cacari Stone et al. (2014) note, partnership dynamics affect the roles of evidence, and civic engagement and political participation. To involve more community residents and organizations in further refining the problem and identifying potential ways to approach it, a community meeting was called by a local agency—the Community Benefits District—which was among several organizations for which the youths' apple map was a catalyst to action. Attended by about sixty residents and representatives of the DPH and local community-based organizations (CBOs), the meeting generated considerable interest. As a convener commented, "we had various topics for the community to give input on, but converting the corner stores from something negative into having a positive influence on the neighborhood had the greatest support" (Flood et al., 2015, p. 660). This desire for ownership, coupled with the shared goal of creating broader awareness and understanding of the problem to effect change, culminated in the formalization and naming of the Tenderloin Healthy Corner Store Coalition.

The coalition's regular organizational and individual members met monthly, sometimes joined by an architect interested in healthy retail and members of a local mosque and of the Arab American Grocers Association. Described by an early coleader as a "very, very, very diverse" group, the coalition sometimes experienced tensions based, in part, on this diversity. Yet it quickly emerged as a highly effective organization because of its strong inclusive leadership and its members' unifying belief that "food is a health equity issue" (Gomez et al., 2013). Finally, and commenting on the collaborative, community-driven process, a participant noted that for regular coalition meetings, members "drop [personal or organizational] agendas at the door" and focus on activities they are conducting in support of their collective goal.

The "Politics Stream" and the Coalition's Research and Advocacy Contributions

Building on the early apple map data, and lessons learned from the Bayview work, the coalition further honed in on the goal of improving access to healthy foods and decreasing availability of tobacco and other unhealthy products in a form that made sense within the community: turning corner stores into community assets through conversion to healthy retail.

To make the case for action promoting healthy retail, food justice leaders led in gathering more data on the needs and concerns of local residents to be shared locally and with policy makers. A 2012 multilanguage survey of 640 residents revealed that most participants shopped outside the neighborhood for staples (e.g., produce, dairy, meat and poultry, and grains), representing close to 50 percent of their total grocery expenditures. Extrapolating from these figures, TNDC staff members estimated that the neighborhood was losing some $11 million in revenue each year (Gomez et al., 2013). These stark realities, and the fact that close to 80 percent of respondents reported that they *would* buy healthy food locally if it were available and affordable, were seen by coalition members as underscoring the need for healthier, more comprehensive food options locally, which could also strengthen the local revenue base.

The Vietnamese Youth Development Center (VYDC) and the coalition held a joint press conference in December 2012 sharing their survey findings and those of the earlier apple map study to help leverage support for change (Estrada & Mathews, 2012). Coverage included a piece on local public radio featuring the voices of several involved youth and an article in a district supervisor's newsletter. As another policy maker remarked, "The fact that local people provided actual numbers and facts from work on-the-ground made a difference," because any proposed policy measure "has to have support from the community."

Community support, however, also needed to come from local merchants, who could be resistant to a policy measure that might discourage the selling of what many perceived as their most profitable items: tobacco and alcohol. The coalition, SFDPH, and a nonprofit design and architecture firm specializing in grocery store retailers, Sutti & Associates, educated merchants about the strong profit margins on dairy, bread, meat, and fresh produce (25 to 50 percent, and sometimes exceeding 100 percent for precut fruit and salads), compared to 15 to 25 percent on tobacco and alcohol (PolicyLink, 2013, p. 8). They also reminded merchants of the voluntary nature of the proposed program.

A key legislative aide further noted that to get buy-in from all stakeholders, "we sent different iterations of the [proposed] legislation around to the Arab American Grocers' Association (AAGA), the coalition, and others to talk through the language of the measure." This inclusive approach proved critical with a particularly important player: the AAGA, representing 450 stores in the city, many of them in the Tenderloin and Bayview Districts, which eventually endorsed the proposed ordinance.

Merchants also were involved with DPH, the coalition, San Francisco Office of Economic and Workforce Development (OEWD), and other partners in working out details of the legislation. The final product of this collaborative effort was the Healthy Retailer Incentive Ordinance, which would provide technical assistance with redesigns and other benefits for selected stores that, in turn, would commit to changes (e.g., shifting their business plan) to meet the definition of a healthy retailer in the legislation. That definition included devoting at least 35 percent of selling space to healthy foods and no more than 20 percent to alcohol and tobacco combined while removing specified amounts of their cigarette and alcohol advertising and paying minimum wage to workers (www.sfsbdc.org/HealthyRetailSF).

To make the proposed healthy retail measure politically attractive and feasible (Kingdon, 2003), the roles of different players were clearly laid out and the need for only a small monetary investment from the city highlighted. OEWD would house the program and contribute just $60,000 annually for the physical and business operations, technical assistance, and equipment. OEWD would work closely with the DPH in running the program, with the latter also contributing community engagement resources and materials. The fact that the coalition had already brought in a small foundation grant in support of healthy retail, including funding for an initial pilot store conversion, further underscored the commitment of diverse stakeholders to assisting the city in this endeavor. This bundling of resources supported the HealthyRetail SF (HRSF) model, which emphasized community engagement, physical redesign of stores, and improved business operations.

Detailed methods were described in the legislation for ensuring store and program accountability, monitoring, and evaluation, including, in addition to point-of-sale data, "report cards" to be completed by the FJLs in each participating store biweekly. Further, and prior to the legislation's passage, a fifty-four-item Standards for Health and Sustainability Tool (http://southeastfoodaccess.org/138) introduced by DPH and piloted in the Bayview was revised minimally and conducted by the coalition's FJLs in two-thirds of the Tenderloin's seventy-plus corner stores. The FJLs' strong relationships with local store owners and managers helped achieve this high level of participation. Findings were made accessible to residents and merchants through an eleven-page Tenderloin Corner Store Shopping Guide, which included a color picture of each store, its data-based rating on a one- to four-star scale, and a summary of its "healthy highlights" (e.g., low-fat dairy, no tobacco, and acceptance of Electronic Benefits Transfers or food stamps). In addition to capturing baseline data for studying changes in the stores over time, the initial findings (e.g., that the majority of stores received a rating of just one to two stars, with only one receiving four stars) provided additional evidence of the need for the proposed legislation.

The importance of sustaining trusting relationships with participating stores and growing community engagement while building the evidence base for policy change (Cacari Stone et al., 2014; Minkler, 2014) remained evident in this second phase of the policy-making process. The FJLs, for example, shared copies of the shopping guide first with the merchants as part of individualized feedback packets and one-on-one education. They then distributed the shopping guide at a large community forum attended by about 150 residents and others, with tabling by twelve CBOs, a nutritious meal along with recipes provided by a coalition member organization, and speeches by a supervisor and another's legislative aide about the proposed healthy retail ordinance and how it would benefit the neighborhood.

The "Policy Stream" and a Window of Opportunity

In the final stream of the policy-making process, the FJLs and other coalition members, together with their counterparts in the Bayview, spoke with policy makers in person and at hearings before the full board of supervisors and relevant subcommittees to advocate for the healthy retail legislation. Reflecting on the importance of their testimony at a land use hearing shortly before a vote of the full board of supervisors, a policy maker commented on how coalition members' words seemed to resonate with some members of the board who had not paid much attention to the issue of lack of access to healthy foods. As he noted, "It also brought up things not apparent [to them]. So much publicity about [the city's] great restaurants, the food culture, but hearing from people who couldn't get healthy food in their own neighborhood was something else."

A supervisor cosponsor of the legislation later reflected that "the coalition was extremely influential in drafting, refining, and then passing the healthy retailer ordinance" in part because it "brought members in to educate the legislators [and] had very clear ideas in working with our staff on what the measure should look like." Their collective work paid off, and on September 1, 2013, the board of supervisors unanimously passed the Healthy Food Retailer Incentive Program Ordinance, which was then signed into law by the mayor.

In retrospect, a policy "window of opportunity" (Kingdon, 2003) may have helped with the legislation's passage. As a policy maker noted, city hall–based priorities of redevelopment, reducing community violence, and "doing something" about growing inequalities and hunger in this affluent city provided an ideal environment for getting the absence of healthy retail in the city's poorest neighborhoods on the policy agenda in the *problem stream*. In the *politics stream*, the design of a low-cost measure, with the ability to bring together multiple stakeholders and public-private partnerships, and with grounding in scientific evidence and strong community engagement, was promising. Finally, in the *policy stream*, a progressive board of supervisors, several of whose members prioritized food insecurity; a mayor concerned about the city's poor but also the needs of small business; and effective media and policy advocacy (see for example, Lagos, 2013) proved critical.

Policy Implementation, Monitoring, and Evaluation

Passing legislation, and particularly municipal ordinances that may "lack teeth," must be followed by timely implementation, including detailed measures for monitoring, evaluating, and suggesting course corrections where needed (Bardach, 2005; Breckwich Vasquez et al., 2007). Soon after the ordinance's passage, the HRSF program infrastructure, including a refined model and five implementation steps, was established, along with staffing and the creation of a centralized resource center (see www.Healthyretailsf.org). A HRSF program advisory committee also was established to review progress to date and offer guidance to OECD and DPH in program decision making. Importantly, three representatives of the coalition were invited to join the advisory committee, meeting quarterly in city hall with government representatives and other key stakeholders.

Implementation of HRSF included the conversion of nine corner stores by the end of 2016, five of them in the Tenderloin, and technical assistance to an additional six stores receiving more limited improvements. But successfully translating the ordinance into practice further included engaging more than four thousand community residents in nutrition education and healthy retail efforts, food advocate training and workforce development, the strengthening of healthy retailer skills and collaborations, and the development of new local partnerships with other demand-side projects, for example, a free municipal healthy food voucher program (www.EatSF.org). Finally, implementation also involved sharing promising practices and preliminary findings through sponsorship of a Bay Area convening; media advocacy including at least fourteen press events in 2014–2015 alone; and coalition member presentations at state, national, and international professional meetings. Several articles for peer-reviewed journals also were begun, with academic, community, and health department partners as coauthors.

Ongoing efforts at monitoring and evaluating progress and outcomes of the work on the levels of the corner store, the coalition, the neighborhood, and municipal policy (HRSF) were put into place. These included the FJLs' observational assessments in two-thirds of the Tenderloin's corner stores again in 2014, 2015, and 2017, enabling analysis of changes over time. The addition of ten new observational items on tobacco advertising, availability, and display, including e-cigarettes and small cigars beginning 2014, also enabled additional data collection as new tobacco control legislation was passed and then enforced.

The major hypothesis of this case study research was that the coalition's work and HRSF implementation activities and events would have a ripple effect among other Tenderloin corner stores. We thus expected to see improvements in aggregate corner store assessment scores not only in the five Tenderloin stores participating in HRSF but also in many of those that applied but weren't accepted into the program or expressed no interest in healthy retail. Initial data suggest that this ripple effect was indeed taking place. From the 2013 baseline through 2015, the number of stores with a poor composite healthy retail assessment score (one to two stars) decreased from forty-three to twenty-five, and the number of stores with a good rating (three or four stars) increased from thirteen to thirty. Subsequent interviews with the owners or managers of fifteen stores not participating in the program further supported a ripple effect, with most reporting that they had made some healthy changes (e.g., offering some fresh fruit or reducing cigarette advertising). Reasons given typically included wanting to stay competitive, hoping to get into HRSF in the future, and not infrequently, because "my customers deserve it."

Comparison of baseline point-of-sale data from the first four Tenderloin HRSF stores with data from their monthly POS printouts, collected quarterly thereafter, also showed promise. The average units of produce sold per month in these stores increased from 6,025 at baseline to 7,489 by month six and beyond in the program. One store that did not sell any produce at baseline increased average monthly units sold to 1,438 between months six and ten. The stores decreased absolute units of tobacco sold per month, although tobacco as a percent of total sales in a fourth store remained similar. More data are needed to examine fluctuations in sales because of the seasonality of some items, store launches and other community events, and the passage and enforcement of new state and local tobacco legislation (e.g., placing more restrictions on e-cigarette advertising and display, increasing excise tax on cigarettes, and increasing minimum age from eighteen to twenty-one). These and other initial findings, however, are encouraging. Further, as a DPH partner commented, tools like the biweekly store report cards, although helpful for data analysis, also are critical to the program in other ways, "[enabling] FJLs to help merchants receive feedback and problem solve, while tracking changes."

Data collection on the coalition and its functioning also are yielding useful findings. Although many of the facilitating factors contributing to the coalition's work are discussed previously, detailed analysis of these and of key challenges faced are still under way. In the meantime, however, some of the striking obstacles that surfaced should be underscored. Among these are severe limitations in fiscal and human resources that constrain the amount that can be accomplished by the coalition and by HRSF. Although the conversion of five Tenderloin stores to healthy retail in 2014–2016 is impressive, against the background of need, five corner stores out of about seventy remain a drop in the bucket. Additionally, as some merchants noted, practices such as the recent and well-intentioned distribution of fresh fruits and vegetables by local volunteer programs may result in customers' not purchasing these items in the stores, with stores in turn seeing fresh produce go bad. One further commented that by failing to require that "food stamps" be spent primarily on healthy foods, this critical government program was thwarting the sale and consumption of healthier fare. Finally, merchant incentives from the tobacco and sugary drink industries to display ads or in other ways promote their products also were seen as barriers to healthier retail.

A major strength of the coalition was its emphasis on building individual and community capacity and receipt of a large three-year Tobacco-Related Disease Research Program grant by the academic PI in 2014, with two-thirds of the funding subcontracted for the coalition, further contributing to such capacity building. The grant enabled a doubling of the time of coalition coleaders, increased the number of FJLs from four to eight, and funded more multilingual community materials and outreach to more broadly and deeply engage additional residents. The grant also made possible more rigorous quantitative and qualitative data collection and analysis and added a coalition participatory evaluation subcommittee to help study the functioning of the partnership and its contributions to achieving project aims. As FJLs and other coalition members and staff members enhanced their skills in research and evaluation, they made new contributions to the work and increased their confidence in the importance of the lived experience, community trust, and social networks they brought to bear.

Although coalition leaders and DPH staff members facilitated important capacity building in areas such as testifying and media advocacy among their members, challenges also emerged in this area. As coalition members commented, for example, although being able to testify at hearings was "huge," in reality, conflicting family and other obligations, mobility limitations, and the frustrating tendency for hearings to be cancelled or delayed for hours without notice are often major barriers to participation. With policy makers and other stakeholders reaching out to the FJLs and other coalition members for testimony and support on other issues related to healthy retail (e.g., a soda tax and new tobacco control measures), the importance of addressing such barriers, for those who wish to increase their civic participation in this way, is underscored.

CONCLUSION

At their Health Equity Summit in 2013, the California Department of Public Health and the California Tobacco Control Program emphasized the importance of "endorsing a paradigm shift in how to look at equity. For example, supporting and building communities' ability to engage in reducing inequities at the state and local level; identifying creative ways to eliminate inequities; and measuring equity differently. . ." (Butler et al., 2013, p. 5).

In this chapter, we examined how a neighborhood coalition and its partners demonstrated this "paradigm shift" through their focus on CBPR and policy change to address food justice and inequities in exposure to tobacco and other unhealthy products in low-income neighborhoods. We further illustrated how the coalition and other actors helped affect each stream of the policy-making process, culminating in their work on helping to pass, implement, and evaluate HealthyRetail SF.

The power of youth voices and participation in CBPR as a catalyst for change emerged early in this case study and has also been widely demonstrated in studies with homeless youth (Garcia et al., 2013) and those in other low-income and marginalized communities (Berg, Coman, & Schensul, 2009; Ozer, Lavi, Douglas, & Wolf, 2015; Wilson et al., 2007; see Chapter 8).

The role of the coalition's "partnership dynamics" in strengthening the evidence base and civic engagement for change (Cacari Stone et al., 2014) was also well illustrated in our case study. Respectful, interactive trainings of the coalition's FJLs in research methods and related areas, co-led by a DPH partner and later supplemented by additional trainings in participatory evaluation with UC Berkeley researchers, emphasized the bidirectional nature of learning and data collection, interpretation, and dissemination.

As in other CBPR efforts (Minkler, 2014), there were multiple challenges of time and resources, including some that involved clashes between grant deliverables and preexisting community priorities. Additionally, rapid gentrification of the neighborhood, although positive in bringing in a stronger local revenue base and new customers for stores stocking healthier fare, also raised questions about whether a project such as HRSF may inadvertently contribute to further squeezing out of low-income residents and small businesses. Although the community engagement leg of the HRSF model is key in buffering against the displacement of local residents and increasing community pride, more attention to gentrification and how it might equitably be addressed should be explored.

Cacari Stone et al.'s (2014) model of CBPR as a strategy for policy change and Kingdon's (2003) three streams of the policy-making process proved useful conceptual frameworks for studying the processes and outcomes of the coalition and of the HRSF program it helped craft and bring to fruition. As this case study has illustrated, the use of multiple methods of evaluative data collection (e.g., interviews with policy makers and other stakeholders, focus groups, archival review, and ongoing participant observation) "can together improve a partnership's assessment of its contributions to changing a policy or the policy environment" (Minkler, Garcia, Rubin, & Wallerstein, 2012, p. 46).

Another takeaway from this case study was the imperative of *community-led* data gathering and high-level involvement in all phases of the project. FJLs had trusting relationships with, and therefore much greater access to, merchants than outside academics or health professionals. It was that trust and access that enabled the FJLs' detailed observational assessments in two-thirds of stores three years in a row, with more to follow. Indeed, one merchant commented that when strangers want to write down what he's stocking, "I throw them out."

Local members of the coalition also knew what to ask, how to ask it, and which organizations to go through in getting hundreds of residents to take part in a survey of their shopping habits and concerns. Their sharing of findings proved critical in reaching the media, the broader public, and policy makers. Further, and whether educating merchants, helping lead large community forums, or speaking out at municipal hearings and helping advise the city on implementation and sustainability, community leadership is the life blood of efforts like this one.

The imperative of doing your homework before pushing for a policy measure that requires broad-based support from diverse constituents (Minkler, 2014) also was demonstrated. For merchants who often saw alcohol and tobacco as important sources of income, for example, the FJLs' ability to understand and discuss the profit margins on these products, compared to the much more favorable margins for fresh produce, was critical. Similarly, the coalition, DPH, and other partners' working out in advance the means for monitoring implementation and measuring progress and outcomes helped underscore for policy makers that this was a well-thought-out proposal to which key supporters continue to contribute well beyond the implementation phase. Particularly in uncertain or difficult economic times, the importance of accenting for government, potential funders, and other key players the sustainability of a new project also is critical. As noted, ongoing collaboration between DPH and the coalition, and later with academic partners, helped raise the foundation and other support for HRSF beyond the modest resources available through the city.

Local leadership development, community capacity building, and increased visibility through the media and professional and academic channels helped keep the coalition and the city's HRSF program in focus. Together with organizations such as SEFA (now the Healthy

Southeast Coalition) in the Bayview and DPH, the Tenderloin Healthy Corner Store Coalition and its partners remain viable and thriving contributors to the fight against inequities in who can access healthy food and who has greater neighborhood saturation with tobacco, alcohol, and other unhealthy offerings. "Food insecurity *is* a civil rights issue," just as tobacco control is a health equity issue, if poor neighborhoods are no longer to bear the brunt of disproportionate exposure to the advertising and availability of these products. Policy-focused CBPR can play an important role in helping study and address such injustices and building community capacity and visibility as key players in helping make change happen.

QUESTIONS FOR DISCUSSION

1. Thinking back on the "three stages in the policy-making process" illustrated in this chapter (the problem, politics, and policy stages), discuss whether and how you see this model as relevant to your own work or other policy-focused CBPR with which you are familiar.
2. Some argue that having community residents take the lead in data collection may compromise the rigor of the research. Discuss this concern, and describe one to two ways in which the key data collection role of local FJLs in this case study may have improved research quality and utility.

ACKNOWLEDGMENTS

The authors gratefully acknowledge our fellow members of Tenderloin Healthy Corner Store Coalition and, particularly, the FJLs, without whom this work would not have been possible. We thank, as well, the Tenderloin Neighborhood Development Corporation, the San Francisco Department of Public Health, the SF Office of Economic and Workforce Development, and Sutti & Associates for their support, and the Food Guardians and Bayview Heal Zone for paying the way for healthy retail efforts in the Bayview neighborhood. The Tobacco-Related Disease Research Program provided funding for much of the research and policy analysis described in this study, with additional support from the California Endowment and an American Heart Association postdoctoral fellowship. We are deeply grateful to Metta Fund, San Francisco Foundation, and Dignity Health for their early and continuing support of the coalition and to Patricia Wakimoto and Gladis Chavez for their assistance. Finally, we owe deep thanks to the residents and merchants of the Tenderloin and to former Supervisor Eric Mar for their contributions to making healthy retail an increasing reality in San Francisco food swamps and beyond.

REFERENCES

Bardach, E. (2005). *A practical guide for policy analysis: The eightfold path to more effective problem solving*. New York, NY: Chatham House.

Berg, M., Coman, E., &. Schensul, J. J. (2009). Youth action research for prevention: A multi-level intervention designed to increase efficacy and empowerment among urban youth. *American Journal of Community Psychology, 43*(3–4), 345–359.

Birkland, T. A. (2015). *An introduction to the policy process: Theories, concepts and models of public policymaking* (3rd ed.). New York, NY: Routledge.

Breckwich Vásquez, A., Lanza, D., Hennessey Lavery, S., Facente, S., Halpin, H. A., & Minkler, M. (2007). Addressing food security through public policy action in a CBPR partnership. *Health Promotion Practice, 8*(4), 342–349.

Butler, D., Aboelata, M., Cohen, L., & Spilker, S. (2013). Advancing health equity in tobacco control. *Proceedings*. Health Equity Summit, June 25–26. Sacramento, CA: California Department of Public Health and California Tobacco Control Program.

Cacari Stone, L., Wallerstein, N., Garcia, A. P., & Minkler, M. (2014). The promise of community-based participatory research for health equity: A conceptual model for bridging evidence with policy. *American Journal of Public Health, 104*(9), 1615–1623.

City Data. (2015). Tenderloin neighborhood in San Francisco, CA, 94702, 94703, 94109 detailed profile. www.city-data.com/neighborhood/Tenderloin-San-Francisco-CA.html

Coleman-Jensen, A., Gregory, C., & Singh, A. (2014). Household food security in the United States in 2013. *USDA-ERS Economic Research Report* (*173*).

Estrada, J., & Mathews, G. (2012, December 3). Finding the good apples in the Tenderloin: Tenderloin youth and new community coalition launch healthy retail program. Unpublished press release.

Farley, T. A., Rice, J., Bodor, J. N., Cohen, D. A., Bluthenthal, R. N., & Rose, D. (2009). Measuring the food environment: Shelf space of fruits, vegetables, and snack foods in stores. *Journal of Urban Health, 86*(5), 672–682. doi:10.1007/s11524-009-9390-3

Farley, T. A., & Sykes, R. (2015). See no junk food, buy no junk food. *New York Times* (March 21): A19.

Feeding America. (2014). Hunger in America. Retrieved from www.feedingamerica.org/hunger-in-america/our-research/hunger-in-america/

Flood, J., Minkler, M., Hennessey Lavery, S., Estrada, J., & Falbe, J. (2015). Healthy retail as a strategy for tobacco control and food justice: A case study of collective impact. *Health Education and Behavior, 42*(5), 654–668.

Garcia, A. P., Cardenas, Z., Porter, C., Grills, C., & Minkler, M. (2013). Engaging homeless youth in community-based participatory research: A case study from skid row, Los Angeles. *Health Promotion & Practice, 15*(1), 18–27.

Gomez, A., Loresca, E., Myer, F., Payan, K., Sanseau, E., & Selpides, P. (2013). *Healthy foods at the corner store: A community project by the Tenderloin Healthy Corner Store Coalition* (Unpublished report for the PRIME program). Berkeley: University of California, Berkeley, Joint Medical Program.

Hennessey Lavery, S., Smith, M. L., Esparza, A. A., Hrushow, A., Moore, M., & Reed, D. F. (2005). The community action model: A community-driven model designed to address disparities in health. *American Journal of Public Health, 95*(4), 611–616.

Kingdon, J. W. (2003). *Agendas, alternatives, and public policies* (2nd ed.). New York, NY: Longman.

Lagos, M. (2013). Measure to help corner stores sell healthy fare. *San Francisco Chronicle* (July 7).

Milio, N. (1998). Priorities and strategies for promoting community-based prevention policies. *Journal of Public Health Management and Practice, 4*(3), 14–28.

Minkler, M. (2014). Enhancing data quality, relevance and use through community-based participatory research to improve data relevance, quality and use to effect change. In N. Cytron, K. Petit, & G. T. Kinglsey (senior eds.), *What counts? Harvesting data for American's communities* (pp. 245–259). San Francisco, CA: Federal Reserve Bank of San Francisco and the Urban Institute.

Minkler, M., Garcia, A., Rubin, V., & Wallerstein, N. (2012). *Community-based participatory research: A strategy for building healthy communities and promoting health through policy change*. Oakland, CA: PolicyLink. Retrieved from www.policylink.org/sites/default/files/CBPR.pdf

Ozer, E. J., Lavi, I., Douglas, L., & Wolf, J. P. (2015). Protective factors for youth exposed to violence in their communities: A review of family, school, and community moderators. *Journal of Clinical Child & Adolescent Psychology*, pp. 1–26.

PolicyLink. (2013). Economic and community development outcomes of healthy food retail. *PolicyLink*, p. 8. Retrieved from www.policylink.org/sites/default/files/FINAL_HER_ECONOMIC_WHITE_PAPER_FINAL_1%2018%2013.PDF

San Francisco Department of Public Health. (2012). *Community health status assessment: City and county of San Francisco*. Retrieved from www.cdph.ca.gov/data/informatics/Documents/San%20Francisco%20CHSA_10%2016%2012.pdf

Wilson, N., Dasho, S., Martin, A., Wallerstein, N., Wang, C., & Minkler, M. (2007). Engaging young adolescents in social action through photovoice: The Youth Empowerment Strategies (YES!) project. *Journal of Early Adolescence, 27*(2).

CHAPTER

22

CRIMINAL JUSTICE REFORM THROUGH PARTICIPATORY ACTION RESEARCH

SANETA DEVUONO-POWELL, MEREDITH MINKLER, EVAN BISSELL, TAMISHA WALKER, LAVERN VAUGHN, ELI MOORE, AND THE MORRIS JUSTICE PROJECT

WITH AN ESTIMATED 2.3 million of its people behind bars, the United States has the highest incarceration rate in the world (Wagner & Rabuy, 2016). Despite a recent decline, the more than quadrupling of the number of people in jail or prison from 1980 to 1990—driven by such factors as a proliferation of new felony designations, mandatory minimum sentencing, increased criminalization of drug violations, and the political capital gained through "tough-on-crime" policies and narratives—set the stage for the unfortunate "incarceration capital" designation the country holds today (Alexander, 2010). The Trump administration, led by Attorney General Jeff Sessions, has committed to increasing, rather than decreasing, arrests for minor drug and other offenses as well as the length of prison and jail terms. This policy stands in sharp contrast to the Obama administration's mandating that federal prosecutors evaluate "the unique facts and circumstances of each case" and "select charges and seek sentences that are fair and proportional based upon this individualized assessment" (Dominguez, 2017, p. 1). Further, the Trump administration's criminal justice policy builds on and reflects historical systems of racialized confinement including reservations, slavery, and internment camps.

Although white males born in the United States in 2001 had a one in seventeen chance of imprisonment, the predicted odds increased to one in six for Latino males and to an astonishing one in three for Black males (The Sentencing Project, 2013). Similar racial disparities in rates of incarceration exist for women, although the gap has declined since 2001 (Mauer & Sabrina Jones, 2013). Just 15 percent of people detained can afford to pay bail and more than half of individuals in jail are below the poverty line (Wagner & Rabuy, 2016). Indeed, low income helps explain why less than two hundred thousand of the 11 million jail admissions a year are of people who have actually been convicted (Wagner & Rabuy, 2016).

Prisons and jails are only one part of the criminal justice apparatus. It also encompasses interlocking systems and institutions, including immigration, juvenile detention centers, probation, parole, policing, and punitive aspects of child services, welfare, public housing, and third-party policing. The impact of these systems extends beyond the individual, affecting families and entire communities (Alexander, 2010; Gaber & Wright, 2016). Forty-four percent of African American women have an incarcerated family member (Lee, McCormick, Hicken, & Wildeman, 2015), and an estimated 10 million children experience parental incarceration during their lives (Pew Charitable Trusts, 2010). By 2012, three in ten Americans were under community supervision, leading to estimates that close to a third of US adults have some criminal justice record (US Bureau of Justice, 2012).

In this chapter, we summarize evidence that the criminal justice system constitutes a major public health problem. We then highlight such positive developments as the momentum for change created by Black Lives Matter and efforts to "realign" government funds away from prison and jail expansion toward community-based organizations (CBOs) and resources for prevention and successful reentry. Although situating such efforts within a public health framework, we argue that many widely heralded reform efforts focus too narrowly on individual behavior change and fail to engage those most directly affected by mass incarceration and police brutality in broader systems change. We present two contemporary case studies, driven respectively by formerly incarcerated individuals in Richmond, California, and residents of the Bronx, New York, fighting aggressive policing. Both partnerships consciously use the term *participatory action research (PAR)* rather than *CBPR* because of the former's explicit emphasis on the centrality of action in the research process. As discussed further on, however, the terms *PAR* and *CBPR* often are used interchangeably, and they share common principles and commitments such as addressing issues that matter locally, engaging community members throughout the research process, and using findings to help effect change (see also Chapters 1 and 2). We examine how these two projects collected meaningful insider data and worked for community and policy-level change while promoting personal transformation among participants. Finally, we discuss the lessons learned and their potential relevance for other CBPR-PAR efforts addressing criminal justice reform.

MASS INCARCERATION AND THE PUBLIC'S HEALTH

Increasingly, private and public discourse has focused on reforming our criminal justice system. The United States spends more than $80 billion on incarceration annually—more than six times the expenditures of other OECD countries (National Association of State Budget Officer, 2013)—yet remains one of the most violent developed countries in the world (Pew Charitable Trusts, 2011). Harsher sentencing laws had limited effect on crime rates from 1990 to 2000 and no effect since 2000 (Roeder, Eisen, & Bowling, 2015). The rehabilitative failures of incarceration also have been documented, with close to half of those released re-incarcerated within three years (Pew Charitable Trust, 2011). Further, educational and other programs that have shown lowered recidivism and greater cost savings have, with few exceptions, received little support (Anderson, 2015; Fine & Torre, 2006).

Incarceration also exacerbates negative health outcomes and poses public health risks (Binswanger, Krueger, & Steiner, 2009; Gaber & Wright, 2016). Since 2000, suicide has been the leading cause of death in local jails (Noonan, Rohloff, & Ginder, 2015). Living in neighborhoods with high incarceration rates—even for those who have never been incarcerated—puts one at significant risk for major depressive disorder and general anxiety disorder (Hatzenbuehler et al., 2015).

In many of the largely Black and Latino low-income neighborhoods, coercive and lethal policing also are concentrated. Similar to high rates of incarceration, the impact of police brutality and killings on communities imposes stressors and can erode social cohesion. The need for hypervigilance in such neighborhoods can contribute to depression and other mental health problems as well as to HIV risk-taking, obesity, and a range of chronic diseases (Sewell & Jefferson, 2016).

MOVING TOWARD A BROADER PUBLIC HEALTH APPROACH

Despite strong public outcry epitomized by Black Lives Matter, residents of Ferguson and many other groups across the country, the lack of judicial interest in prosecuting or convicting police who kill people of color is a stark indicator of institutional bias and the insecurity people of color often experience within the criminal justice system. Further, and despite limited recent, high-profile examples of police being held accountable, the continuing norm of institutional bias also reflects how a fear of the non-white "other" helps define notions of crime and "reasonable" police action. Further, it shines a spotlight on the need to address historical racism in any public health approach to arenas such as criminal justice (see Chapter 4).

Actions for reform of the criminal justice system have resulted in some important victories; between 2001 and 2009 the rate of growth in the prison population declined significantly (Mauer & Sabrina Jones, 2013). By 2013, seventeen states—supported by the Department of Justice and led by governors and legislators of both parties—had directed funding away from prison construction and toward evidence-based programs and services, including treatment and supervision (Goode, 2013). States from California to Florida have reduced sentences and eliminated enhancements for drug offenses. Laws that promulgate "collateral consequences" of felony convictions also are being challenged and changed (Mauer & Jones 2013; Sewell & Jefferson, 2016; Travis, 2002). These include the role of police in public housing (*Davis v. City of New York*); private housing (*Ligon v. City of New York)*; the exclusion of those carrying felony convictions from public housing and private rental housing, food stamps, and many jobs (US Department of Housing and Urban Development Office of Public and Indian Housing, 2015); and the growth of the "ban-the-box" movement to prohibit employers from asking applicants about prior convictions.

A diversity of states, cities, businesses, and universities also has responded to the pressure of grassroots movements to divest from prisons and prison construction. In 2015, San Francisco supervisors unanimously voted to return $80 million of state funds for the construction of a new jail. Columbia University was the first to divest from private prisons in 2015, an important step despite the small percentage of people held in private prisons nationwide. Californians are also organizing to ensure that savings generated by recent laws and rulings reducing the incarcerated population are not spent on the construction of new jails but go toward alternatives such as treatment programs or community supervision.

Concurrently, movements against police brutality have grown locally and nationally through the frequent use of direct action, increased documentation, and data collection and dissemination. Most visible is the aggregate actions of Black Lives Matter, whose ideological and political interventions challenge systemic anti-Black racism (see https://policy.m4bl.org/). Although challenges to police misconduct have been made for decades, increased community documentation of police violence and direct action responses have helped move the issue onto the policy agenda (Kingdon, 2003). This includes "The Counted," the most reliable database to date of fatal killings by police (*The Guardian*, 2015), which documented 863 such killings in 2016 and 1,134 the preceding year. Responses to community activism have also included requiring dashboard or lapel cameras on police, the right to have a lawyer at bookings in police departments, justice department investigations of municipal police departments, and consent decrees mandating changes in policing practices.

As noted previously, however, such encouraging developments are now being accompanied by a return to more punitive measures under the Trump White House, with many more (and longer-term) jail and prison terms for minor offenses. Overturning criminal justice reforms under the Obama administration, the Justice Department's "Charging and Sentencing Policy" under President Trump stated that "prosecutors should charge and pursue the most serious, readily provable offense" and invoke the most severe penalties possible (Dominguez, 2017, p.1).

Further, and independent of the often draconian measures of the Trump administration, many reform efforts have continued to focus downstream, emphasizing changing criminal behavior without acknowledging structural issues of racism and violence. Hybrid programs also have gained traction, most notably the widely heralded CeaseFire program (also called Cure Violence), which began in Chicago more than twenty years ago and now is operating in two dozen cities and several other countries, including Canada, the United Kingdom, and Iraq (www.cureviolence.org). CeaseFire involves former gang members and felons whose "street cred" enables them to reenter their communities as "interrupters" of retaliatory fights and other violence before it happens. Rigorous early research in three Chicago communities showed a reduction in violent crime of 41 to 73 percent over a three-year period (Skogan, Harnett, Bump, & Dubois, 2009).

A hallmark of CeaseFire's efforts is the involvement of local police, who typically accompany the interrupters on night walks and in other capacities. Such partnerships, however, are fraught for some communities distrustful of law enforcement. In some instances, local community groups have pulled out of CeaseFire, concerned that the decreases in violence may be largely a result of increased arrests facilitated by the program's strong police presence. Further, CeaseFire limits its members to the downstream role of interrupters on the ground. They are not engaged in discussions of the root causes of violence and mass incarceration, let alone invited to participate in developing and promoting upstream changes in policy for more-lasting, population-level health and social outcomes (personal communication from G. Slutkin, November 4, 2015).

To facilitate efforts to move upstream in the fight against mass incarceration and police violence, a broader public health approach is needed that will ensure access to resources for living, such as healthy food, education, adequate housing, and health care. But a public health approach also includes changing upstream, political economic factors, such as structural violence and racism. Nancy Krieger's (2011) "ecosocial approach" is a helpful tool in this regard. Ecosocial analysis recognizes that "people literally embody, biologically, their lived experience and the societal and ecological context of the material and social world in which we live" (p. 214). "Social trauma," exemplified by incarceration and aggressive policing, is one of the pathways of embodiment toward ill-health (p. 215).

Finally, a broader, ecosocial and community-partnered approach to prevention and public health can advance solutions that are "rooted in community wisdom—the combined knowledge, assets, intuition, and skills of community members" and will "alter policies, institutional practices, and physical environments to catalyze norms change" to support "equity, health, and safety" (Cohen, 2017). The following two case studies showcase how community-driven PAR is a strategy for helping develop and implement policies that promote, rather than thwart, social justice in the critical arena of criminal justice reform.

THE SAFE RETURN PROJECT

Just being involved with Safe Return, the impacts of how things change for people who are coming home. The changing attitude of people, telling our story, and watching a whole room of people in tears; it really was the best job I have ever had, where I felt the most useful and made an impact.

L. V.

Based in Richmond, California, the Safe Return Project is rooted in the region's unique history. With 107,000 residents, Richmond has seen not only high levels of violence and incarceration but also robust community organizing and engagement in progressive politics.

In 2010, the Safe Return (SR) Project was formed as a response to city and county discussions about realignment of funds. The project's founders were concerned that the populations that would be most affected by these changes—currently and formerly incarcerated people and their families—were not included in the conversation. The goal of Safe Return was to engage formerly incarcerated residents in PAR, leading to action on issues that affected their lives. In the seven years since its inception, Safe Return has conducted research, published reports, and advocated for and seen policy changes to improve the lives of those coming home from prison and jail (www.safereturn.org; deVuono-Powell, 2016).

SR began with a strong commitment to community-driven PAR with three organizations—the city of Richmond's Office of Neighborhood Safety, the nonprofit Contra Costa Interfaith Supporting Community Organization (CCISCO), and a research organization, the Pacific Institute. With funding from The California Endowment and two nonprofits, the partners hired a team of eight individuals who had recently returned from prison or jail to work part-time at a living wage. Organizational partners engaged the team in more than seventy-five hours of initial trainings that promoted trust and a sense of community and helped members develop skills that would facilitate community research, organizing, and advocacy. The meetings began with discussions about salient issues that team members faced in adjusting to life outside. Topics, such as how to deal with conflict, trauma, and legal challenges, were used to develop other tools and skills that informed their research and their understanding of what issues and concerns they shared with other members of the team. Concurrently, the group began to conduct informal interviews with community members and city officials and to develop the survey instrument they would later use to understand the issues faced by other formerly incarcerated people when they came home. As part of developing the survey instrument, the team was further trained in conducting interviews and other research methods. Although no formal institutional review board (IRB) process was required, team members also were taught about ethical considerations in conducting research and how to reflect these in their work.

Using their survey instrument, team members interviewed 450 Richmond residents and 101 adults who were on probation or parole. Among their findings were that fully 70 percent of those released in the last three to eighteen months had unstable housing and 78 percent were unemployed, compared to 16.5 percent citywide (Safe Return, 2011).

To create awareness and get policy makers' attention, the team published research findings, stories, and recommended action steps in a fifteen-page report, *Speaking Truth on Coming Home* (Safe Return, 2011), which was presented at a community meeting attended by 150 community residents and six public officials. In response to a major identified problem—job applications requiring felons to indicate their status—the SR team played a leading role, with other stakeholders, in helping craft and pass "ban-the-box" legislation in Richmond. SR team members did their homework, finding out that the municipal government was Richmond's third largest employer, which itself required "the box" on job applications. During this first *problem stage* in the policy-making process, SR and its allies helped create increased awareness of the adverse consequences of "the box" on the economic well-being of many of Richmond's residents, families, and neighborhoods.

In the subsequent *politics stage,* SR worked with city council members and the city attorney's office to develop a policy that was politically attractive (e.g., low cost and popular). The proposed measure would prohibit the city, or employers with city contracts, from asking about criminal history, not only on job applications but also at any point in the hiring process. During the *politics* and subsequent *policy* stage, SR and its allies continued to testify, meet with key stakeholders, and secure public and media support for the ordinance, in part by arguing that it would be among the most comprehensive in the country (Safe Return, 2011). The ban-the-box measure passed two years after SR began its efforts, and Safe Return continues to be acknowledged as a major player in this successful campaign.

The SR team also partnered with local service providers and government officials to advocate for and address another of its priority issues: creating a "one-stop shop" for reentry services. To make such a center politically feasible, SR helped lead the fight to prevent county funds from being used for jail expansion, instead making them available for substance abuse and other health and social services for people at risk of incarceration or re-incarceration. In 2015, the city celebrated the opening of the Richmond Reentry Success Center—a comprehensive center that was something every member of the Safe Return team had wished for when they were released. SR continues to work on strategies to help formerly incarcerated people. Led by one of its first formerly incarcerated members, the project now runs a biannual leadership academy for cohorts of thirty recently released individuals, who are committed to developing their personal skills and helping effect systems change.

Although not without challenges, including member and staff turnover and fund-raising difficulties for this nontraditional organization, the effective work of Safe Return is a result of its full engagement of participants and their ability to bring their lived experience and insider knowledge to the table. Further, and although not a traditional research project that needed to conform to IRB requirements and the like, the collaborative of community organizers with Pacific Institute researchers and city staff members created a promising model of ethically informed on-the-ground research that other communities have shown interest in adapting (deVuono-Powell et al., 2016).

THE MORRIS JUSTICE PROJECT

Dear NYPD, This is the Morris Justice Project . . .
This is our home! We live here. 50% of us were asked to show I.D. outside our homes. We raise our children here. 75% of community members who took our survey were stopped by the police. 25% of those were stopped for the 1st time when they were 13 or younger . . .

On the side of a twenty-story public housing building in the South Bronx, a giant bat signal illuminates the night. The projection flashes statistics and text as members of the Morris Justice Project read an open letter detailing their findings about the New York Police Department's (NYPD's) racially targeted practices of "stop-and-frisk" policing in the neighborhood. As the data performance gains momentum, with people leaning out of windows and slowing on the sidewalk, police show up and shut down the event. Such is the nature of public science and PAR focused on aggressive policing practices by the nation's largest police department in a heavily policed New York neighborhood.

The Morris Justice Project (MJP) is a PAR collective of South Bronx residents, academics from the City University of New York (CUNY) Graduate Center, John Jay College, as well as lawyers, artists, and activists. MJP's core collective is composed of about twelve people—parents and grandparents, youth, faculty members, and students. The group operates with no formal structure or consistent funding source. MJP formed to gather neighborhood thoughts and experiences on aggressive police practices in order to speak back to the police and intervene against harassment of area residents.

MJP's process is rooted in the organizing call for "no research about us, without us" (Charlton, 1998) or what Arjun Appadurai (2006) has called the "right to research." Consistent with the philosophy of PAR (Cornwall & Jewkes, 1995), this notion expands conventional conceptualizations of expertise, insisting that those who have been traditionally the objects of research be repositioned as architects of research—designing, conducting, interpreting, and reporting the findings (Appadurai, 2006). Following this, at each stage of research, MJP members work collaboratively and iteratively.

MJP was formed in 2011 after neighborhood mothers sought to respond, in part through a successful lawsuit, to frequent police harassment of their sons because of NYPD's stop-and-frisk practice. Known colloquially as "broken windows" policing, stop-and-frisk, as practiced by the NYPD, required police officers to meet a quota of stops and resulted in disproportionate harassment of Black and Latino residents. The mothers were introduced by their lawyers to researchers at the Public Science Project (PSP; publicscienceproject.org). A PAR research center at the CUNY Graduate Center, the PSP was interested in partnering with the mothers, and the Morris Justice Project was formed. Community activists, including MJP, saw a major victory in the 2014 decision in *Floyd v. City of New York*; how the NYPD practiced stop-and-frisk was shown to exhibit racial bias and was found to be in violation of the 4th and 14th amendments of the US Constitution.

MJP employs and develops context-specific participatory research methods for a forty-two-block neighborhood defined by the group. After outlining this geographic area, the partnership went through an iterative process of developing a community survey, accountable to the expertise of area residents and the university IRB. The survey was systematically distributed by members throughout the neighborhood and attracted 1,030 respondents. The survey process created opportunities for additional neighborhood residents to join, and this expanded group analyzed the results from the surveys through a "stats-'n-action" collaborative data analysis process (Stoudt & Torre, 2014). MJP members then designed a "back-pocket" report, which could be folded up and put in one's back pocket, for ease of distribution on neighborhood streets (see morrisjustice.org). This back-pocket report included a summary of quantitative and qualitative findings, an overview of the project, sample demographics, and a comparative analysis of their Bronx neighborhood with a whiter, more affluent neighborhood in lower Manhattan. The findings cast in stark relief the highly disproportionate policing of the MJP neighborhood, with 75 percent of residents surveyed, for example, reporting that they personally had been stopped by police prior to age twenty-six.

Given limited public space in the neighborhood, MJP next designed a strategy to share and gather research that it calls *sidewalk science*. Sidewalk science actions are iterative practices of sharing and collecting data through temporary installations on street corners, school fences, outside the adjacent Yankee Stadium, and other slivers of public space (Stoudt & Torre, 2014). Consistent with PAR-CBBR's emphasis on translational research to educate and help inform policy and community change, during summer 2014 after stop-and-frisk was found unconstitutional in the way it was practiced, MJP created posters (see Photo 22.1), stickers, letters, and interactive displays installed throughout the neighborhood that connected stop-and-frisk and the broader, but lesser known, police strategy in which it sits—order-maintenance policing or broken windows policing. This also included the collection of new data about resident visions of a safe and healthy neighborhood (see Photo 22.2).

Sidewalk science actions create what MJP's María Elena Torre (2010) calls "contact zones," in which connection across difference generates knowledge across and through those differences. As a result, the zones become a container for communication, relationship building, debate, and data collection. As highly visible actions in a heavily policed area, these actions are reclamations of public space and an assertion of the need for community safety beyond policing. Although data are aggregated and confidential, participation may bring increased police or community attention. To address this, MJP works in larger groups, partners with lawyers while in public, and members text and call each other at the end of meetings and actions to make sure everyone is home safe.

The role of MJP actions in contributing to outcomes is based on using its sidewalk science, data collection, and other participatory research methods in multiple policy, legal, and organizing arenas. As only one player in a broad movement to challenge police practices, it is

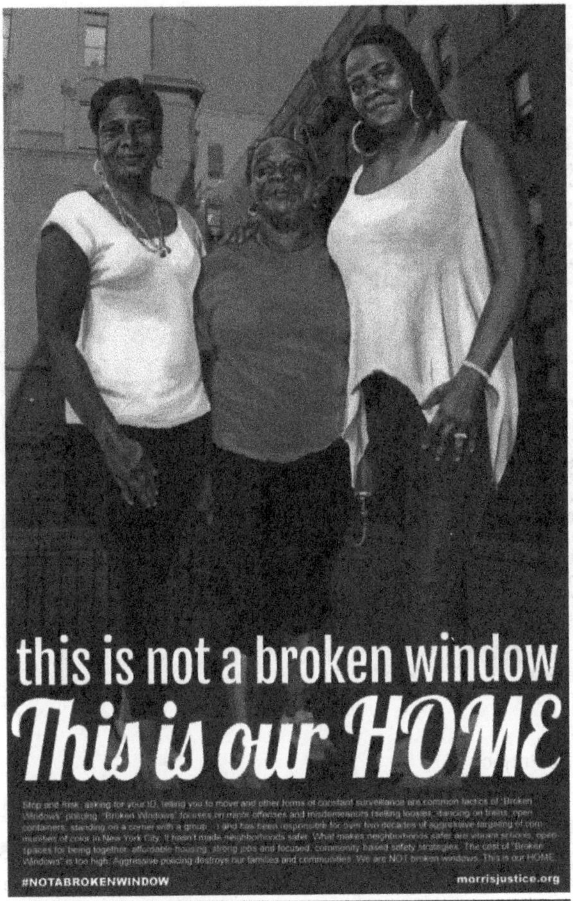
this is not a broken window
This is our HOME
#NOTABROKENWINDOW
morrisjustice.org

PHOTO 22.1
Source: María Elena Torre.
Photo Credit: Morris Justice Project

difficult, and perhaps unnecessary, to trace linear or direct policy, legal, and political outcomes precipitated by MJP's work. MJP members, however, actively speak about their findings at local town halls, rallies, and block parties as well as through various media (Pabon, 2013; Tuttle & Schneider, 2012). As MJP has expanded its audience, it embarked on a series of academic papers, including a twelve-coauthored journal article on the potential of PAR for policy making that was created through a process of interviews, group writing, and editing (Stoudt et al., 2015). MJP has been invited to present in close to a dozen academic and professional gatherings across the United States, including keynotes and presentations in venues ranging from Bronx Community College to a 2015 Citizen Science Forum at the White House.

The work of MJP included its key role in the coalition Communities United for Police Reform (CPR) (changethenypd.org), founded in 2011 to build public support for police reform legislation and legal challenges to aggressive policing. As a member, MJP infused

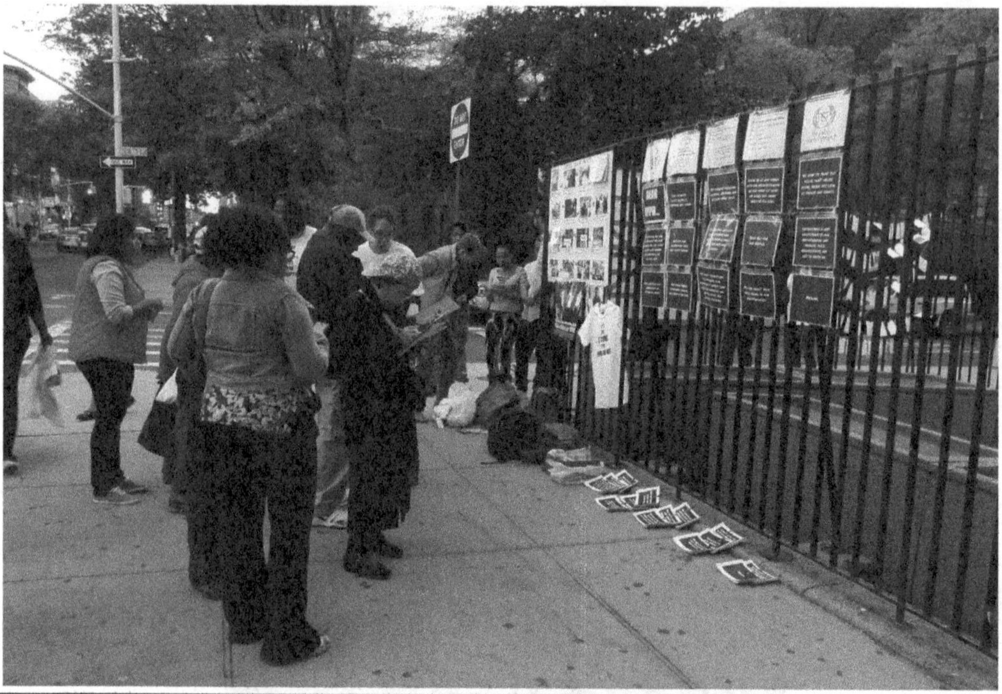

PHOTO 22.2

Photo Credit: Morris Justice Project

data and research into demonstrations, policy discussions, council votes, press conferences, and press releases, including compiling reports on court hearings for the stop-and-frisk case (see morrisjustice.org/watching-floyd). This work contributed to the passage of the Community Safety Act legally ending discriminatory profiling and providing independent oversight of the NYPD. The appointment of a MJP member to the judge's community advisory board tasked with overseeing the joint remedial reform process of stop-and-frisk further underscored the visibility of and respect in which MJP and its work was held.

MJP's prioritization of resident expertise in all stages of research, its responsive iterations of research forms, and emphasis on sharing back research from where it was gathered have informed other studies. Researchers for Fair Policing (RFP), to which two of MJP's academic researchers also belong, drew from MJP's process in its survey development on youth experiences with policing in New York. As a result of its impressive work, RFP went on to gain representation on President Obama's Task Force on 21st Century Policing. Finally, and although MJP is focused on a local area, it also worked with the law firm assisting the city of Toronto, Canada, in reforming its "carding" policy, which was resulting in racially discriminatory profiling. As part of its police reform efforts, Toronto further adapted the work of MJP for a study on carding abuse in its communities of color (Meng, 2014).

Such developments are encouraging, as is the dramatic drop in New York City's officially recorded police stops, from 685,724 in 2011 to 22,939 in 2015 (New York Civil Liberties

Union, 2015). However, significant concerns remain that the decline doesn't capture the *actual* stops experienced by residents and that formal reform efforts tend to tokenize resident participation. Nearly a year after the successful legal challenge to how NYPD practiced stop-and-frisk, the widely publicized murder of an unarmed Black man, Eric Garner, at the hands of police and the officers' acquittal, made horrifically clear how much work remains. The reform of policing is not an end, but conversely, as an MJP researcher recently commented, "We are just beginning with this." MJP recognizes that deep, lasting change necessitates critical analysis and action on schools, surveillance, gentrification, and the structures that create the social conditions of the South Bronx, particularly in the current sociopolitical climate.

CONCLUSION

The criminal justice system encompasses a complex set of institutions, policies, and dynamics, reflected in community policing, incarceration, and surveillance and how judicial systems define and punish crimes. It is therefore easy to lose sight of the upstream causes of the overlapping issues of mass incarceration and aggressive, sometimes lethal, policing in low-income, mostly Black and Latino communities. As discussed in this chapter, many new efforts at reforming some of the most obvious failures of the criminal justice system are gaining traction. Unfortunately, many of these strategies that gain mainstream acceptance are focused on downstream efforts that do little to address deeply rooted causes of and contributors to these problems.

Health professionals and academic health researchers increasingly have recognized the need to study and help address criminal justice reform, as illustrated in recent special issues of the *Journal of Urban Health* (April 2016) and the *Journal of Health Care for the Poor and Underserved* (Spring 2016). Further, as Smith and Braithwaite (2016) suggest in their "Call to Action," academic health researchers concerned with criminal justice reform should include participatory research as one of six top priorities.

Both partnerships explored in this chapter intentionally chose to use the term *participatory action research* in place of CBPR, given the former's more explicit emphasis on the centrality of action as part of the research process. Yet as noted, CBPR and PAR share a core set of values and principles, key among them beginning with an issue of local relevance and importance, engaging residents throughout the research process, building capacity, and using study findings to help effect change, often including change on the policy or systems level (see Chapters 1 and 20). In the United States, research labeled *CBPR* is more likely to be university funded or negotiated than *PAR* and to include the formal development and approval of an IRB protocol to help ensure that the partnership upholds high ethical standards in research. Yet even when there is no university or related partner, PAR (or CBPR) efforts are committed to ethical practices in survey and other data collection, maintaining confidentiality when appropriate, and so on.

The efficacy of CBPR and PAR for studying and helping address a wide range of health problems is well established. But with some important exceptions (e.g., deVuono-Powell, Schweidler, Walters, & Zohrabi, 2015; Freudenberg, Rogers, Ritas, & Nerney, 2005) its application in the criminal justice context is relatively underdeveloped. Conceived by three Oakland, California, community-based organizations (deVuono-Powell et al., 2015), reports on how trained community researchers conducted more than one thousand interviews with formerly incarcerated persons, family members, and other stakeholders in fourteen states and close to three dozen focus groups. Among their findings were that apart from immediate expenses, the costs to families of a member's incarceration often equal the annual household income, with pronounced gender differences. Fully 83 percent of family members responsible for a member's legal and other fees while incarcerated were women.

Through the two studies highlighted in this chapter, we examined how the use of PAR produced community-driven and evidence-based research and advocacy while employing novel means of community education and personal transformation, contributing to policy and community change. Efforts by Safe Return and MJP to carry a participatory ethos through all aspects of the work emphasize a political and epistemological challenge to dominant forms of research and knowledge production, particularly those that have supported mass incarceration and aggressive policing.

As these two examples illustrated, although typically cast as the "other," formerly incarcerated residents and those living in Black and Latino neighborhoods most affected by aggressive policing have a critical role to play. Community team members' knowledge and personal experiences frequently reveal deeper insights into the problems faced, connect the research with others affected by aggressive policing or incarceration, and build innovative educational- and systems-level movements for change.

Understanding the role of policy as a catalyst for promoting what the Prevention Institute describes as the "norms of equity, health and safety" (www.preventioninstitute.org/about-us/our-approach) was also demonstrated in the two case studies. For MJP, community-led education, research, and action with artists, lawyers, and other actors helped people think differently, and more deeply, about root causes of aggressive policing, including systemic racism and exclusionary forms of leadership and decision making. Their work helped catalyze change by contributing to policies that privilege "equity, health and safety," regardless of one's color or zip code. Finally, Safe Return and the Morris Justice Project offer not only lessons on reforming the failed criminal justice system but also how "upstream" intervention can occur, as well as what it can help achieve.

Among these lessons are the need to do the following:

- Prioritize the leadership and knowledge of those most directly affected by unjust and inequitable systems.
- Design data collection processes that are rigorous enough to capture complex collateral consequences of practices, such as mass incarceration and aggressive policing, and produce data outcomes relevant to those affected by the system.
- Create a research process that simultaneously focuses on policy and legal avenues to change as well as contributing to the capacity, leadership, and healing of community researchers.
- Produce accessible and creative means of disseminating knowledge created through the research to diverse audiences, from community residents through policy makers, toward the end of equity-focused sustainable change.
- Increase financial and other support for community-level, CBPR-PAR groups and partnerships to thrive and contribute their gifts to helping study and address problems that matter locally and beyond. In the case of projects such as MJP and Safe Return, because those conducting this critical work tend to live in largely Black and Brown heavily policed neighborhoods, support should include helping ensure that their participation does not contribute to increased surveillance and harassment—and engaging the media and other sectors to shine a spotlight on such harassment, if and when it occurs.

Despite the Trump administration's efforts to roll back recent reforms at the federal level (Dominguez, 2017), we are encouraged that many policy makers, particularly on the state and local levels, are finally grappling with the criminal justice system and related problems that contribute to violence, including police violence, and the unrelenting cycle of poverty and loss they exacerbate. Particularly in efforts to effect authentic and sustainable change, the engagement of affected community members as leaders and key PAR-CBPR partners in disrupting policy as usual cannot be overstated.

QUESTIONS FOR DISCUSSION

1. You are an academically trained researcher, have access to seed funding for a CBPR project, and have reached out to a community group about possibly doing a project together to address your mutual concerns with lethal policing. Members seem interested but have only heard of participatory action research and wonder what the differences are between PAR and CBPR. How would you react if they want to use the term *PAR,* but your funder is a firm believer in the lexicon of CBPR?
2. Many groups and individuals address issues such as inequities in incarceration and other aspects of the criminal justice system through direct advocacy and organizing. What role does research have in relation to these issues? Why include research instead of just action?
3. How do the case studies address upstream factors related to the criminal justice system? Why do the authors critique CeaseFire as a downstream approach?

ACKNOWLEDGEMENTS

We gratefully acknowledge the members of the Safe Return Project and the Morris Justice Project, and the many other participants in and supporters of their work. For the Safe Return Project, special thanks go to Richard Boyd and Sam Vaughn, and to others interviewed for this chapter. We also are deeply grateful to The California Endowment and the Robert Wood Johnson Foundation for their major support. For the Morris Justice Project, we thank the following members of MJP for ongoing conversations about this work and guidance on this chapter: Paul Bartley, Fawn Bracy, Anthony Downs, Cory Greene, Prakriti Hassan, Nadine Sheppard, Brett Stoudt, María Elena Torre, and Jacqueline Yates.

Finally, our deep thanks go to Black Lives Matter, the Sentencing Project, and the numerous other individuals and organizations who have made imperative ending police brutality and mass incarceration. Angela Glover Blackwell, Leonard Cavise, and Larry Cohen are among those to whom we are especially grateful for insights and contributions.

REFERENCES

Alexander, M. (2010). *The new Jim Crow: Incarceration in the age of mass incarceration.* New York, NY: The New Press.

Anderson, N. (2015, July 31). A diploma really is a crime-stopper. Feds aim to fund inmate education. *Washington Post.*

Appadurai, A. (2006). The right to research. *Globalisation, Societies and Education, 4*(2), 167–177. http://doi.org/10.1080/14767720600750696

Charlton, J. I. (1998). *Nothing about us without us: Disability oppression and empowerment.* Berkeley: University of California Press.

Clear, T., Frost, N. A., Carr, M., Dhondt, G. D., Braga, A., & Warfield, G. (2014). *Predicting crime through incarceration: The impact of rates of prison cycling on rates of crime in communities.* Washington, DC: US Department of Justice.

Cohen, L. (2017). Prevention institute: Our approach. Retrieved January 31, 2017, from www.preventioninstitute.org/about-us/our-approach

Cornwall, A., & Jewkes, R. (1995). What is participatory research? *Social Science & Medicine, 41*(12), 1667–1676. http://doi.org/10.1016/0277-9536(95)00127-S

deVuono-Powell, S., Schweidler, C., Walters, A., & Zohrabi, A. (2015). *Who pays? The true cost of incarceration on families.* Oakland, CA: Ella Baker Center, Forward Together, Research Action Design. Retrieved from http://whopaysreport.org/who-pays-full-report/

deVuono-Powell, S., Vaughn, L., Walker, T., Moore, E., & Minkler, M. (2016). Home with a purpose: A history of the Safe Return Project. The Haas Institute for a Fair and Inclusive Society. Retrieved from http://haasinstitute.berkeley.edu/sites/default/files/safereturncasestudy_publish.pdf

Dominguez, I. (2017). AG Sessions issues retrograde charging policy, seeks return to 20th century's so-called war on drugs and the age of mass incarceration. *Washington Post* (May 12), p. 1.

Fine, M., & Torre, M. (2006). Intimate details: Participatory action research in prison. *Action Research, 4*(3), 253–269.

Freudenberg, N., Rogers, M. A., Ritas, C., & Nerney, M. (2005). Policy analysis and advocacy: An approach to community-based participatory research. In B. A. Israel, E. Eng, A. J. Schulz, & E. A. Parker (Eds.), *Methods in community-based participatory research for health* (pp. 349–370). San Francisco, CA: Jossey-Bass.

Gaber, N., & Wright, A. (2016). Protecting urban health and safety: Balancing care and harm in the era of mass incarceration. *Journal of Urban Health, 93*(Suppl 1), 68–77. doi:10.1007/s11524-015-0009-6

Goode, E. (2013, July 25). U.S. prison populations decline, reflecting new approach to crime. *New York Times.* Retrieved from www.nytimes.com/2013/07/26/us/us-prison-populations-decline-reflecting-new-approach-to-crime.html

Hatzenbuehler, M. L., Keyes, K., Hamilton, A., Uddin, M., & Galea, S. (2015). The collateral damage of mass incarceration: Risk of psychiatric morbidity among nonincarcerated residents of high-incarceration neighborhoods. *American Journal of Public Health, 105*(1), 138–143.

Kingdon, J. W. (2003). *Agendas, alternatives, and public policies* (2nd ed.). New York, NY: Longman Press.

Krieger, N. (2011). *Epidemiology and the people's health: Theory and context.* Oxford, UK: Oxford University Press.

Lee, H., McCormick, T., Hicken, M. T., & Wildeman, C. (2015). Racial inequalities in connectedness to imprisoned individuals in the United States. *Du Bois Review, 12*(2), 269–282.

Mauer, M. (2013). *The changing racial dynamics of women's incarceration.* Washington, DC: The Sentencing Project. Retrieved from www.sentencingproject.org/publications/the-changing-racial-dynamics-of-womens-incarceration/

Mauer, M., & Sabrina Jones, M. (2013). *Race to incarcerate: A graphic retelling* (3rd ed.). New York, NY: The New Press

Meng, Y. (2014). Racially biased policing and neighborhood characteristics: A case study in Toronto, Canada. *Cybergeo: European Journal of Geography.* Retrieved May 23, 2017, from https://cybergeo.revues.org/26165

National Association of State Budget Officer. (2013). State spending for corrections: Long-term trends and recent criminal justice policy reforms. Retrieved from www.nasbo.org/sites/default/files/pdf/State%20Spending%20for%20Corrections.pdf

New York Civil Liberties Union. (2015). Stop-and-frisk data. Retrieved from www.nyclu.org/content/stop-and-frisk-data

Noonan, M., Rohloff, H., & Ginder, S. (2015). *Mortality in local jails and state prisons, 2000–2013 statistical tables.* Bureau of Justice Statistics. Retrieved from www.bjs.gov/index.cfm?ty=pbse&sid=76

Pabon, J. (2013, April 22). South Bronx continues to organize against "stop & frisk." *Huffington Post.* Retrieved May 24, 2016, from www.huffingtonpost.com/julio-pabon/stop-and-frisk-south-bronx_b_3123403.html

Pew Charitable Trusts. (2010). *Collateral costs: Incarceration's effect on economic mobility.* Washington, DC: The Pew Charitable Trusts. Retrieved from www.pewtrusts.org/~/media/legacy/uploadedfiles/pcs_assets/2010/collateralcosts1pdf.pdf

Pew Charitable Trusts. (2011). State of recidivism: The revolving door of America's prisons. Retrieved from www.pewtrusts.org/en/research-and-analysis/reports/0001/01/01/state-of-recidivism (p. 2).

Roeder, O., Eisen, L., & Bowling, J. (2015). What caused the crime decline? Brennan Center for Justice. Retrieved from www.brennancenter.org/publication/what-caused-crime-decline

Safe Return. (2011). Speaking truth on coming home: Research findings and recommendations on reentry in Richmond. Retrieved from www.pacinst.org/wp-content/uploads/sites/21/2013/02/reentry_report3.pdf

Sewell, A. A., & Jefferson, K. A. (2016). Collateral damage: The effects of invasive police encounters in New York City. *Journal of Urban Health, 93*(Suppl 1), 42–67.

Skogan, W., Harnett, S. M., Bump, N., & Dubois, J. (2009). *Evaluation of CeaseFire—Chicago*. Washington, DC: National Institute of Justice.

Smith, S. A., & Braithwaite, R. L. (2016). Introduction to public health and incarceration: Social justice matters. *Journal of Health Care for the Poor and Underserved, 27*(2A), 1–4.

Stoudt, B. G., & Torre, M. E. (2014). The Morris Justice Project. In P. Brindle (Ed.), *Sage cases in methodology*. Thousand Oaks, CA: Sage Publications.

Stoudt, B. G., Torre, M. E., Bartley, P., Bracy, F., Caldwell, H., Downs, A., Greene, C., Haldipur, J., Hassan, P., Manoff, E., Sheppard, N., & Yates, J. (2015). "We come from a place of knowing": Experiences, challenges, advantages and possibilities of participating in Morris Justice Project. In C. Durose & L. Richardson (Eds.), *Re-thinking public policy making: Why co-production matters*. Bristol, UK: Policy Press.

The Guardian view on killings by US police: Why we must keep counting (2015, December 31). *The Guardian*. Retrieved from www.theguardian.com/us-news/2015/dec/31/the-counted-killings-by-police-editorial

The Sentencing Project. (2013). Report of the Sentencing Project to the United Nations Human Rights Committee regarding racial disparities in the United States criminal justice system. Retrieved from http://sentencingproject.org/wp-content/uploads/2015/12/Race-and-Justice-Shadow-Report-ICCPR.pdf

Torre, M. E. (2010). *The history and enactments of contact in social psychology*. Ann Arbor, MI: UMI Dissertations Publishing.

Travis, J. (2002). Invisible punishment: An instrument of social exclusion. In M. Mauer & C.-L. Meda (Eds.), *Invisible punishment: The collateral consequences of mass imprisonment* (pp. 15–36) New York, NY: The New York Press.

Tuttle, R., & Schneider, E. (2012, October 8). Stopped-and-frisked: "For being a f**king mutt" [Video]. *The Nation*. Retrieved from www.thenation.com/article/stopped-and-frisked-being-fking-mutt-video/

US Bureau of Justice Statistics. (2012). Survey of state criminal history information systems, 2012. US Department of Justice, Office of Justice. Retrieved from www.ncjrs.gov/pdffiles1/bjs/grants/244563.pdf

US Department of Housing and Urban Development Office of Public and Indian Housing. (2015). Notice PIH 2015–19 guidance for public housing agencies (PHAs) and owners of federally assisted housing on excluding the use of arrest records in housing decisions. Retrieved from https://portal.hud.gov/hudportal/documents/huddoc?id=PIH2015–19.pdf

Wagner, P., & Rabuy, B. (2016). Mass incarceration: The whole pie 2016. Prison Policy Initiative. Retrieved from www.prisonpolicy.org/reports/pie2016.html

CHAPTER 23

GLOBAL HEALTH POLICY

SLUM SETTLEMENT MAPPING IN NAIROBI AND RIO DE JANEIRO

JASON CORBURN, IVES ROCHA, ALEXEI DUNAWAY, AND JACK MAKAU

IN COMMUNITIES ACROSS the Global South, the urban poor are organizing to map the physical and social conditions in which they live and using visualization to advocate for improved health. There is a long tradition in urban public health of mapping social conditions, exposures, and morbidity and mortality, ranging from John Snow's historic mapping of cholera cases and resultant removal of a contaminated water pump in nineteenth-century England to the twenty-first-century use of geographic information system (GIS) science to analyze and model potential interactions among biophysical, built, and social environmental factors across time and space (Brown, McLafferty, & Moon, 2010). Community-based organizations (CBOs) are increasingly partnering with universities and others to combine their local knowledge of place with computer-aided data collection and mapping tools. One result is that community-driven mapping is shaping global health interventions and policy making in new ways because map making is including new participants in the action research process and revealing information by and about communities previously ignored in global health discourses.

In this chapter, we suggest that map making is as much a process as a product and that both help community members and researchers organize and prioritize information, make visible key data, challenge professional characterizations of whether or not a place is "healthy," and contribute to the important narratives of healthy policy making. Using case studies of community-driven mapping from Rio de Janeiro, Brazil, and Nairobi, Kenya, respectively, we highlight how map making can support CBPR and vice versa only when the process reflects norms of democratic science. These include a commitment to transparency, an openness to critical scrutiny, a skepticism toward claims that too neatly support reigning values, a willingness to listen to countervailing opinions, a readiness to admit uncertainty and ignorance, and a respect for evidence gathered by local and professional experts (Corburn, 2009).

Ensuring that map making is a democratic process owned and controlled by community members requires that local people, not outside researchers, define the geographic or other boundaries over what counts as part of the "community." The collaborative partnerships and knowledge generated through action research must be oriented toward existing community organizing goals, focus on mapping assets and hazards, and aim to highlight issues that may be ignored or given scant attention by outsiders, particularly policy makers. In this process, mapping can facilitate learning about place and health equity relationships by researchers and community members, particularly if the process is ongoing and dynamic, rather than a static, one-time effort. Finally, map making that extends CBPR must capture the broad, often cumulative, determinants of health in places and communicate this complexity easily and widely to residents and others beyond the community's boundaries.

PLACE AND MAPPING IN A RELATIONAL VIEW

Mapping is necessary (but perhaps insufficient) for capturing the complexities of places that influence health inequities and thus can lead to interventions that more fully characterize the determinants of health. Much work in public health, defined as "built environment and health," in fact tends to conflate neighborhood characteristics (often using static variables) with place (Ellaway et al., 2012; Kimbro & Denney, 2013). These studies aim to explore for significant "neighborhood effects" on well-being using a subset of quantitative variables. When little or no statistical influence is found, they often conclude that individual biology, behaviors, or genes must be responsible for health status, not "neighborhood characteristics." In neighborhood-effects research, the most proximate scale is used often because of the relative ease in accessing administrative data (i.e., census or health surveys). However, this may miss community knowledge or forces outside the neighborhood or local place, such as national and international policies, which can influence local access to a health-promoting good, such as affordable food.

Distance under the relational view ought to include physical and social relations and view populations and places embedded within networks. This concept of distance is important for health promotion, and although distance typically is seen as posing a barrier for people without close proximity to needed health or social services, the converse may also be true. The poor, for example, may not access a service that is physically close to them, especially if they perceive it as not being culturally appropriate or affordable or if traveling far away from one's home might reduce the chances of being stigmatized for being treated for a disease in one's community (Popay, Williams, Thomas, & Gatrell, 1998).

In the relational view of place taken here, there are mutually reinforcing relationships between places and people and the position of places relative to each other. Further, the place effects on health ought to be understood as a result of endogenous and exogenous processes operating at a variety of spatial scales, not just the neighborhood scale (Cummins, Curtis, Diez-Roux, & Macintyre, 2007). Healey (2007, pp. 3–4) describes the relational approach as emphasizing

> . . . the dynamic diversity of the complex co-location of multiple webs of relations that transect and intersect across an urban area, each with their own driving dynamics, history and geography . . . This involves moving beyond an analysis of the spatial patterns of activities as organised in two-dimensional space, the space of a traditional map. Instead, it demands attention to the interplay of economic, socio-cultural, environmental and political/administrative dynamics as these evolve across and within an urban area.

CBPR mapping can reveal the "double construction" of places: first through material and physical building (the buildings, streets, parks, etc., of the "built environment") and second through the shaping of social processes that assign meanings, interpretations, narratives, perceptions, feelings, and imaginations within places. CBPR projects have a natural affiliation for the relational view and frequently capture the multiple features and meanings in places (Cashman, Adeky, & Allen, 2008; Rambaldi et al., 2006).

Importantly, these meanings are contingent and contested, constantly being constructed and reconstructed as, for instance, when new population groups and cultures move into a place. Differences in social processes, such as power, inequality, and collective action, are often revealed through the construction and reconstruction of the material forms and social meanings of places, and a nuanced understanding of these processes is required for health equity planning (Emirbayer, 1997; Escobar, 2001). The contingent and contested characteristics of place meanings suggest an anti-essentialist view of places or the notion that there is no one single set of place characteristics, meanings, or relationships that will make all cities and neighborhoods healthy. Such a perspective further underscores the necessity of understanding the history of places and the biographies of people living there if health equity is to be seriously understood, sought, and achieved.

RIO DE JANEIRO CASE STUDY

The *Mapeamento Digital Liderado por Adolescentes e Jovens* (Youth-Led Digital Mapping) was a joint initiative implemented between 2011 and 2015 by UNICEF and a Brazilian non-governmental agency (NGO), the *Centro de Promoção da Saúde* (Center for Health Promotion, CEDAPS).[1] The project directly involved 550 people in nineteen poor communities throughout the country and invited youth to explore and map socio-environmental health risks as a tool for advocacy and community mobilization. In doing so, the mapping process aimed to help youth move from passive observers into arbiters of local knowledge and principal agents of local social transformation.

Three mapping methodologies were used. The first employed mobile phones to identify and geo-locate specific health risks, uploaded to a Google Maps–based interactive platform. The second built a non-cartographic but symbolic spatial representation of important community areas. Finally, the third used an aerial kite-and-camera rig to modernize outdated satellite images and validate the existence and true size of neighborhoods. Together, these methodologies elevated community expertise in the definition of place and provided an alternate epistemology that drove local community mobilization and government action.

Throughout the implementation of the initiative, collaborative engagements among youth, local associations, civil society, and government partners were instrumental in ensuring concrete, integrated results. Using networks built through the mapping process, local community associations spearheaded initiatives to reduce trash levels, in one instance removing two tons of refuse and in another redistributing trash collection points through the neighborhood.

CEDAPS Methodology

The first and primary focus of the youth-led digital mapping was to build an interactive, digital map showing specific socio-environmental health risks in *favelas* (slums) and to subsequently build action plans for communities, civil society actors, and government.[2] In workshops with twenty-five youth at a time, CEDAPS invited participants to interrogate conceptual categories of risk and identify those that were most pressing in their communities. The youth then took pictures of these theme-based risks to populate a map of their environment through an Android application built with the assistance of MIT Media Lab and InSTEDD. The application enabled each user to take a picture, write a tagline and any commentary, and geo-locate the information. When the cellphone connected to the Internet, all the mapped items synchronized with the UNICEF-GIS mapping server.[3] (See Picture 23.1.)

When the group members were younger or averse to using technological tools, CEDAPS used a second technique: the *Mapa Falante* (Talking Map), which is a hand-drawn map offering a symbolic, graphic representation of local points of interest. Although it lacks cartographic rigor, this process allows community residents to register how they think about their neighborhood, to highlight those areas of high risk, community strengths, and potential interventions, thus adding a layer of social meaning—from the perspective of those who experience and live in the territory—to the two-dimensional space of a traditional map.

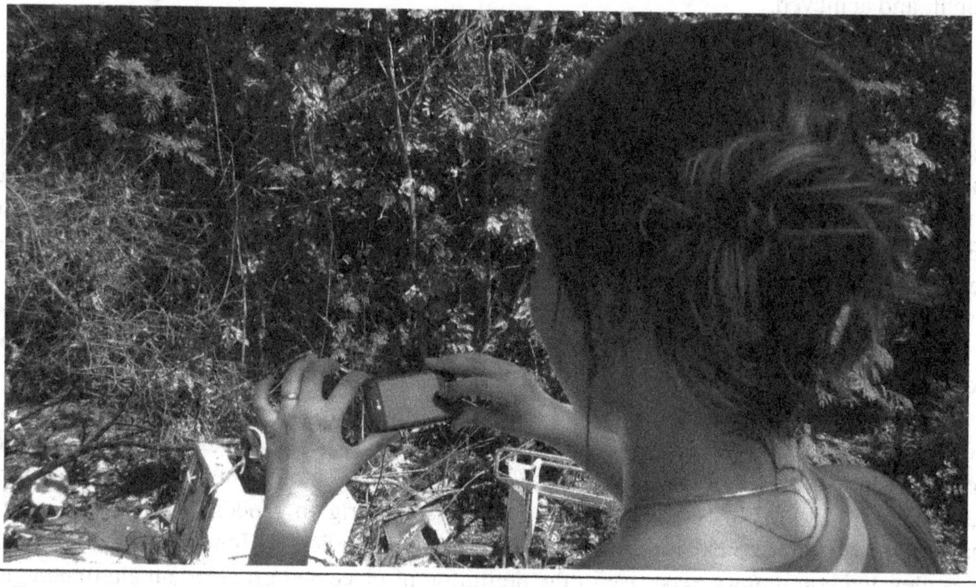

PICTURE 23.1 *Recycle Project: Young Mapper Using "Voices of Youth Maps" App to Document Garbage Accumulation.*
Source: © CEDAPS/Ives Rocha.

The third form of community mapping was an aerial mapping technique developed by the Public Laboratory for Open Technology and Science (http://publiclab.org/) and adapted for this project. Held securely within an aerodynamic capsule, a digital camera was attached to the line of a delta kite and set to take a picture every second as it rose into the air. Once downloaded, the individual photos could be manipulated and stitched together to form a complete picture that was often several years more current than existing Google satellite footage. That picture showed houses and the extension of the community where there had been no previous record, thus providing community residents with concrete evidence, or "proof of place," that could be leveraged to demand government services.

After the digital and aerial mapping, youth participants met with CEDAPS and local partners to define action plans addressing the identified risks in the form of youth-led community mobilizations as well as political advocacy, where they presented their data-backed demands to the municipal government. Taken together, these mapping techniques offered opportunities for youth participants to know and redefine their space. By using their realities as teaching materials, the training aimed to offer participants new perspectives to problematize and debate their surroundings: as the technical coordinator of the initiative noted, "in registering their reality through image and proposing concrete changes, boys and girls see themselves not only as subjects able to critically analyze their reality but also as actors responsible for its transformation" (Rocha, 2014).

Mapping Successes

Of all the themes mapped (poor accessibility, trash accumulation, frayed or knotted electrical lines, risks of housing collapse and landslides, open sanitation, and gender-based violence), only one was present across all communities: the accumulation of trash. The density of housing in *favelas* in Rio de Janeiro, broken only by narrow footpaths, means that these low-income communities are often deprived of effective public trash collection. With no trashcans or dumpsters in sight, refuse accumulates on hillsides, wells, and the public paths snaking between homes—by providing nooks and crannies for bacteria and mosquitos to thrive, the piles of trash contribute to high rates of various preventable diseases, including dengue and Zika.

It should be no surprise then that trash served as a lightning rod for mobilization in multiple communities following the mapping process. In Morro dos Prazeres, a *favela* climbing the hills above the historic Santa Teresa neighborhood, CEDAPS partnered with a local association, Galera.com, to draw attention to a massive trash heap that had caused a landslide earlier that year. Branding their project *Acredite e Faça Acontecer* ("Believe and Make It Happen"), Galera.com invited the government trash collection agency to a clean-up day they organized with residents. With the support of the municipal government, they removed two tons of trash. In partnership with UNICEF and CEDAPS, Galera.com and other local institutions then mobilized the same youth participants to renovate the open space next to the former dump, turning it into a community recreation space (see Picture 23.2). Dozens of other activities similar to these were planned and executed in two other *favelas,* Morro de Macacos and Morro de Borel. In both, the local housing associations distributed trash cans throughout the community and lobbied the municipality to move the dumpster sites where they collect trash to more convenient areas.

In one case in 2015, a public school launched the youth-led digital mapping as an elective course for students. The course was instituted at Ginásio Olímpico Juan Samaranch in the Rio

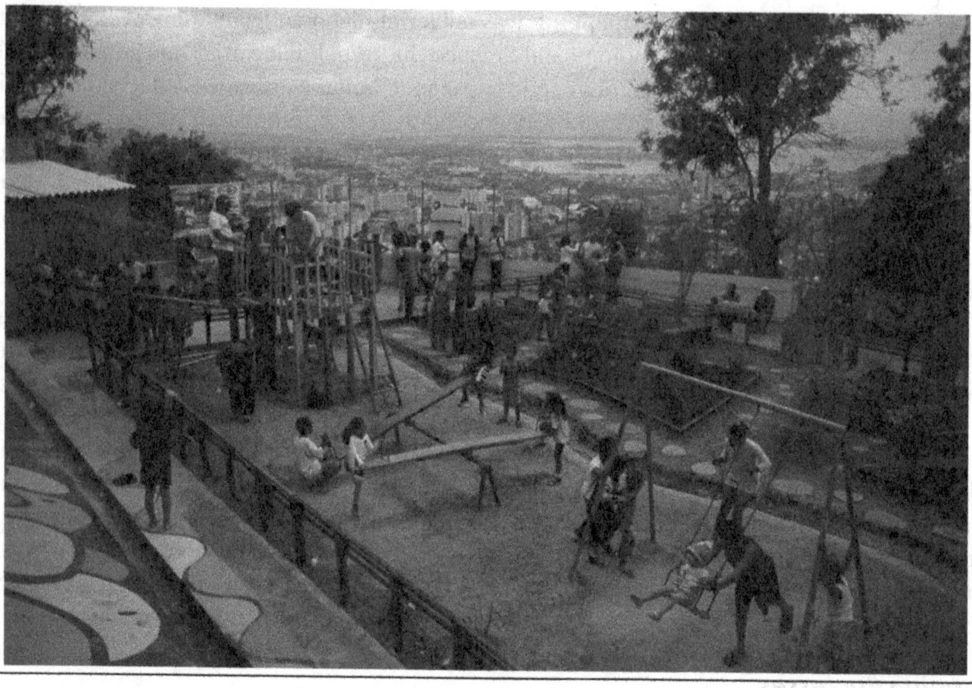

PICTURE 23.2 *Recycle Project: João Tuteia Square—From Dump Site to Recreation Place in Two Years of Mobilization and Action.*
Source: © CEDAPS/Ives Rocha.

Comprido neighborhood through the initiative of the geography teacher. Every week for fifty minutes students carried out each stage of the mapping process. The semester commenced with twelve students and ended with thirty-three, plus a waiting list. As in the mapped *favelas,* the principal problem students identified was the inadequate disposal of solid refuse in the three *favelas* around the school. As part of the mitigation action plan, the students launched an educational campaign themed "a little gesture makes a big difference," which sought to sensitize all five hundred students and the almost eight thousand people who transited around the school daily.

The youth-led digital mapping project also was successful in pushing the municipality of Rio de Janeiro to take limited action. In one instance, youth participants in the Morro de Prazeres took a particularly impactful picture of young girl crossing a deteriorating wood bridge, just steps away from a gaping hole. When the director of the project's government partner saw the picture, he ordered the bridge rebuilt out of concrete.

Lessons from CEDAPS Mapping

Although many lessons were learned from the described youth-engaged mapping and action experiences, five stand out as particularly important:

Location-specific approaches to community issues galvanize mobilization more than higher-level ones. Across all the methodologies used, youth participants were invited to critically consider the pressing issues facing their communities. Of the three types of mapping, the two that elicited the greatest positive responses by participants were the digital map and the Talking Map, through which they highlighted and located the risks that youth face every day. For external partners, the digital map was of most interest, because it provided a traditional geographic perspective and the layer of social meaning ascribed by the community. Youth could not relate as directly to the aerial map, perhaps because non-recognition by government was less immediately pressing than other, more-common injustices.

Local leaders are needed to act as intermediaries to legitimize community knowledge and promote follow-through. The collaborative partnership with local leaders (coming from institutions such as community associations, housing associations, women's associations, and schools) was a critical success factor in three respects. First, they were necessary to secure the buy in of residents; almost always, youth participants needed to overcome the distrust of residents who had witnessed years of frustrated attempts to implement change. Second, strong local institutional backing was necessary for the implementation of the action plans derived by the youth. Such backing, in fact, proved critical in helping keep participants motivated and together beyond the workshop. When such backing was not present, youth engagement fell off, with some groups disbanding. Finally, participants' recognition and power outside the community bridged the gap between residents and government authorities. They helped mitigate one of the most-complex challenges faced: guaranteeing that the voice and self-determination of youth was respected while ensuring a collaborative partnership. Each time the initiative was launched in a new site, the advice and feedback of all local actors was included, including youth and adolescents. Further, because each neighborhood was unique, adjustments were always necessary.

Government involvement is critical, even though it sometimes creates bottlenecks. From the beginning of the youth-led digital mapping, the team partnered with the *Defesa Civil* (Civil Defense), a government body tasked with designing, coordinating, and implementing projects to reduce disasters in the city. This partnership proved critical to the success of the mapping and to the follow-up coordination with government entities, because Civil Defense made contacts, built bridges, and pushed for action. At the same time, there is a large discrepancy between the urgency felt by community residents (particularly youth and adolescents) and the bureaucratic delays involved with making requests of—and getting action from—the city government. In this regard, too, the policy mentorship (see Chapter 20) provided by Civil Defense was valuable in helping youth participants better understand, and not give up on, the politics of helping effect change at the municipal level.

The different epistemologies of government agencies and communities can cause tension and delays. Although the Civil Defense recognized the value of community youth perspectives, the information generated was not considered sufficiently systematic or technical. Thus, despite its support, this organization proved unable to integrate the mapping database in its original form and was forced by internal policy to reevaluate the mapped points, particularly those that spoke about risks of landslides or housing collapse. Although partnership members were still able to organize for action with the assistance of Civil Defense, the data were not used as a foundation of policy decisions. This highlights a common challenge with CBPR, namely, that information generated by communities can be seen as inferior to that generated by technocrats. This perception also underscores the importance of bringing government partners into project design early to help ensure that the information generated will be in a form that meets their needs.

Pilot projects require responsive technical partners and back-up plans. As with any pilot of a new tool, CEDAPS frequently faced challenges in the field while sorting out bugs in the technology. The implementing partnership's success was, in part, because of highly engaged technical partners, whose involvement allowed for rapid iteration and technical support. Even with such assistance, however, delays sometimes were faced when the mapping application was not functional, non-digital methodologies had to be employed, or when a return to the community another day to redo the mapping was necessary.

Despite such limitations, however, this case study provides a useful illustration of the impressive role youth can play as partners in digital and other mapping for information and action, even in extreme resource-poor environments.

CASE TWO: NAIROBI, KENYA: SHACK/SLUM DWELLERS INTERNATIONAL (SDI) IN THE MATHARE VALLEY

In Nairobi, Kenya, close to 65 percent of the population lives in informal settlements, or slums, on about 10 percent of the city's land area. Children under five living in Nairobi's slums are almost three times as likely to die as their counterparts in the rest of the city, and women experience disproportionate health burdens compared to men. For example, more than a quarter of all women and girls in Nairobi's slums reported an episode of diarrhea in the past month, compared to about one-fifth of all Kenyans. More than 36 percent of slum-dwelling women report being physically forced to have sex, and more than one-third report being sexually abused (Swart, 2012). This case study describes work in and with the Mathare informal settlement located about six kilometers from the city center, with about 260,000 people, and composed of thirteen different villages: Mashimoni, Mabatini, Village No. 10, Village 2, Kosovo, 3A, 3B, 3C, 4A, 4B, Gitathuru, Kiamutisya, and Kwa Kariuki.

From 2009 to 2014, Shack/Slum Dwellers International (SDI), an international NGO, partnered with and supported the Kenyan federation of the urban poor, called Muungano wa Wanavijiji (Muungano). SDI and Muungano developed an action-research partnership with the University of California, Berkeley, and the University of Nairobi to document living conditions in Mathare and advocate for change. SDI, established in 1996, is a global network of community-based organizations of the urban poor with its origins in India, but it now has a presence in thirty-three countries in Africa, Asia, and Latin America (http://sdinet.org). In Kenya, SDI supports Muungano, the national federation of the urban poor with hundreds of community-based affiliates. SDI assists Muungano's community-based organizations and the entire federation to organize residents, conduct research, collaboratively advocate and negotiate with governments to deliver life-supporting services, and address issues of tenure security, safety, and social and political exclusion (sdinet.org).

The aims of the Mathare collaboration were to develop and sustain community mobilization that contributed to an alternative development plan and advocacy strategy for the entire informal settlement, not just a specific mapping project. Multiple participatory data gathering and mapping processes were employed, including household enumerations, spatial mapping, designing place-based physical and social improvements, and drafting new plans and policies. In these ways, data gathering and mapping explicitly included different groups: youth documented safety; and women documented food, water, and sanitation locations; and schools were enrolled to capture student and teacher perspectives. Resident planning teams were organized in each village to organize a surveying and field-mapping process (Makau, Dobson, & Samia, 2012).

Making the Invisible Visible

In 2008–2009, the United Nations Environment Programme (UNEP) and the Kenyan National Environment Management Authority (NEMA) proposed to clean up the Nairobi River and its tributaries, citing health and environmental risks. A concern of Muungano and its network of slum dwellers was that tens of thousands of urban poor residents living alongside waterways in Nairobi would be evicted through this river clean-up program (All Africa, 2008; Weru, 2012).

Muungano and the universities designed and implemented a detailed household survey, training and employing residents in data gathering. A separate team generated aerial photos using a camera attached to a balloon that was flown over the entire Mathare settlement. This created more than 5,400 detailed images of the community in much more detail than a Google Earth image could provide. These images were "stitched together" digitally to create a high-resolution "base map" that enabled residents to see their community in a new way. The detailed aerial images highlighted potential health hazards not well documented before, such as the presence of cooking near open drains (see Picture 23.3). These and other findings were discussed in focus groups and directed ground-level mapping teams in their data collection efforts.

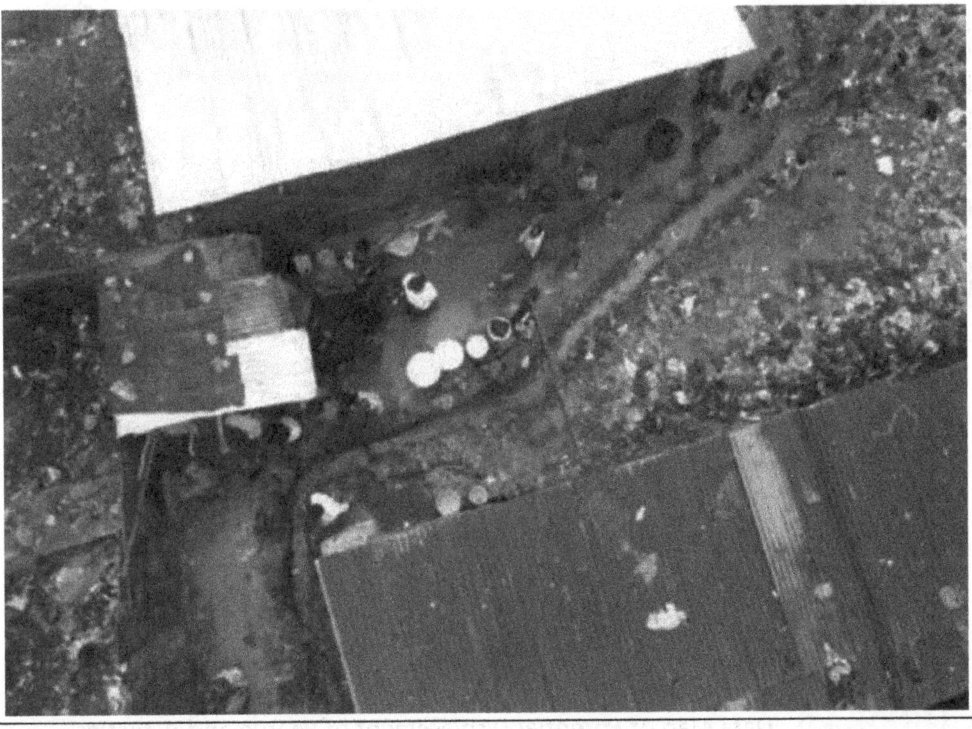

PICTURE 23.3 *Balloon Captured Aerial Image Showing Cooking Pots (Round White Circles Adjacent to Open Drain), Later Found to Contain High Amounts of Human Waste*
Source: Edwin Simiyu. Used with permission.

The community satellite images and focus group discussions over community health priorities were used to inform field-based mapping, where teams of residents and students walked every meter of the community to document the locations of each water point, toilet, electricity power pole, food vendor, dump site, school, community facility, and other assets and hazards. Student interns from the University of Nairobi worked with residents, and university courses, co-led by UC Berkeley and University of Nairobi faculty members and involving tens of students, were organized to conduct participatory mapping and data gathering.

First, data and maps were generated to highlight the number of people and types of community activities that would be displaced by the UNEP river program (Figure 23.1). These data were presented to UN and local government, and residents marched to the Nairobi City Council to prevent evictions. The data visualization combined with community mobilization resulted in a temporary stay of planned evictions in Mathare. One result was a recognition by the state, for the first time, that community residents, working in partnership with universities, could produce policy-relevant data.

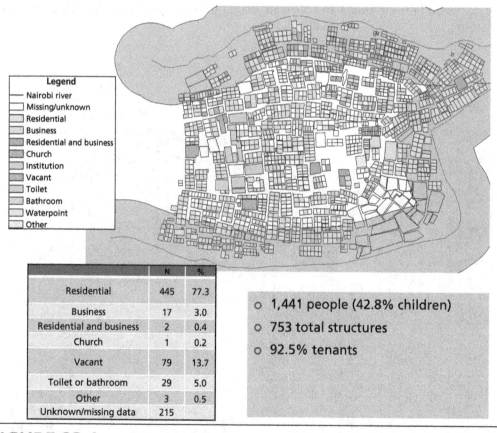

	N	%
Residential	445	77.3
Business	17	3.0
Residential and business	2	0.4
Church	1	0.2
Vacant	79	13.7
Toilet or bathroom	29	5.0
Other	3	0.5
Unknown/missing data	215	

- 1,441 people (42.8% children)
- 753 total structures
- 92.5% tenants

FIGURE 23.1 *Data Map of Potential Displacement of People and Activities*
Source: Muungano wa Wanavijiji. Used with permission.

Sanitation and Women's Health

A second key result of the processes in Mathare was a finding that girls and women were disproportionately burdened from inadequate sanitation. Our map-making processes revealed the uneven access to toilets across Mathare. However, it was survey and focus group data that complemented the spatial mapping to highlight the serious health consequences of the maps. For example, household survey data revealed that more than 83 percent of Mathare residents relied on an unimproved pit latrine and that more than 60 percent used a "flying toilet," defecating into a plastic bag and throwing it into an open dump.

The team also heard in focus groups with Mathare women about the indignity they endured from a lack of private, safe, well-lit, nearby toilets. One women noted:

> Past eight, we can't go out to use the toilet. There is no lighting and the men drinking Chang'aa [local alcohol] on that side, get violent with us, even girls. We are forced to use a bucket . . . a bucket in one room in front of your children, fathers and brothers. Can you imagine? Sometimes we use the "flying toilets" at night but your neighbors don't like this. Without any garbage collection, I wake up at dawn and sneak away to empty the bucket or dispose the bag. There is no dignity in our toilet situation.

Team members also heard in focus groups with girls that they were more likely than boys to miss school because of sanitation-related illness and lack of safe, private, and hygienic toilets at their school. A lack of adequate toilets in schools decreases the attendance of girls especially during their menstrual cycle (Chebbii, 2014). One schoolgirl noted:

> As girls, when we don't have a toilet in school, we are forced to stay with one pad for a whole day. I know many girls who just do not come to school during those days. Even if we have a toilet at school and we have to share them with boys, girls will avoid them and stay home. We do not have a bath place so I know when you have your period you do not want to smell in school, so us girls avoid it.

For girls and women in Mathare, toilets are a relational issue of inadequate infrastructure, safety, economic opportunity, stigma, dignity, and human health.

Collaborative Analysis and Policy

All maps and data were shared in draft form with community planning teams and during in-depth discussions with residents over the meaning of the maps and how the information should be used. For example, maps of the distribution of water points were used to advocate with the Nairobi Water and Sewer Company to install new piped water service to residents. Muungano used the data to not only advocate for piped water but also for a community-run management scheme, so that economic opportunities and oversight responsibilities would go to local residents. The campaign was successful and now acts as the Mathare-Kosovo Water Model and is used in other urban slums across Kenya (Kenya Water Services Trust Fund [WSTF], 2010).

All maps and data contributed to the Mathare Zonal Plan, a comprehensive upgrading plan for the community that was used to advocate for investments and organize disparate improvement efforts (SDI, 2012). Two years after the publication of the report, the World Bank

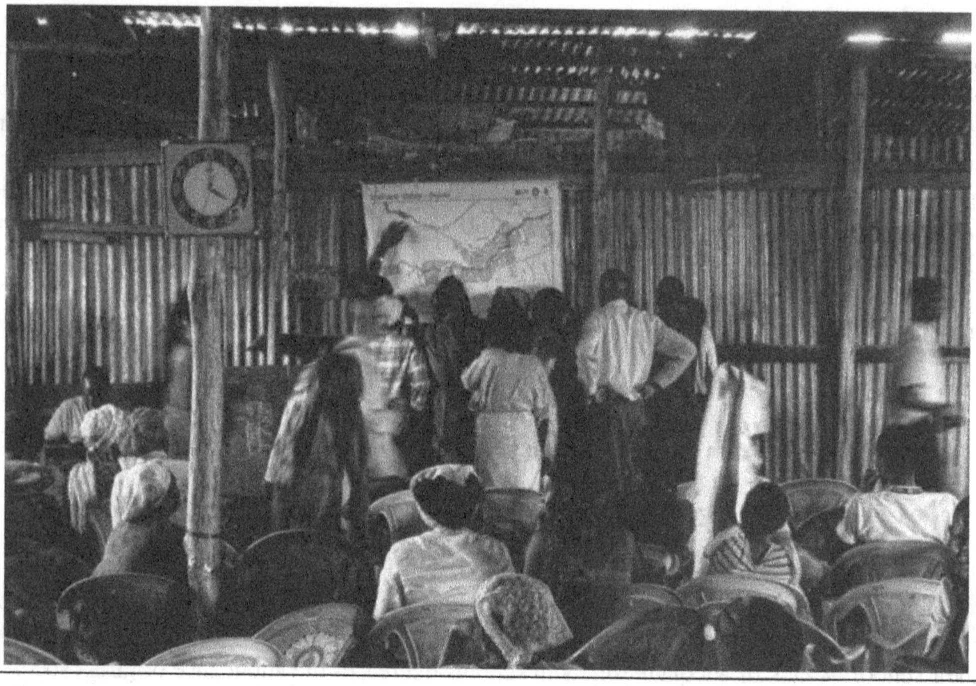

PICTURE 23.4 *Mathare Residents Review Maps During Community Planning Forum.*
Source: Jason Corburn. Used with permission.

approached the university about the spatial data they created for upgrading sanitation, namely, the trunk sewers. The GIS shape files were shared with the bank and the Athi Water Services Board, and by 2014, ten kilometers of the community-designed sewer plan were constructed in Mathare. In January 2015, the president of Kenya, Uhuru Kenyatta, came to Mathare and launched a new project of the National Youth Service (NYS) to upgrade roads. The NYS also used the Mathare Zonal Plan to determine where to formalize and tarmac new roads in Mathare. Although data collection and mapping by slum dwellers continues in Nairobi's informal settlements, the work in Mathare has delivered tangible improvements to the living conditions of residents and has given them "data" to negotiate with the state for greater recognition and health-promoting resources (Picture 23.4).

ONGOING CHALLENGES AND OPPORTUNITIES

In both case studies, it is clear that mapping technologies have expanded beyond desktop GIS, with capacity for community generation of data using free and publicly accessible web-based mapping tools such as Google Maps, MapServer, OpenStreetMap, and GRASS GIS to only name a few (maps.google.com, Mapserver.org, openstreetmap.org, grass.fbk.eu). These web-based tools have made sophisticated mapping available to community and nonprofit groups with limited resources, in part because they have centralized and made freely available very high resolution background geographic data, including satellite data, street photography, and building outlines.

Importantly for CBPR, new social media, sometimes linked to mapping technologies, are reshaping definitions of community and how people see themselves in relationship with their surroundings, neighbors, and institutions by mapping things such as access to food or the responsiveness of government agencies. For example, individuals and community-based organizations have mobilized citizens to send text messages and photos from mobile phones to track a range of community health "field" data that can be located on a map, many with addition geo-referenced data, such as incidents of violence, housing code complaints, dangerous streets and intersections, and pedestrian injuries (see crimemapping.com, www.everyblock.com, www.seeclickfix.com, www.infrastructurist.com/f-this/, www.appsfordemocracy.org/stumble-safely, www.mybikelane.com, healthycity.org). Software developed by groups such as Ushahidi (www.ushahidi.com) are enabling community map makers to track identified community hazards and assets through time (i.e., at what time of day a report was sent) and space (i.e., geographic location)—giving rise to sophisticated "time-space health biographies." These, in turn, are enabling collaborative researchers to suggest that movement, and thus exposure, varies from person to person (e.g., elderly versus adult versus young person) living in the same place.

As suggested throughout this chapter, map making using CBPR should be open to engaging with new technologies while also acknowledging its inherent limitations, because low-cost mapping technology can help achieve multiple important ends:

- Ensuring that community residents are valued coproducers of health knowledge
- Offering a platform for community residents to express what matters to them and share this with a world of potentially new listeners and allies
- Providing new forums for residents and researchers to collaboratively generate innovative solutions for persistent health inequities
- Raising awareness among community members of the benefits and pitfalls of technology, such as the potential for overwhelming residents with too much information and creating a dependency on technology

The cases presented here also raise some challenges for community members, activists, academics, and others attempting to use mapping to extend CBPR for health equity. First, organizing youth on scientific and health issues can be challenging, especially when engaged research projects demand long-term, multiyear commitments and young people may have limited available time (also see Chapter 7). However, one recommendation from our experience is that the mapping process should engage young people early and often, especially as new technologies, web, and social media geared toward youth become commonplace as mapping tools. Partnering with youth can also help ensure that map making is fun, tied to local culture, and even to a broader fund-raising strategy, as CEDAPS recognized. Engaging youth can also support mapping as a strategy to build new organizational capacity, leadership, and power, especially when community members drive the research questions, selection of appropriate data, and interpretation and presentation and use of results.

A second challenge is that the rapid pace of technological change and sophistication may lead some groups to choose to leapfrog and start with the latest, most advanced tools. Our experience suggests that this rarely builds on local knowledge and may create an overdependency of community groups on technology and outside expert advisors. Hence, we suggest that mapping processes are most successful when they build incrementally from smaller to larger scale, from less to more complex, and from lower to higher technology. This trajectory can be rather quick with skilled partnerships and collaborations, as shown by when CEDAPS quickly led from the Talking Map into a digital one. Ultimately, mapping can act as a key piece of an ongoing community-led research program.

A third challenge for mapping processes is to focus on bonding and bridging social capital (Briggs 1998), where bonding helps different CBOs and community members build trust and partnerships among themselves and bridging allows mapping process and outputs to engage with unlikely allies and change agents, such as regulators and academic scientists. Often, the goal of a community mapping effort is to build community alliances and gather local knowledge or challenge an inaccurate characterization of a place done by outsiders, but not both. The cases presented here suggest that a both-and approach be explicit from the outset and designed into the mapping process.

Fourth, linking concrete community health concerns with broader policy frames and campaigns is another challenge of map making. Characterizing one's community by selecting certain features to map always requires value judgments over what to leave out. Instead of viewing this as a weakness or limitation, we suggest that a community map-making process be explicit about their issues and policy objectives from the outset, with place-based health inequities being one logical policy frame.

CONCLUSION: COMMUNITY MAPPING FOR HEALTH EQUITY

Community mapping can act as a core method and process when using a CBPR approach and should be considered by all practitioners interested in building community knowledge and using that knowledge to inform action, leadership, organizing, and ultimately improving the science of assessing health burdens in places. As these two case studies have shown, when mapping processes embody the core principles of CBPR, they can contribute to the following:

- Building a power or organizing base in communities of color
- Reframing community organizing priorities
- Highlighting local knowledge
- Linking the work to health equity
- Demystifying research and environmental regulations
- Changing policy and improving lives

Community mapping is one important tool to organize residents and extend CBPR's emphasis on ensuring that research contributes to action (Israel et al., 1998). As global public health practitioners and social epidemiologists recognize that "place matters" for understanding why some populations in some places get sick more often and die prematurely, community mapping will be increasingly important for gathering information on the features and characteristics of places that influence well-being and moving from research to policy. Capturing hazards and assets is crucial, and a CBPR approach is vital for ensuring residents and researchers engage in a collaborative process for deciding what information to capture, what role different technologies can play, what to display on maps, and how to share visual information within and outside the community. What is crucial is that community members consider mapping as one part of an ongoing global health equity advocacy and policy change strategy.

QUESTIONS FOR DISCUSSION

1. How can map making help community-driven research capture crucial knowledge that other public health research methods might overlook?
2. What roles do public health professionals have in facilitating CBPR mapping processes?
3. How might map making help the poor develop new skills while also improving the scientific evidence based behind public health interventions and policy making?

NOTES

1. CEDAPS is a NGO founded in 1993, based in Rio de Janeiro and active in several states of Brazil. CEDAPS works with two strategies of health promotion: empowering communities in order for them to become active social actors, generating local solutions, and proposing and developing intervention strategies toward building and enhancing community-based public policies. Read more on http://cedaps.org.br/.
2. CEDAPS used the Construção Compartilhada de Soluções Locais (Shared Contribution to Local Solutions) methodology it has developed over years of operation (Edmundo & Nunes, 2014).
3. Map visible at http://rio.unicef-gis.org/.

REFERENCES

All Africa. (2008). Kenya: Slum dwellers along Nairobi rivers face eviction (July). Retrieved from http://allafrica.com/stories/200807090331.html

Briggs, X. S. (1998). Brown kids in white suburbs: Housing mobility and the many faces of social capital. *Housing Policy Debate, 9*(1), 177–121.

Brown, T., McLafferty, S., & Moon, G. (Eds.). (2010). *A companion to health and medical geography*. Malden, MA: Wiley-Blackwell.

Cashman, S. B., Adeky, S., Allen, A. J., III, et al. (2008). The power and the promise: Working with communities to analyze data, interpret findings, and get to outcomes. *American Journal of Public Health, 98*(8), 1407–1417.

Chebbii, S. J. (2014). Menstruation and education: How a lack of sanitary towels reduces school attendance in Kenyan slums. BUWA (October). Retrieved from www.osisa.org/sites/default/files/27–31.pdf

Corburn, J. (2009). *Toward the healthy city: People, places and the politics of urban planning*. Cambridge, MA: MIT Press.

Cummins, S., Curtis, S., Diez-Roux, A. V., & Macintyre, S. (2007). Understanding and representing "place" in health research: A relational approach. *Social Science & Medicine, 65*(9), 1825–1838.

Edmundo, K., & Nunes, N. R. (2014). *Construção compartilhada de soluções locais: Guia de elaboração e gestão de projetos sociais*. Rio de Janeiro, Brazil: CEDAPS.

Ellaway, A., Benzeval, M., Green, M., Leyland, A., & Macintyre, S. (2012). "Getting sicker quicker": Does living in a more deprived neighbourhood mean your health deteriorates faster? *Health and Place, 8*(2), 132–137.

Emirbayer, M. (1997). Manifesto for a relational sociology. *American Journal of Sociology, 103*(2), 281–317.

Escobar, A. (2001). Culture sits in places: Reflections on globalism and subaltern strategies of localization. *Political Geography, 20*(2), 139–174.

Healey, P. (2007). *Urban complexity and spatial strategies: Towards a relational planning for our times*. London, UK: Routledge.

Israel, B., et al., (1998). Review of community-based research: Assessing partnership approaches to improve public health. *Annual Review of Public Health,19,*173–202.

Kenya Water Services Trust Fund (WSTF). (2010). *Formalising water supply through partnerships: The Mathare Kosovo water supply model*. Nairobi, Kenya: Author.

Kimbro, R. T., & Denney, J. T. (2013). Neighborhood context and racial/ethnic differences in young children's obesity: Structural barriers to interventions. *Social Science and Medicine, 95,* 97–105.

Makau, J., Dobson, S., & Samia, E. (2012). The five-city enumeration: The role of participatory enumerations in developing community capacity and partnerships with government in Uganda. *Environment and Urbanization, 24*(1), 31–46.

Popay, J., Williams, G., Thomas, C., & Gatrell, A. (1998). Theorizing inequalities in health: The place of lay knowledge. *Sociology of Health and Illness, 20,* 619–644.

Rambaldi, G., Corbett, J., Olson, R., et al. (2006). Mapping for change: Practice, technologies and communication. *Participatory Learning and Action* (54). London, UK: IIED and CTA.

Rocha, I. (2014). *Mapeamento digital liderado por adolescentes e jovens: Guia do facilitador*. Rio de Janeiro: CEDAPS. Retrieved from www.unicef.org/brazil/pt/guia_mapeamento_pcu1316.pdf

Swart, E. (2012). Gender-based violence in a Kenyan slum: Creating local, woman-centered interventions. *Journal of Social Service Research, 38*(4), 427–438.

Weru, G. (2012). Nairobi rivers pose health, safety hazards. *Daily Nation* (May 26). Retrieved from www.nation.co.ke/News/Nairobi+rivers+pose+health+safety+hazards+/-/1056/1414258/-/39258y/-/index.html

APPENDIX 1

CHALLENGING OURSELVES

CRITICAL SELF-REFLECTION ON POWER AND PRIVILEGE

CHERYL HYDE

One of the more common, and mistaken, assumptions that community practitioners make is thinking that because they are "fighting the good fight," they do not need to address issues regarding their own power and privilege. Yet engaging in practice under the banner of social justice (or any other "right" reason) does not result in an automatic community of shared interests. Nor does it inoculate against the dividends that one might accrue because of race, class, gender, sexual orientation, or other aspect of an individual's cultural identity. Because so much of community practice is relational (see Chapters 4, 5, and 6), I suggest that it is essential for practitioners to undertake in some rigorous self-exploration as part of their broader anti-oppression work. In this appendix, I offer one approach to such critical reflection that I have used in teaching and training efforts.

Similar to many individuals who engage in anti-oppression teaching and practice, I ground much of my thinking in Peggy McIntosh's (1989) classic essay, "White Privilege: Unpacking the Invisible Knapsack." By delineating the many ways in which white individuals benefit from usually unrecognized or unacknowledged everyday expectations, rituals, and processes (e.g., "I am never asked to speak for all the people of my racial group" [p. 11]), McIntosh connects the personal with broader structures that promote or protect racism and then issues a call to action: "A 'white' skin in the United States opens many doors for whites whether or not we approve of the way dominance has been conferred on us. Individual acts can palliate, but cannot end, these problems. To redesign social systems we need first to acknowledge their colossal unseen dimensions. The silences and denials surrounding privilege are the key political tool here" (p. 12).

Part of the power of McIntosh's essay is that the reader needs to contend with the cumulative impact that seemingly minor activities can have on the perpetuation of racism. In demanding that whites dissect their racial privilege, and then take steps to challenge it, she provided a foundation for much of the anti-oppression work that followed. Comparable examinations can happen for other privileges based on class, gender, sexual orientation, and so forth; indeed, there are many, many examples in the literature (for varying approaches see Adams, 1997; Connell, 2005; Gerschick, 1993; Goodman, 2001; hooks, 2000a, 2000b; Tappan, 2006; Wallerstein, 1999).

Although McIntosh's contribution to antiracism work cannot be underestimated, her approach does, I think, fall short in four important ways. First, it does not distinguish between how we see our own privilege and how others might perceive or experience our identity. McIntosh is focused on the former, yet those with whom we interact also bring to the encounters an awareness (or not) of privilege as beneficiaries or as those denied such benefits. Second, she is focused on race and racism, which is understandable but incomplete. Race is not the only attribute that shapes how we negotiate the world. Third, because of this primary focus on race, McIntosh does not capture how different cultural attributes interact and differentially shape privilege. For example, a white middle-class woman and a white working-class woman both hold racial privilege, yet the manifestation of that privilege will present differently because of class. And fourth, even though McIntosh notes that "unseen dimensions" support societal structures, she nonetheless neglects the broad, systemic impact of labor market, educational, residential, and other forms of institutionalized racism (Jones, 2000). Fundamentally, hers is an intrapersonal framework for addressing racism: certainly critical but not sufficient. Grappling with these points, while still employing the essential insights of McIntosh, became the catalyst for the approach that I use.

ONE APPROACH TO CRITICAL SELF-REFLECTION

Before outlining my approach to a critical self-reflection for community practitioners, I want to emphasize, first, that this is a framework that I have found useful as a learner, teacher, trainer, and practitioner. It is not, however, the only model out there, and it is well worth the effort to find a process that works well and authentically challenges you as a community practitioner. Second, two assessments have been constructed for this appendix (see Tables A1.1 and A1.2), but they are adapted from tools that others and I have developed (Axner, n.d.; Burghardt, 2011; Katz, 1978; McIntosh, 1989). These tools work best when the individual pushes him- or herself to honestly complete them and then when a group debriefing can support further exploration and exchange of ideas.

Step 1: Our Complex Cultural Selves

The first step in this process is to understand the basics of one's culture and the impact on identity. Here, I am referring to the values, attitudes, beliefs, practices, and rituals that shape who we

TABLE A1.1 Cultural Identity Inventory

Cultural Dimensions	Manifestations	Interactions	Domination or Subordination	Vantage Points
Indicate for each (note any conflict concerning this identifier)	What values, actions, or messages are associated with the dimension?	Does the effect of this dimension interact with any other dimension? How so?	If dominant—what privileges do you have? How have you responded? If subordinate—what have you been denied? How have you responded?	How do you understand this aspect of yourself? How do you think or experience the way others see you?
Gender				
Race				
Class				
Sexual orientation				
Citizenship				
Religion				
Physical or mental ability				
Other?				

are and how we act, all of which flow from the various groups of which we are members. The primary cultural dimensions that I focus on are race, gender, citizenship status (in the United States), sexual orientation, class, religion, and physical or mental ability. There may be other dimensions that are important to an understanding of the cultural self (e.g., region of the country or level of education), but I find that these are the significant ones and serve as important springboards to self-awareness.

So turn to the Cultural Identity Inventory (Table A1.1) and consider the first three columns: "cultural dimensions," "manifestations, and "interactions." For each dimension, indicate what you are (note any conflicting messages or challenges to this self-identification) and whether there are any important values, messages, or actions associated with that dimension. For example, if you are a lesbian, did you receive messages of acceptance or condemnation? Or if you are a male, were you told that certain emotions or displays of emotion were not manly (i.e., unacceptable)? As you start this inventory, you may be able to see how different affiliations influence one another, for example, how messages about being female are shaped by one's religion. You should note these connections as they became apparent. What should begin to become apparent is that we are more than just one or two cultural attributes. The foundation of our cultural selves is the complex whole that is generated from these dimensions.

Review and reflect on your inventory. Consider these questions:

1. What are your overall reactions to this information (any affirmations, surprises, points of confusion)?
2. Does any dimension stand out as particularly important to your overall cultural identity and why?
3. What have you learned about yourself? What next steps in this process do you see yourself taking?

It also is important to understand that the level of influence exerted by these dimensions on one's cultural self might not be the same and can vary over time. You might even want to note if a particular dimension is exerting a relatively strong (or weak) effect on you and why. If we imagine these dimensions arrayed in a pie chart, some wedges will be larger than others, and, sometime in the future, these wedges could be resized. This is one reason why it is unwise (and even foolish) to assume that you know a person's culture based on just one or two characteristics. What is important to you may not be as significant to another, because that individual is perhaps more concerned with, or influenced by, a different cultural dimension. There is fluidity to the components of one's identity, depending on specific challenges of a given time and place as well as negotiating daily life.

Step 2: Privilege and Power

Within each of these dimensions there is a dominant and a subordinate group (see Table A1.1, column 4). A dominant group is one that as a group has access to economic, social, political, and civic privileges. This access is temporal and systemic, and the privileges may be consciously sought or unconsciously acquired. The point is not whether each individual in a given group always (and knowingly) enjoys privilege or even wants it (or asked for it). It is about the societal group, which, through its collective activity, turns that privilege over time into societal power. So in twenty-first-century America, the privileged groups include men, whites, the middle and upper classes, heterosexuals, citizens, the able-bodied, and Christians. Continuing with the Cultural Identity Inventory, indicate whether you are a member of the dominant or subordinate group for each cultural dimension in column 4.

Individuals who find themselves mostly or exclusively in dominant-status groups are not bad or evil. Rather, by virtue of these group memberships, they have benefited from various societal "perks," whether they asked for them or not. But once such privilege is revealed, these individuals have an obligation to question, challenge, and otherwise act in good faith to work toward the dismantling of a system that generates such disproportionate rewards based on group membership. And the key here is taking action; wallowing in guilt or engaging in excessive hand-wringing does nothing to contribute to anti-oppression work (indeed, such responses just further underscore one's privileges).

Conversely, the individuals who find themselves mostly or exclusively in subordinate-status groups do not have license to claim victimhood and then withdraw from any constructive action. The tasks for those with less privilege is to understand the injuries, hidden or explicit, that group subordination may have caused (for an excellent analysis of this, see Sennett and Cobb's [1972] classic work, *The Hidden Injuries of Class*). How, for example, has one addressed internalized oppression? Individuals from subordinate-status groups also need to take action against oppressive structure and processes, though their paths to, and strategies for, that action will likely differ from the work that dominant-group individuals undertake.

For most of us, however, it isn't a matter of being in either all-dominant or all-subordinate groups. Instead, our cultural identities are composed of a mix. So we might have access to racial or gender privilege, yet be in subordinate groups for religion and sexual orientation. To further complicate this understanding, as noted, not all dimensions have equal weight on our overall identity. We should not, however, let this complexity become an excuse for not owning the privilege that we may have. Yes, I may need to contend with a disability or gender discrimination, yet I also need to be mindful that as a white, professional person, I benefit from race and class privilege. Moreover, these societal dividends provide me with some resources with which to address or cope with subordination that results from membership in other groups. It is essential that we push ourselves to understand the implications of this complexity.

Step 3: Understanding Different Vantage Points

A final factor that I consider in this particular approach to understanding cultural identity focuses on how we see ourselves versus how others perceive us. Although it is tempting to think that we have primary or sole control over the making of our cultural identity, we do not. When we interact with, or are simply in the presence of, others, our cultural identity is being shaped by that individual's ideas, beliefs, attitudes, experiences, and so forth. This may not always be fair, but in relationship building, we are always negotiating the perceptions and reactions of others and hopefully in the process can address any misperceptions.

Referring again to the Cultural Identity Inventory, column 5, push yourself to consider your subjective (self-)understanding of each cultural dimension and then the understandings of others. If you are white, how do you view this and how do you experience others viewing that? If you have a disability that is not readily apparent, how do you understand this and how might others (if at all)? The point of this aspect of the inventory is to understand that how you move through life does not necessarily correspond with how others see that journey. What you think might be central to your identity may not even register with someone else. Conversely, what you minimize (such as racial privilege) may be of central import to others. Making the genuine effort to understand how others experience you is critical to relationship building and essential if you want to deconstruct and challenge your own societal privileges.

Step 4: Synthesis and Next Steps

Now comes the difficult work—digesting and then acting on what you have uncovered by virtue of doing this inventory. Consider these three questions: (1) What are your overall reactions to this inventory? (2) Does any dimension stand out as particularly important to your overall cultural identity and why? and (3) What have you learned about yourself and what next steps in this process do you see yourself taking? In other words, the inventory, in itself, does not constitute anti-oppression work. It is the precursor to anti-oppression actions. If you have pushed yourself to be honest and reflective thus far, then you have laid a foundation for considering what you need to do. Perhaps education is needed—if so, how will you go about getting it? Maybe an important relationship needs to be repaired—how might you take the steps to make amends? Or perhaps the inventory revealed that some skills, such as assertiveness training, are needed—where will you obtain this? Did you become aware of new potential problems or challenges for other groups, and if so, how might you respond?

It is tempting, and perhaps even human nature, to try to minimize the inventory messages that we don't want to know. It is not easy to think of oneself as "privileged," particularly if we don't ask for it or believe we use that privilege to our advantage. Often, we become more focused on those parts of our identity associated with subordinate-group membership and then don't see the privilege we might have. We also run the risk of becoming paralyzed by building an identity of victimization. Self-awareness, flexibility, empathy, and openness are essential, but perhaps most important is understanding that anti-oppression work takes time (Burghardt, 2011; hooks, 2003). Be patient with yourself and others as more authentic relationships are built.

CONNECTING TO COMMUNITY PRACTICE

Community practitioners would be wise to take a page from the training manual of most clinical social workers, therapists, and counselors who are trained to be cognizant in the "use of self." Use of self may be defined as the knowledge and skill sets employed by the practitioner in such a way that he or she becomes an instrument to facilitate change (Heydt & Sherman, 2005). Within the parameters of the therapeutic relationship, the practitioner is able to model and reflect transformative possibilities for the client. Yet this approach is not without its dangers, and considerable self-awareness is necessary if the practitioner wishes to minimize unnecessarily complicated or messy relationships with clients. As part of this training, these practitioners learn to recognize and address the emotions generated in the therapeutic relationship; identify what client actions might "push buttons"; negotiate expectations of the client, including the maintenance of "appropriate" boundaries; and work through resistance and reluctance. The cultural selves of practitioner and client significantly affect these dynamics as cultural variations in seeking help, dealing with authority and power, and building relationships come into play (Heydt & Sherman, 2005; Reupert, 2007). Thus, the use of self is actually the use of the cultural self.

How does this translate to community practice? The strategic use of self is concerned with relationship building that encourages constructive change, which in many respects is the core of community practice. In order to be an effective community organizer or other practitioner who can build the relationships necessary for increasing community capacity, that individual needs to understand how his or her cultural identity affects facilitating and sustaining relationships. The assumption is that if one does not acknowledge or address the affect of privilege, then one risks poisoning this critical aspect of practice. Moreover, the ability to build authentic connections rests on how well one understands oneself. Many practitioners want to move quickly to finding commonalities, but the realities of oppression—including the personal side—need to be addressed first (Burghardt, 2011). Time, patience, and humility are essential ingredients in this process.

Building on the insights from the Cultural Identity Inventory, one needs to turn to making connections between that awareness and community practice. For this, another assessment is suggested (see Table A1.2). Adapted from Axner's (n.d.) exercise, the goal is to identify how one's cultural identity helps and hinders one's community practice abilities and then extend these findings by determining what one needs to continue with his or her development. This information is then linked to an emerging use of self. By systematically engaging in this self-assessment, one will not only understand how cultural attributes of the practitioner become part of practice (for better or worse) but also begin to think strategically about how to maximize the assets and minimize the concerns.

TABLE A1.2 Assessment: Connecting Cultural Identity to Community Practice

Cultural Dimension	As Strength or Asset to My Community Practice	As Challenge or Concern to My Community Practice	What Do I Need to Continue My Development?
Gender			
Race			
Class			
Sexual orientation			
Citizenship			
Religion			
Physical or mental ability			
Other?			

Note the ways in which the different components of your cultural identity have influenced you as a community practitioner. Specifically, record how that attribute has (1) given you strengths or assets and (2) provided challenges or concerns.

A. Indicate what you need to continue your development (i.e., how can you build on your strengths or address concerns?).

B. How does this assessment inform your cognizance of "use of self"?

Adapted from M. Axner, *Diversity and Community Strengths* (Lawrence, KS: Work Group for Community Health and Development, University of Kansas, 2011); Community Tool Box, http://ctb.ku.edu/en/tablecontents/sub_section_tools_1170.aspx. Used with permission from the Work Group for Community Health and Development, University of Kansas.

SUMMARY

Community practitioners typically are concerned with, and adept at analyzing, the power structures and processes that affect their constituencies. In this appendix, I have challenged practitioners to look at a more personal aspect of power—the privileges derived from membership in dominant-status groups. I have argued that one's cultural identity largely is determined by these memberships, and I have highlighted the need for reflecting on the multiple and often intersecting identities we hold (woman, Latina, middle class, etc.). With a more comprehensive understanding of our cultural identities, including the ways in which the various dimensions can change and be challenged over time, we are better situated to build authentic relationships with constituents and community members. In more fully understanding how we benefit from oppressive systems, we are more likely to find the tools to dismantle the attendant structures and processes. This is a critical aspect of "fighting the good fight" and takes time, self-patience, and an openness to continued learning. In doing so, we forge better bonds with our partners and allies and, ultimately, create better communities for us all.

REFERENCES

Adams, M. (1997). Pedagogical frameworks for social justice education. In M. Adams, L. A. Bell, & P. Griffin (Eds.), *Teaching for diversity and social justice: A sourcebook* (pp. 30–43). New York, NY: Routledge.

Axner, M. (n.d.). Diversity and community strengths. Community Tool Box. Retrieved from http://ctb.ku.edu/en/tablecontents/sub_section_tools_1170.aspx

Burghardt, S. (2011). Why can't we all just get along? Building effective coalitions while resolving the not-so-hidden realities of race, gender, sexuality, and class. *Macro practice in social work for the 21st century* (pp. 176–214). Thousand Oaks, CA: Sage.

Connell, R. W. (2005). *Masculinities* (2nd ed.). Berkeley: University of California Press.

Gerschick, T. (1993). Should and can a white, heterosexual, middle-class man teach students about social inequality and oppression? In D. Schoem, L. Frankel, X. Zuniga, & E. Lewis (Eds.), *Multicultural teaching in the university* (pp. 200–207). Westport, CT: Praeger.

Goodman, D. J. (2001). *Promoting diversity and social justice: Educating people from privileged groups.* Thousand Oaks, CA: Sage.

Heydt, M. J., & Sherman, N. E. (2005). Conscious use of self: Tuning the instrument of social work practice with cultural competence. *Journal of Baccalaureate Social Work, 10*(2), 25–40.

hooks, b. (2000a). *Feminist theory: From margin to center* (2nd ed.). Boston, MA: South End Press.

hooks, b. (2000b). Where *we stand: Class matters.* New York, NY: Routledge.

hooks, b. (2003). *Teaching community: A pedagogy of hope.* New York, NY: Routledge.

Jones, C. P. (2000). Levels of racism: A theoretic framework and a gardener's tale. *American Journal of Public Health, 8,* 1212–1215.

Katz, J. (1978). *White awareness.* Norman, OK: University of Oklahoma Press.

McIntosh, P. (1989). White privilege: Unpacking the invisible knapsack. *Peace and Freedom* (January/February), 10–12.

Reupert, A. (2007). Social worker's use of self. *Clinical Social Work Journal, 35,* 107–116.

Sennett, R., & Cobb, J. (1972). *The hidden injuries of class.* New York, NY: W. W. Norton.

Tappan, M. B. (2006). Reframing internalized oppression and internalized domination: From the psychological to the sociocultural. *Teachers College Record, 108*(10), 2115–2144.

Wallerstein, N. (1999). Power between evaluator and community: Research relationships within New Mexico's healthier communities. *Social Science and Medicine, 49,* 39–53.

APPENDIX 2

GUIDING CBPR PRINCIPLES

FOSTERING EQUITABLE HEALTH CARE FOR LGBTQ+ PEOPLE

MIRIA KANO, KELLEY P. SAWYER, AND CATHLEEN E. WILLGING

With transphobia and homophobia, a lack of knowledge can be just as damaging as a slur.[1]

Although often focused on ethnic-racial minorities, community-based participatory research (CBPR) approaches are equally beneficial to address health inequities faced by other vulnerable communities that face stigma and social marginalization. In 2014, we received a PCORI Pipeline to Proposal award to address health inequities faced by lesbian, gay, bisexual, transgender, and queer (LGBTQ+) people in urban and rural areas of New Mexico. The community-academic partnership was formalized as the New Mexico LGBTQ+ Health Collaborative (the collaborative), a fifteen-person advisory board of health care advocates, patients, providers, and health services researchers from across the state, whose stated purpose is to improve quality of care for LGBTQ+ people based on their lived experiences. To promote community-partnered research, optimal stakeholder communication, and better health care, the collaborative authored *Guidelines for Healthcare Research with LGBTQ+ Individuals and Communities in New Mexico* (see online resource at http://hsc.unm.edu/programs/nmcareshd/docs/LGBTQ-guidelines.pdf).[2]

This appendix provides a brief overview of this process and our key principles for positive and productive partnerships.

Compared to their heterosexual, cisgender[3] counterparts, LGBTQ+ people are more likely to suffer from mental health and substance abuse problems, eating and body-related disorders, sexually transmitted diseases, poor diet and exercise, and are less likely to benefit from preventative services (Hembree et al., 2009; McNair & Hegarty, 2010). Recent reviews of existing guidelines to promote LBGTQ+ competence across clinical services have highlighted insufficient inclusion of LGBTQ+ patient and provider perspectives in their design and implementation (McNair & Hegarty, 2010).

Historical discrimination within health care services, including from cultural stigma concerning sex and gender atypicality, have generated distrust by LGBTQ+ people of medical institutions and research enterprises (Eckstrand & Sciolla, 2015). Over the last fifty years, LGBTQ+ people have experienced denial of treatment for HIV/AIDS (Wright, 2013), invasive and damaging genital surgeries and hormone treatments to normalize sex and gender in babies with ambiguous genitalia (Kessler et al., 1998), and ongoing damaging "reparative therapies" (Berger, 1994). Such commonplace experiences, also embedded in discriminatory laws, policies, and care-giving practices, pathologize sexual and gender difference and alienate LGBTQ+ patients.

DEVELOPING LGBTQ+ GUIDELINES

These guidelines were created to promote bidirectional learning, effective communication, and trust among members of the LGBTQ+ community, health care providers, and health services researchers to inspire health equity and catalyze social change. The collaborative developed a series of semi-structured interview questions, UNM HRPO (14–077), to guide one-on-one discussions, and a collection of vignettes from LGBTQ+ individuals from New Mexico tapped to discuss relational and participatory needs of sexual and gender minority research participants from rural and urban areas of the state.

In 2015, a contracted ethnographer interviewed twenty LGBTQ+ New Mexicans. Participants were twenty-seven to sixty-five years old, with a range of gender, sexual, and ethnic-racial-cultural identities. Most resided in Albuquerque, but many were originally from rural and tribal communities. Many had explicit interests in health research, with specialties of nursing, mental health, and surgery. Other participants were students, advocates, activists, and self-described "regular" members of an LGBTQ+ community.

Interview participants and members of the collaborative cited examples of research and health care–related encounters that were "homophobic," "transphobic," "biased," "discriminatory," and "insensitive." Many suggested that such encounters could be avoided if researchers and clinicians had greater exposure to and more information about LGBTQ+ communities and more effective training in inclusive communication practices within health care and research. For Native American or Hispanic participants, issues of research misconduct were brought to the fore, as were calls to use CBPR, with special attention to negative historical relationships between the community and local universities in research. One participant stressed having ongoing relationships with communities:

> We would love to work with researchers on [LGBTQ+] issues, as long as the researcher will stick around, and give something back to the community. Some have come in to research the trans community. They gather information and just disappear. How does that help our community? It just reinforces stigma, our sense of outsiderness, and negative feelings about research and privilege on the part of academics.

The following three themes were considered essential in building research relationships with LGBTQ+ communities.

Be Aware of the Link between Historical Trauma and Individual Experiences of Trauma

Historical trauma theories posit that past violence and assaults (e.g., the colonization of the Americas and slavery) have undermined physiological and psychological health, leading to personal trauma among many in these same communities today. They also contend that historical oppression has led to a "weak mainstream political will to ameliorate [these disparities]" (Chávez et al., 2008, p. 96). Although theories of historical trauma have been developed to explain the colonization of Indigenous peoples and internment and genocide of Jewish peoples, persons contributing to these guidelines were adamant that they be applied to past violence and attempts to oppress LGBTQ+ populations.

The "humanity" of LGBTQ+ people has been defined historically in opposition to sexual and gender roles considered "normal" by a dominant Western standard. Medical pathologization of LGBTQ+ people, through the *Diagnostic and Statistical Manual of Mental Disorders,* has been a source of historical trauma and contributes to gender- and sexuality-based social trauma and violence. Collaborative members and participants provided insight into how such trauma is internalized for LGBTQ+ individuals. One participant explained:

> We are already pretty unhealthy in our community: smoking, substance use, obesity . . . but there has to be a high level of understanding as to why that is. Systemic things and hardcore trauma have created this. Please, don't just tell people not to smoke, or to exercise more. This really starts at healing from trauma.

Although LGBTQ+ communities and their allies may be well aware of endured traumas that lead to health disparities, one participant observed, "The roots are not widely understood by health care professionals." Constant reinforcement of traumatic experiences can lead to internalized trauma and "minority stress" for LGBTQ+ individuals excluded from benefits and protections offered to heterosexual and cisgender people (Meyer, 2003). This context must be understood by researchers to build strong and lasting partnerships with community members.

Understand the Intersectional and Diverse Identities and Experiences of LGBTQ+ Individuals with Whom You Are Working

Although the umbrella term *LGBTQ+* is often used as a cohesive category, it encompasses a broad spectrum of diversity. Some LGBTQ+ individuals may experience gender and sexuality as stable, identifying with certain categories throughout their lives, and others will experience fluidity, occupying different categories during their lifetimes.

"Sexual diversity means more than gay or straight," stated one participant, adding that "poly and kinky people can sometimes still feel stigmatized or sensationalized and not as free to speak about their sexual lives and relationships." A second addressed the "B" in LGBTQ+, clarifying that "bisexual people have traditionally been largely ignored and often feel marginalized and judged within the LGBTQ community [and research]." A third expressed concerns in terms of cisgenderism and binary bias (versus inclusion) within LGBTQ+ health care and research:

> I worry about non-binary folks . . . a lot of our work deals with more binary trans people, and these folks get left behind more than anyone else; a lot of times it's butch lesbians [and those with] non-normative gender presentations who get the weirdest, most uncomfortable reactions.

For CBPR to be successful in LGBTQ+ communities, recruitment, data collection, and analysis must include diversity along the sexual and gender minority continuum while remaining mindful of intersecting identities. Partnering with community leaders, advocates, and LGBTQ+ persons allows researchers to understand how gender and sexuality intersect with race, economic position, regional and rural-urban locales, age, (dis)ability, and local contexts. For some, residency in rural areas, economic disadvantage, and even tribal affiliation, can intersect to create isolation and compound disparities in health and access to care. Others may find rural residency preferable, experiencing resilience through kinship networks from the local culture.

When working with LGBTQ+ people, investigators may encounter unique challenges, and as a participant remarked, "We have to get creative to address the intersectionality of New Mexico's queer communities: for trans people living on the streets, we have to find out how to reach these individuals." Describing the reticence some sexual- and gender-minority Native Americans have in participating in research, one participant said, "Being labeled in general is difficult for Native people—we had our names thrust upon us. So even adding 2S (Two-Spirit) onto acronyms is challenging and not particularly accurate for a lot of us." She added, "Maybe that's why we don't get more Native [research] participation; with colonization and sovereignty struggles—with the US governmental system that was pushed upon us."

When Working in LGBTQ+ Communities, Using Preferred Terminology and Maintaining Respectful Attitudes Are Important

For nonheterosexual and gender-nonconforming people, sexualized and gendered labels and categories are not merely descriptive, they are deeply social and political identities. Identity labels and pronouns are hotly debated within and outside LGBTQ+ communities. As one participant explained, "Researchers should probably be aware of the internal politics and tensions . . . In activist circles we pay great attention to language and pronouns."

Persons sharing the same identities may identify differently from each other, and individuals who vary in identities or attraction may use the same label. For example, a cisgender women who sleeps with other cisgender women may identify as a lesbian, while another may identify as queer. A transgender man in a relationship with a cisgender man may identify as gay, as do many cisgender men in relationships together. A transgender woman in a relationship with a cisgender man may also identify as gay.

Mislabeling someone may cause harm or repeat patterns of trauma. Gender-nonconforming contributors to these guidelines cited ignorance or misuse of pronouns as a major source of misunderstanding and harm in interactions with researchers and health care providers. One participant used an example of seeking gynecological care to illustrate why it is important to be aware of pronoun use. Already uncomfortable as a trans man and confronting past body and identity-related trauma, he had put off seeking such care until the situation became life-threatening. At the appointment where he learned that he would need an emergency hysterectomy, nurses repeatedly referred to him as "Miss." He said, "It added more trauma to the experience." Participants unanimously agreed that a good rule of thumb is for researchers and health providers to talk to research partners, ask what they call themselves, and avoid assuming identifications based on how they present themselves.

QUICK TIPS FOR FOSTERING EQUITABLE RESEARCH PARTNERSHIPS WITH LGBTQ+ COMMUNITIES

- Begin by developing meaningful partnerships with community members and understand the needs of the community in which you are conducting research.
- Partner with leaders, advocates, and community members to define research questions and culturally sensitive research methodologies.
- Incorporate inclusive, community-preferred language in consent documents and research instruments. Acceptable pronouns may include *they, them, ze, zhe, zir, hir, her,* and *him.*
- Use open-ended demographic forms: let participants dictate preferred names, pronouns, labels, behaviors, what they call their relationships, and why.
- Understand historical trauma within the LGBTQ+ community *and* how this trauma interacts with other axes of historical trauma and oppression.
- Train all CBPR team members (e.g., researchers, providers, and community members) in LGBTQ+ competency.
- Know the relationship between the community and your research institution (power dynamics are often long-standing between institutions and communities).

Our experiences suggest that CBPR is an effective method for developing positive, respectful, and long-term relationships with members of the LGBTQ+ community. The CBPR approach provides a space for people with multiple intersecting identities to work together to inform research projects with potential to create sustainable and equitable health care experiences for LGBTQ+ people while simultaneously advancing the science of health disparities.

ACKNOWLEDGMENTS

These guidelines were made possible through support by the Community Engagement Core of NM CARES HD (http://hsc.unm.edu/programs/nmcareshd/cec.shtml#tabs1-toolkits).

See research guidelines for Latino border communities at this same website: http://hsc.unm.edu/programs/nmcareshd/docs/CECFINALGuidelinesHealthResearchBorderPromotores10.03.15.pdf.

Spanish version for Latino border communities: http://hsc.unm.edu/programs/nmcareshd/docs/CECFINALInvestigacionsaludFronterizasPromotores10.03.15.pdf.

The authors thank members of the New Mexico LGBTQ+ Health Collaborative, Edward Fancovic, Rebecca Dakota, Greg Gomez, Barbara Cichosz, Amber Royster, Cameron Crandall, Nathaniel Sharon, Beverly Gorman, Adrien Lawyer, Alma Rosa Silva-Bañuelos, and Robert Sturm for their expert recommendations.

NOTES

1. K. Sawyer, personal communication with research participant (September 15, 2015).
2. Also see "Acknowledgments" for guidelines for Latino border communities.
3. *Cisgender* refers to individuals whose sex assigned at birth aligns with their gender identity.

REFERENCES

Berger, J. (1994). The psychotherapeutic treatment of male homosexuality. *American Journal of Psychotherapy, 48*(2), 251–261.

Chávez, V., Duran, B., Baker, Q. E., Avila, M. M., & Wallerstein, N. (2008). The dance of race and privilege in CBPR. In M. Minkler & N. Wallerstein (Eds.), *Community-based participatory research for health: From process to outcomes* (2nd ed., pp. 91–106). San Francisco, CA: Jossey-Bass.

Eckstrand, K. L., & Sciolla, A. F. (2015). History of health disparities among people who are or may be LGBT, gender non-conforming, and/or born with DSD: A resource for medical educators. In A. D. Hollenbach, K. L. Eckstrand, & A. Dreger (Eds.), *Implementing curricular and institutional climate changes to improve health care for individuals who are LGBT, gender nonconforming, or born with DSD* (pp. 10–21). Washington, DC: Association of American Medical Colleges.

Hembree, W. C., Cohen-Kettenis, P., Delemarre-van de Waal, H. A., Gooren, L. J., Meyer, W. J., III, Spack, N. P., Tangpricha, V., & Montori, V. M. (2009). Endocrine treatment of transsexual persons: An Endocrine Society clinical practice guideline. *The Journal of Clinical Endocrinology and Metabolism, 94*(9), 3132–3154.

Meyer, I. H. (2003). Prejudice, social stress, and mental health in lesbian, gay, and bisexual populations: Conceptual issues and research evidence. *Psychological Bulletin, 129*(5), 674–697.

McNair, R. P., & Hegarty, K. (2010). Guidelines for the primary care of lesbian, gay, and bisexual people: A systematic review. *Annals of Family Medicine, 8*(6), 533–541.

Wright, J. (2013). Only your calamity: The beginnings of activism by and for people with AIDS. *American Journal of Public Health, 103*(10), 1788–1798.

APPENDIX 3

QUALITY CRITERIA OF THE INTERNATIONAL COLLABORATION FOR PARTICIPATORY HEALTH RESEARCH (ICPHR)

MICHAEL T. WRIGHT

Participatory approaches to health research are increasingly drawing the attention of funders, decision makers, researchers, and civil society worldwide. There is a great diversity among these approaches in terms of intention, theory, process, and outcome. Community-based participatory research (CBPR) is an important contribution to these approaches from North America; in other parts of the world there are other traditions of participatory research going by different names (e.g., *participatory action research, participatory research, action research, collaborative inquiry*). This diversity reflects the large variety of people, places, and issues involved in participatory health research (PHR) in many different countries and under widely varying conditions. PHR is often viewed as being a means for achieving positive transformation in society in the interest of people's health, for example, by changing the way health professionals are educated, the way health care institutions work, and the politics and policies affecting the health of society.

The International Collaboration for Participatory Health Research (ICPHR, www.icphr.org) was created in 2009 as a place to bring together international learning about the application of participatory research approaches to address health issues (Wright et al., 2009, 2010). After some debate, the ICPHR chose *PHR* as a neutral umbrella term that can encompass different national and regional traditions. Through consolidating existing knowledge and reaching agreement on common terminology and principles, the ICPHR seeks to strengthen the role of PHR in intervention design and decision making on health issues and thus to provide a means for people most affected by health problems to influence how these problems are addressed in society. This includes developing guidelines for conducting and evaluating PHR, describing which forms of theory and evidence are produced by this approach, and finding a means for conducting systematic reviews of the PHR literature in order to contribute to the body of international knowledge on health.

Some examples of the projects initiated by members of the ICPHR include the following: a position paper on ethics has been published on the website and ethics case studies are being collected from members in several countries for a book publication. ICPHR members are also developing position papers on empowerment, the training of professionals in participatory research, and the relationship between PHR and implementation science. An international conference on impact in PHR was held in Germany, resulting in special issues in two journals examining the various effects of participation over the course of PHR projects. The ICPHR has also developed a continuing education course that has been offered in English, German, and Portuguese and is being piloted in an online version. And the project Kids in Action is drawing people of all ages together from several countries who are interested in children's participation in health research.

In its first position paper (ICPHR, 2013) the ICPHR sought to identify some of the central characteristics of participatory approaches to health research that cut across various cultures. The paper has since been translated into several languages and is used for promoting critical thinking in the teaching and practice of PHR. Many people engaged in PHR find the position paper too long and complicated to be used in their work. To address this problem, Tina Cook from the United Kingdom distilled the eleven primary characteristics into short statements that are meant to describe the unique qualities of PHR. These statements are not necessarily specific to research on health issues but rather can be applied to participatory research more generally.

ENSURING QUALITY: INDICATIVE CHARACTERISTICS OF PARTICIPATORY (HEALTH) RESEARCH

The following criteria can be used when reflecting on the quality of participatory research projects.

Participatory

The goal of PHR is to maximize the participation of those whose life or work is the subject of the research in all stages of the research process, including the formulation of the research question and goal, the development of a research design, the selection of appropriate methods for data collection and analysis, the implementation of the research, the interpretation of the results, and the dissemination of the findings. Such participation is the core, defining principle of PHR, setting this type of research apart from other approaches in the health field. Whatever model is used to describe participation in the research process, the goal of PHR is to provide the opportunity for all participants to be equitably involved to the maximum degree possible throughout the research.

Locally Situated

PHR is grounded in the reality of daily life and work in a specific place and time. The issue being researched must be located in the social system, which is likely to adopt the changes that result from the research process. This is the strength of PHR and results in the further development of local knowledge. It is this local dimension that often presents the greatest challenge to funders and policy makers as well as to those who assume that their generalized knowledge ("scientific" or "professional" knowledge, in the usual sense) is superior.

A Collective Research Process

In PHR the research process is typically conducted by a group representing the various stakeholders taking part in the study. This group can include engaged citizens, members of civil society (e.g., nongovernmental organizations), health and social welfare professionals, health organizations, academic researchers, and policy makers. Any one of these stakeholders can initiate and lead a study. The title *participatory researcher* or *coresearcher* is not reserved for the academics but rather designates all members of the research group. The leadership role consists of facilitating a shared decision-making group process for developing, implementing, analyzing, and disseminating the research.

PHR Projects Are Collectively Owned

Consistent with the previously named principles, the ownership of the research lies in the hands of the group conducting the study. The group needs to decide how best to report on the findings of the research in order to meet the set goals.

Aims for Transformation through Human Agency

PHR follows the explicit goal of creating positive social change as a result of the research process for those persons whose life or work is the focus of the research. Typical research goals are as follows:

- Improving the health of a specific group of people
- Addressing the social determinants of health by improving living standards
- Addressing the political determinants of health by changing repressive or restrictive policy
- Improving the quality of services by addressing organizational issues

A quality criterion for PHR is supporting transformation processes that go beyond the span of the research project so as to contribute to lasting change in the interest of better health. Sustainable change is promoted, for example, by involving a broad coalition of stakeholders in the research, setting up structures for sustained learning and action as part of the research process, and providing skills training for local people to carry on the initiatives launched during the research once the project is completed.

Promotes Critical Reflexivity

Critical reflexivity means considering how power and powerlessness affect the daily lives and practice of those whose life or work is the focus of the research. It requires professionals to question their roles and their knowledge based on power differentials between themselves and service users and based on the expertise gained through life experiences and the social disadvantages faced by people without professional health qualifications.

Produces Knowledge That Is Local, Collective, Cocreated, Conversational, and Diverse

Knowledge produced by health research is typically by and for an academic audience. Often highly technical in methodology and reporting, the knowledge can be difficult to diffuse to policy makers, practitioners, community leaders, and others who could use the information to make change. Knowledge produced through PHR is accessible to different audiences, especially for whom the work has direct impact.

Strives for a Broad Impact

An explicit intention of PHR is to bring about social change. Social learning (learning together and from each other) is a fundamental dimension of the PHR process, and the continual cycle of "look, reflect, act" underpins the dynamics of developing a connected knowing. Interactive processes engage people in transformative learning, that is, changes in the way they see the world and themselves. This generates an intention of being able to act based on their experience during the research and the research findings, thus having a wider impact.

Produces Local Evidence Based on Broad Understandings of Generalizability

The generation of local evidence can accumulate over time, strengthening the ability of local participants to take effective action. Transfer of interventions from one locality to the next is about understanding the contextual conditions in the new setting, how they differ from the setting in which the knowledge was produced, and reflecting on the consequences.

Follows Specific Validity Criteria

- *Participatory validity:* extent to which stakeholders take an active part in research process
- *Intersubjective validity:* extent to which the research is viewed as being credible and meaningful by the stakeholders from a variety of perspectives
- *Contextual validity:* extent to which the research relates to the local situation
- *Catalytic validity:* extent to which the research is useful in presenting new possibilities for social action
- *Ethical validity:* extent to which the research outcomes and the changes exerted on people by the research are sound and just
- *Empathic validity:* extent to which the research has increased empathy among the participants

Is a Dialectical Process Characterized by Messiness?

As knowledge and action strategies generated by PHR arise out of a collective research process characterized by dialogue among participants with different perspectives on the subject under study, this does not necessarily result in a consensual view. It may reveal and promote several different views resulting in different ways of addressing the issue at hand. The occurrence of this messiness is a fundamental characteristic of PHR and its nonlinear, multifocused research process and outcomes that cannot be characterized prior to the study. The rigor in PR lies in the extent the research is facilitated so as to make possible new, transformative insights that offer fresh approaches for action.

REFERENCES

International Collaboration for Participatory Health Research (ICPHR). (2013, May). *Position paper 1: What is participatory health research?* Berlin, Germany: International Collaboration for Participatory Health Research. Retrieved from www.icphr.org/uploads/2/0/3/9/20399575/ichpr_position_paper_1_defintion_-_version_may_2013.pdf

Wright, M. T., Gardner, B., Roche, B., von Unger, H., & Ainlay, C. (2010). Building an international collaboration on participatory health research. *Progress in Community Health Partnerships: Research, Education, and Action, 4*(1), 31–36.

Wright, M. T., Roche, B., von Unger, H., Block, M., & Gardner, B. (2009). A call for an international collaboration on participatory research for health. *Health Promotion International, 25*(1), 115–122.

APPENDIX 4

CULTURAL HUMILITY

REFLECTIONS AND RELEVANCE FOR CBPR

VIVIAN CHÁVEZ

The words humanity *and* humility *come from being tied to the earth and the soil. Unpretentious. Being able to tell the truth and acknowledging that to tell the truth is to allow suffering to speak. There is no real talk or engagement with the truth about our lives, individually, collectively, nationally, or globally without allowing suffering to speak.*

CORNEL WEST, KEYNOTE, AMERICAN PUBLIC HEALTH ASSOCIATION MEETING, DENVER (2010)

In their seminal essay, "Cultural Humility versus Cultural Competence," Tervalon and Murray-Garcia (1998) reframed the discourse of health disparities and institutional inequities in medicine. The authors defined *cultural humility* as "a lifelong commitment to self-evaluation and critique, to redressing the power imbalances in the physician-patient dynamic, and to developing mutually beneficial and non-paternalistic partnerships with communities on behalf of individuals and defined populations" (p.123). Cultural humility is a rich multifaceted construct that reflects key dimensions of CBPR thinking, behavior, and actions and recognizes the pervasiveness of culture in every research encounter (see Box A4.1). Now cited in 894 related publications, cultural humility is recognized as a resource in a number of fields including public

Box A4.1 Principles Guiding Cultural Humility That Resonate with Principles of CBPR

- Lifelong learning and critical self-reflection
- Recognize and change power imbalances
- Develop mutually beneficial partnerships
- Institutional accountability

health (Chávez et al., 2008; Fleckman et al., 2015; Minkler, 2012; Rajaram & Bockrath, 2011; US Department of Health and Human Services, 2009; Wallerstein & Duran, 2010; Yonas et al., 2006); psychology (Gallardo, 2014; Hook et al., 2013;); social work (Fisher-Borne, Cain, & Martin, 2014; Hyde, 2012; also Appendix 1; Ortega & Coulborn, 2011); nursing (Faronda, Baptiste, Reinholdt, & Ousman, 2016); community development (Rice, 2007; Ross, 2010); and spiritual formation (Owen et al., 2014).

Although definitions play an important role in enhancing collaboration between and within disciplines, solidarity, more than cognitive understanding, is required. Cultural humility is an embodied approach that expands the frame from traditional understandings of race and ethnicity to include the culture of building alliances between groups and individuals from diverse backgrounds, genders, sexual orientation, (dis)ability, educational levels, immigration status and other socioeconomic and social-identity indicators. "Humility, and not so much the discrete mastery traditionally implied by the static notion of competence, captures most accurately what researchers need to model" (Tervalon & Murray-Garcia, 1998, p. 120). Cultural humility takes into account the fluidity of culture and challenges individuals and institutions to address inequalities (Fisher-Borne et al., 2014). The concept came out of the social injustices experienced by Rodney King in 1992 when people all over the world watched videotaped images of an African American man brutally beaten by the Los Angeles police. "At Children's Hospital, Oakland, we started talking about our own private Rodney Kings, the circumstances where families felt they were not being taken care of in a respectful way. That was a big part of our work, being certain that we were living up to the principles; that given the composition of the faculty and given the composition of the patients, the faculty (alone) could not teach about the issues of culture and race, difference and income" (see Chávez, 2012 [video]). As the National Partnership for Action to End Health Disparities (2015) notes, cultural competence is part of the evolutionary process toward cultural humility. Ultimately, "experiencing with the community the factors at play in defining health priorities, research activities and community-informed advocacy activities require that we recognize that foci of expertise with regard to health can indeed reside outside of the academic center" (Tervalon & Murray-Garcia, 1998, p. 122).

Faronda and her colleagues (2016) provide a concept analysis for cultural humility based on use of the term in articles published between 2009 and 2014. They note that the movement toward cultural humility implies social and personal transformation and not only skills and information about various cultures. "Cultural humility involves a change in overall perspective.

Cultural humility is a way of being. Employing cultural humility means being aware of power imbalances and being humble in every interaction with every individual" (Faronda et al., 2016, p. 214). On a similar note, Rajaram and Bockrath (2011) advocate for integration of reflective inquiry of researcher's social location in systems of privilege and oppression to extend beyond mastery of knowledge and communication skills to a deeper understanding of the underlying sociopolitical and economic processes of power and privilege that create, support, and maintain existing health disparities.

TEACHING CBPR WITH CULTURAL HUMILITY

Strong CBPR partnerships reflect three levels of cultural humility: intrapersonal, interpersonal, and institutional. Through community dialogue, the relationship-based character of cultural humility has the potential to open courageous conversations and offer healing to communities of practice. At the intrapersonal level, researchers, teachers, and students of CBPR engage in critical self-reflection and awareness of biases and limitations. They commit to a lifelong learning process that includes "not knowing" and deference to multiple sources of knowledge. This key aspect of the model is difficult given academic training in having "expert knowledge" at all times. The place of humility is a full-bodied experience that requires recognition of how each of us is socialized by the cultures of the university, health department, hospital, or other professional workplaces. We embody structures and may contribute to making invisible and exploiting others through our positions of privilege without intention because of lack of awareness. Instructors are prepared to design classroom activities that provoke emotional responses necessary to expand students' comfort zone and explore bias in an open environment without reacting or defending.

The interpersonal level is the level of partnership in which issues of race, ethnicity, class, gender, disability, and other forms of hierarchy present in academia and the health professions risk being replicated at community gatherings, one-on-one, or in CBPR partnerships. Building alliances across differences and having a commitment to redress power imbalances need an action plan and adequate time dedicated to develop, implement, and evaluate the intended actions. Approaching community members as peers starts with recognizing students as colleagues and partnering with them in their education. Even when CBPR researchers come from working class backgrounds or are people of color, of the same gender identity, religion, age group, and so on, we must be aware of the varied historical experiences of powerlessness, poverty, racism, trauma, and privilege. Peer learning promotes a culture of collaboration and cooperation that takes practice and is a key component of the hidden or implicit curriculum for CBPR.

At the institutional level, organization(s) sponsoring CBPR recognize and value the dynamic terrain of culture. Currently, a third of the US population is composed of racial-ethnic "minorities," and in some communities the word *minority* itself is a misnomer. The institution is thus committed to an ongoing examination of staffing patterns and equitable hiring, training, and advancement practices that are representative and drawn from the communities being served. Antidiscrimination policies are followed, updated, and revised to reflect culturally appropriate language. There is a supportive environment for professional development in the areas of unlearning oppression and examining privilege.

CONCLUSION

Humility is an elusive concept with ethical dimensions emphasized by spiritual practices worldwide. An expanded definition of health includes spirituality as the fourth dimension of health (World Health Organization, 1991) and emphasizes *social engagement* and *mindfulness.* Freire was a deeply spiritual human being who believed in humility to be an act of solidarity (Boyd, 2012; Darder, 2000). Freire's solidarity was not simply a cognitive decision but a spiritual transformation that brings one into identification and common struggle with those who have less power. Freire himself said, "dialogue cannot exist without humility" (Freire, 1970, p. 79). Given the centrality of authentic dialogue and collaboration between partners in CBPR to understand, study, and address community-identified problems, cultural humility is a basic requirement.

"Definitions are vital points for the imagination," says bell hooks, in *All about Love* (2000, p. 14). "A good definition marks our starting point and lets us know where we want to end up. As we move toward our desired destination we chart the journey, creating a map." Reversing the starting point, I end with an open-ended definition of cultural humility and an invitation for readers to keep finding its meaning, particularly in relation to CBPR. Genuine, high-level CBPR can move cultural humility from idea to embodied practice. Cultural humility is a daily practice of self-study, openness to understanding others' cultures, and developing skills to deal with and redress power imbalances. Often, it means changing organizational policy to reflect these commitments while building relationships based on mutual trust and a shared commitment to equity and social justice.

REFERENCES

Boyd D. (2012). The critical spirituality of Paulo Freire. *International Journal of Lifelong Education, 31*(6), 759–778.

Chávez, V. (2012). *Cultural humility: People, principles & practices* [Video]. CES4Health.info. Retrieved from www.ces4health.info/find-products/view-product.aspx?code=XT4NJRJP

Chávez, V., Duran, B., Baker, Q., Avila, M., & Wallerstein, N. (2008). The dance of race and privilege in community-based participatory research. In M Minkler & N. Wallerstein (Eds.), *Community-based participatory research for health: From process to outcomes* (2nd ed.). San Francisco, CA: Jossey-Bass.

Darder, A. (2000). *Teaching as an act of love: Reflections on Paulo Freire and his contributions to our lives.* Unpublished manuscript. Retrieved September 1, 2016, from www.darder.org/publications/darderarticles

Faronda, C., Baptiste, D. L., Reinholdt, M., & Ousman, K. (2016). Cultural humility: A concept analysis. *Journal of Transcultural Nursing, 27*(3), 210–217.

Fisher-Borne, M., Cain, J. M., & Martin, S. (2014). From mastery to accountability: Cultural humility as an alternative to cultural competence. *Social Work Education: The International Journal, 334*(2).

Fleckman, J., Corso, M., Ramirez, S., Begalieva, M., & Johnson, C. (2015). Intercultural competency in public health: A call for action to incorporate training into public health education. *Frontiers in Public Health, 3,* 210.

Freire, P. (1970). *Pedagogy of the oppressed.* New York, NY: Herder and Herder.

Gallardo, M. (2014). *Developing cultural humility: Embracing race, privilege and power.* Thousand Oaks, CA: Sage.

Hook, J., Davis, D., Owen, J., Worthington, E., & Utsey, S. (2013). Cultural humility: Measuring openness to culturally diverse clients. *Journal of Counseling and Psychology, 60*(3), 353–366.

hooks, b. (2000). *All about love.* New York, NY: Harpers Collins.

Hyde, C. (2012) Challenging ourselves: Critical self-reflection on power and privilege. In M. Minkler (Ed.), *Community organizing and community building for health and welfare* (3rd ed.). Rutgers, NJ: Rutgers University Press.

Minkler, M. (Ed.). (2012). *Community organizing and community building for health and welfare* (3rd ed.). New Brunswick, NJ: Rutgers University Press.

National Partnership for Action to End Health Disparities. (2015). *Cultural competency; What is it and why is it necessary.* Southeastern Health Equity Council. Retrieved September 1, 2016, from http://region4.npa-rhec.org/in-the-spotlight/resourceguidewhitepaper

Ortega, R., & Coulborn, F. (2011). Training child welfare workers from an intersectional cultural humility perspective: A paradigm shift. *Child Welfare, 90*(5), 27–49.

Owen, J., Jordan, T., Turner, D., Davis, D., Hook, J., & Leach M. (2014). Therapists' multicultural orientation: Client perceptions of cultural humility, spiritual/religious commitment, and therapy outcomes. *Journal of Psychology and Theology, 42*(1).

Rajaram, S., & Bockrath, S. (2011). Cultural competence: New conceptual insights into its limits and potential for addressing health disparities. *Journal of Health Disparities Research and Practice, 7*(5), 82–89.

Rice, M. (2007). A post-modern cultural competency framework for public administration and public service delivery. *International Journal of Public Sector Management, 20*(7), 622–637.

Ross, L. (2010) Notes from the field: Learning cultural humility through critical incidents and central challenges in community-based participatory research. *Journal of Community Practice, 18,* 315–335.

Tervalon, M., & Murray-Garcia, J. (1998). Cultural humility versus cultural competence: A critical distinction in defining physician training outcomes in multicultural education. *Journal of Healthcare for the Poor and Underserved, 9*(2), 117–125.

US Department of Health and Human Services. (2009). Transforming the face of health professions through cultural and linguistic competence education: The role of the HRSA Centers of Excellence. Retrieved from www.hrsa.gov/culturalcompetence/cultcompedu.pdf

Wallerstein, N., & Duran, B. (2010). Community-based participatory research contributions to intervention research: The intersection of science and practice to improve health equity. *American Journal of Public Health, 100*(Suppl 1), S40–S46.

World Health Organization. (1991). Issue 9290211407. Chapter 4: The Spiritual Dimension. Retrieved from http://new.worldlibrary.net/wplbn0000152157-world-health-organization-publication--year-1991--issue-9290211407--chapter-4-by-world-health-organization.aspx?

Yonas, M., Jones, N., Eng, E., Vines, A., Aronson, R. E., Griffith, D. M., White, B., & DuBose, M. (2006). The art and science of integrating undoing racism with CBPR: Challenges of pursuing NIH funding to investigate cancer care and racial equity. *Journal of Urban Health, 83*(6), 1004–1012.

APPENDIX 5

FUNDING IN CBPR IN US GOVERNMENT AND PHILANTHROPY

LAURA C. LEVITON AND LAWRENCE W. GREEN

Although academic-community partnerships can thrive and grow based on mutual commitment to address community priorities and health inequities, actual funding for CBPR and community-engaged research remains essential. Resources are needed for program implementation, research costs, and opportunities for community members to be involved in the research enterprise. Sharing budgets, between universities and community agencies or associations, is in fact one of the identified promising practices that best exemplify power sharing and collaborative decision making. The history and growth of federal and foundation funding illustrates this importance.

GOVERNMENT

The US federal government has supported the use of CBPR in grants, contracts, centers, and systematic reviews for close to three decades. Although it has never been the dominant approach to research and evaluation, multiple government agencies have recognized the importance of CBPR for its underlying democratic and social justice underpinnings and for its utility in engaging communities to obtain better data, analysis, and interpretation of findings. It remains to be seen how federal policies in the new administration might include CBPR. The Community-Campus Partnerships for Health at https://ccph.memberclicks.net/ tracks federal opportunities for funding in CBPR-related projects.

Mercer and Green (2008) reported on the history of US federal CBPR funding in the second edition of this book.[1] As they noted, there was a gradual shift in community participation from "downstream to upstream involvement of people in the continuum of research to policy and practice" (p. 400). Initially, people's engagement in research had a decided utilitarian point of view. People's cooperation in implementing programs produced superior results; then it emerged that community-engaged advocacy and planning had better outcomes, and today it is abundantly clear that community participation is important to the meaningful translation of research in local circumstances. By 2016, some agencies have added requirements in their application guidelines for community participants in research to be identified and others require letters of commitment from representatives of the community organizations or groups participating.

The first significant milestone for CBPR involved the Prevention Research Centers (PRCs) funded by the Centers for Disease Control and Prevention (CDC). When Congress created the PRCs in 1988, it mandated that each university-based PRC was to engage its communities in collaborative development and execution of research projects (Mercer & Green, 2008). In 1998 an Institute of Medicine (now National Academy of Medicine) committee evaluated the experience of the thirteen centers funded during that first decade. "The broad mission of the Prevention Research Centers . . . can be achieved only through the sustained cooperation of a diverse array of professionals and nonprofessionals who have roles in influencing the health of communities, who have competing goals and priorities, and who have little history of engaging in long-term cooperative efforts" (Green, 1997, p. v). Though community participation was found to be a shortcoming of most centers, the committee recommended additional funding of PRCs with requirements for community engagement. The PRCs, in turn, became a major source of subsequent grant applications to CDC for CBPR projects in the following decade.

In 1995, the National Institute of Environmental Health Sciences (NIEHS) became the first of the National Institutes of Health to support CBPR by that name when it funded fifteen CBPR projects at about $6.1 million per year (Mercer & Green, 2008). Among the NIH Institutes, NIEHS had been under the greatest pressure to undertake PR, owing to public concern about the reliability of environmental research—a skepticism brought on by Love Canal and other pollution disasters in which residents perceived government scientists as protecting industry or failing to represent community knowledge, concerns, and perspectives in their environmental research.

From 2002 through 2005, NIEHS sponsored a federal interagency working group (IWG) on CBPR, with active participation from eleven federal agencies. The purpose of this IWG was to strengthen communication among federal agencies with an interest in supporting CBPR methodologies in biomedical research, education, health care delivery, or policy. One of the IWG's most important products was a funding announcement titled "Community Participation in Research," cosponsored by the NIH, AHRQ (Agency for Healthcare Research and Quality), and CDC. The goal was to support research on health promotion, disease prevention, and health disparities that was jointly conducted by communities and researchers. In 2008 this announcement was replaced with two NIH announcements of funding for "community participation in research targeting the medically underserved," and a co-funding initiative by NIH and CDC for "community participation in research" (Mercer & Green, 2008).

Since that time, federal funders have increased their investments in CBPR, including multiple National Institutes of Health, at least five areas of CDC, the US Department of Agriculture

(USDA, for prevention of obesity), Environmental Protection Agency (EPA), Housing and Urban Development (HUD), Health Resources and Services Administration (HRSA), and the AHRQ.

Beginning in 2006, applications for the NIH Clinical Science Translational Research Awards required community-engagement cores, which opened new initiatives within schools of medicine and academic health centers. Since 2010, the Patient Centered Outcomes Research Institute (PCORI) has mandated greater stakeholder involvement in research, including patients and families. Similarly, the Affordable Care Act (ACA) focus on eliminating disparities relies on community-engaged research to align academic health centers with community priorities and build bidirectional capacity, especially among hard-to-reach populations. NIH funding of interdisciplinary team science centers has increased community partner involvement as part of these teams. A specific Program Announcement (PA-13–209) from the National Institute of Nursing Research is succeeding to advance the science of measures and metrics of community engagement.

A collaboration of the Indian Health Service and NIH, the Native American Research for Centers in Health (NARCH), is now on its tenth call and has spurred the generation of CBPR and tribal participatory research grants in Indian country to such an extent that multiple institutes launched an RO1—https://grants.nih.gov/grants/guide/pa-files/PAR-14–260.htm—that has successfully encouraged Native scholars and others working in Indian country to apply for RO1 intervention grants, all with a CBPR focus.

The consequences of participatory research for health-related goals now extend beyond those key agencies when one considers the "Health in All Policies" approach: that health is affected by a variety of systems and policies that might benefit from CBPR. Consider these examples:

- Problem-oriented policing prevents violent crime, uses data, and is best done with community participation in problem-solving (National Institute of Justice, www.crimesolutions.gov/PracticeDetails.aspx?ID=32).
- The Federal Reserve promotes community development investments in low- to moderate-income communities. Community development corporations (CDCs) and community development financial institutions (CDFIs) finance important changes in the built environment that are conducive to health, often use data for selection of investments, and are best done with community participation (www.federalreserve.gov/communitydev/cdf.htm).

PHILANTHROPY

The W.K. Kellogg Foundation led the way in philanthropic contributions to CBPR in the early 1990s, with its Community Health Scholars program (Chapter 19). In the present day, foundations of all sizes use CBPR approaches on a regular basis, including some of the largest, such as the Kresge and Annie Casey Foundations, and smaller ones with a consistent commitment to CBPR, such as the Liberty Hill Foundation of Los Angeles. Grantmakers in Health (www.gih.org/) and the Foundation Center (http://foundationcenter.org/) can help the reader find resources for CBPR projects.

Some of the strongest proponents of CBPR in the present day are the health-focused conversion foundations, such as the California Endowment, the Colorado Trust, and the Portland-based Northwest Health Foundation. This is understandable given that these foundations use what is arguably public money, derived from converting nonprofit insurance companies and health care institutions to private, for-profit organizations. As such, the founding documents for their very existence often stipulate community involvement. As part of their mission, therefore, many conversion foundations feel a distinct requirement to be responsive to underserved and marginalized communities. CBPR offers a good vehicle for doing so.

For illustration, we will focus on the CBPR investments of the Robert Wood Johnson Foundation (RWJF). RWJF is not a conversion foundation: similar to other private foundations it is accountable only to its board of trustees and the Internal Revenue Service. At over $10 billion in assets, in 2017 it is among the largest private foundations in the country and the largest domestic foundation devoted to improving health and health care. RWJF sometimes supports CBPR, although it is usually for a utilitarian motivation, as opposed to viewing CBPR as a central vehicle for democratic process or social justice in research and evaluation. Nevertheless, some past investments in CBPR are noteworthy. For example, the Clinical Scholars Program recently had a training specialization on CBPR. The evaluation of the RWJF Allies Against Asthma was based in CBPR (Butterfoss et al., 2006). The African American Childhood Obesity Research Network (AACORN; http://aacorn.org/) uses CBPR as part of its founding principles. Salud America!, the research network to prevent childhood obesity in Latino children, formulated its entire research agenda by consulting a nationwide network of Latino community leaders and researchers about their communities' priorities, and community partners were required for each project (Leviton & Lavizzo-Mourey, 2013—the results of initial funding can be seen in a special 2013 supplement of the *American Journal of Preventive Medicine*).

RWJF is now shifting its focus to "Building a Culture of Health" to improve the upstream social, economic, and environmental forces creating health (www.rwjf.org/en/culture-of-health/2015/11/measuring_what_matte.html). This new focus is compatible with the principles of CBPR. Although CBPR will not likely be the primary approach used in research and evaluation, it has an important new place at the table. For example, RWJF's new predoctoral program, Health Policy Research Scholars (www.healthpolicyresearch-scholars.org), will train using the principles of CBPR. Interdisciplinary Research Leaders (www.interdisciplinaryresearch-leaders.org) involve cross-disciplinary teams that must include a community partner and will focus on actions to address these upstream factors affecting health. New "research pillar programs" (www.rwjf.org/en/how-we-work/grants/grantees/r-e-l-signature-programs.html) fund efforts to cast light on actionable changes in systems, policies, and the environment that can better address the drivers of health.

In sum, the Culture of Health and other foundation initiatives have the opportunity to demonstrate the importance of community voice as equal partners within the research enterprise. Foundations are important stakeholders, along with the public sector, in ensuring resources are available for partnerships to be effective in their research and actions for a more healthful and equitable society.

NOTE

1. We gratefully acknowledge the contributions of Shawna Mercer to the information provided in this appendix.

REFERENCES

Butterfoss, F. B., Gilmore, L. A., Krieger, J. W., Lachance, L. L., Lara, M., Meurer, J. R., Orians, C. E., Peterson, J. W., Rose, S. W., & Rosenthal, M. P. (2006). From formation to action: How allies against asthma coalitions are getting the job done. *Health Promotion Practice, 7*(2), 34S–43S.

Green, L. W. (1997). Preface. In M. A. Stoto, L. W. Green, & L. A. Bailey (Eds.), *Linking research and public health practice: A review of CDC's program of Centers for Research and demonstration of health promotion and disease prevention.* Washington, DC: National Academy Press.

Leviton, L. C., & Lavizzo-Mourey, R. (2013). A research network to prevent obesity among Latino children. *American Journal of Preventive Medicine, 44*(3S3), S173–S174.

Mercer, S. L., & Green, L. W. (2008). Appendix B: Federal funding and support for participatory research in public health and health care. In M. Minkler & N. Wallerstein (Eds.), *Community-based participatory research for health: From process to outcomes* (2nd ed., pp. 399–406). San Francisco, CA: Jossey-Bass.

APPENDIX 6

REALIST EVALUATION AND REVIEW FOR COMMUNITY-BASED PARTICIPATORY RESEARCH

WHAT WORKS, FOR WHOM, UNDER WHAT CIRCUMSTANCES, AND HOW?

JUSTIN JAGOSH

Realist methodology (including realist evaluation and realist review) is a relatively new approach that can help in the study of how CBPR partnerships achieve research and improvement goals. The complex dynamics of partnership relations play a significant role in determining outcomes. Key efforts include building and strengthening trust and overcoming mistrust; establishing equitable roles and decision making; determining the research agenda; consenting on who will own data; converging on research methods, ethics, and analysis; accepting or challenging academic and institutional demands and restrictions; and resolving concerns over potential stigma from research evidence.

In a large systematic realist review of the CBPR literature conducted from 2009 to 2013, I worked with a team of CBPR and realist methodology experts at the University Center for

Participatory Research at McGill (PRAM) to understand what benefits, if any, accrue from participatory research.[1] The use of realist methodology was found to be beneficial in conceptualizing how CBPR outcomes accrue and in testing causal pathways from collaboration to outcomes. Resulting publications include a rationale for using a realist review for participatory research (Macaulay et al., 2011); protocol to identify, select, appraise, and synthesize literature (Jagosh et al., 2011); results (Jagosh et al., 2012, 2015; Macaulay et al., 2014); and reflections for CBPR assessment (Jagosh et al., 2014).

This appendix provides a brief overview of how realist methodology can be applied to CBPR assessment.

WHAT IS REALIST METHODOLOGY AND WHY IS IT ADVANTAGEOUS?

Realist methodology is a theory-driven inquiry that has the goal of understanding "what works, for whom, under what circumstances, and how" (Pawson, 2013; Pawson & Tilley, 1997). Realist evaluation is for primary data collection and analysis, whereas realist review (also known as *realist synthesis*) is a secondary, literature-based analysis. Realist methodology uses the context-mechanism-outcome (CMO) configuration to provide explanatory insight and theory for the nature of programs and how they work in context.

A realist line of inquiry involves a series of iteratively derived steps:

1. Establishing initial research or evaluation questions that involve inquiry along the lines of what works, for whom, under what circumstances, and how.
2. Constructing candidate program or middle-range theories that provide a hypothesis or set of hypotheses that may explain how the program (or aspects of the program) work, given

Definitions

Context: Any element in the environment, background, physical setting, or socio-demography that, although not formally a part of the program, has a causal impact on outcomes

Mechanism: The host of resources created or offered through a program and the responses to those resources by program participants

Outcomes: The interaction of contextual elements with the mechanisms; outcomes can be proximal or final, intended or unintended

Middle-range theory: An implicit or explicit explanatory theory that can be used to explain specific elements of the program or how program logic manifests in implementation; *middle-range* means that it can be tested with the observable data and is not abstract to the point of addressing larger social or cultural forces (i.e., grand theories); this theory is sought at the outset and examined iteratively throughout the review (Jagosh et al., 2015) variations in context. The theories can be formulated by the researchers or adopted from the preexisting theoretical and empirical literature.

3. Developing data collection protocols. For realist evaluation, this means determining who to include in the study sample and developing survey instruments and qualitative guides. For realist synthesis, this involves tools to identify, select, and appraise the literature.
4. Analyzing data using context-mechanism-outcome configurations.
5. Synthesizing and integrating data analysis with program and middle-range theory. The product of the evaluation or synthesis is an evidence-informed program or middle-range theories about what works, for whom, under what circumstances, and how.

The advantage of using realist methodology for CBPR is to help unpack the complex causal pathway from the relationship and activities of academic, community, and other stakeholders to the intended and unintended outcomes. The success of CBPR relies heavily on relationship dynamics given numerous influences from the research setting, geopolitical history of collaboration, and preexistence (or not) of social capital, human resources, support infrastructure, and other assets (Trickett & Ryerson Espino, 2004). Members of CBPR projects often experience shifting perceptions of power and ownership over the duration of a project, especially in long-term partnerships. Thus, applying empirical measurement to understand the dynamics of collaboration and testing their causal impacts on outcomes is challenging because, in realist terms, the underpinning causes of outcomes happen through the relatively intangible and shifting thoughts, feelings, and motivations of CBPR stakeholders over time. Alternatively, realist methodology is advantageous because it offers program and middle-range theory development and testing of CMO configurations that produce evidence-informed CBPR theories to guide future partnership development and work processes. These theories should be subject to ongoing scrutiny and testing in new contexts and conditions.

For example, a written memorandum of understanding (MOU) is commonly introduced in early stages to establish roles and responsibilities. Such early agreements may help establish trust for certain communities at certain times, but alternatively they can foster mistrust if community members are not ready to engage at that level or if such contracts are pushed preemptively without providing time and space to discuss what equity in partner roles means. A realist investigation of the impact of an MOU could start by constructing potential theories about how an MOU might work in a context that may rival or complement each other. Then those theories would be used to gather and analyze evidence for a clearer understanding of when, at what point, for which communities, and in what circumstances that the MOU would serve to strengthen coalitions or otherwise create mistrust.

Similarly, the process of choosing research topics can affect partnership functioning and outcomes. If academic researchers approach communities with predetermined funding or topics, this may affect community buy in and have a ripple effect on outcomes. If the predetermined topic coincides with community interests, there may be increased community motivation. If the topic has less community relevance, however, community partners may perceive they are "doing a favor" for academics, which may affect their investment.

EXEMPLIFYING REALIST METHODOLOGY WITH THE PRAM REVIEW

The PRAM review was conducted with a core team of researchers and decision-making partners. Our research questions were as follows:

1. What benefits or constraints emerge from the collaborative undertaking of health-related research by researchers and those affected by the issues under study or by those who would apply the research results?
2. How can the collaborative research process be theorized and evaluated?
3. How do variations in the program's context and mechanisms influence the process and outcomes of collaborative health research (Jagosh et al., 2012)?

The first stages of the review involved identifying, selecting, and appraising key literature from the CBPR field using a series of iteratively developed identification, selection, and appraisal tools (Jagosh et al., 2011). Concurrent with that effort was locating a suitable middle-range theory that could explain how CBPR creates impacts. After an extensive literature search and vetting numerous theories (Jagosh et al., 2014), we settled on "partnership synergy," originally not developed for CBPR, which is defined as combining perspectives, resources, and skills of a group of people to "create something new and valuable together—a whole that is greater than the sum of its individual parts" (Lasker, Weiss, & Miller, 2001, p. 184). We found that the theory was broad enough to account for the heterogeneity of CBPR partnerships but specific enough to help explain why partnerships form and how they produce outcomes over time.

Our findings advanced understanding of partnership synergy within CBPR and demonstrated that genuine forms of CBPR that involved equitable co-governance of all stakeholders tended to (1) generate culturally sound and logistically appropriate research; (2) increase recruitment and retention of study participants; (3) develop capacity of community and academic stakeholders; (4) create productive conflicts, disagreements, and resolutions; (5) increase synergy and trust among partners over time; (6) sustain projects during funding gaps; and (7) produce systemic changes and unanticipated projects and activity (Jagosh et al., 2012). The theory of partnership synergy provided a conceptual currency that served to explain how long-term partnerships were able to achieve these impacts through relationship trust that was established, tested, and maintained over time. We came to refine the theory of partnership synergy by adding a dimension of time to show that the kinds of outcomes achieved from long-term maturation of working relationships was much greater than at the outset of collaboration (Jagosh et al., 2015).

An additional feature of our refinement of the theory of partnership synergy was incorporating the concept of the ripple effect inspired from the work of Hawe, Shiell, and Riley (2009). We linked CMO configurations to each other, with the outcomes of one CMO configuration becoming the context for a subsequent phase in the partnership in a ripple-effect pattern (Jagosh et al., 2015). The advantage of using this is that it served to explain how trust and synergy were built over time and in stages.

CHALLENGES TO USING THE REALIST APPROACH

The main challenge of using realist methodology is that it takes much longer than a traditional review because of the time required to account for complex context-mechanism-outcome interactions and to locate middle-range theories that can explain the data. The heterogeneity within the CBPR literature presents a further challenge to constructing relevant middle-range theories and incorporating different types of partnerships within one review. Another challenge is in understanding mechanisms. For our review, we defined *mechanisms* as the *resources* offered by partnerships and how they were *responded* to by all stakeholders, which we determined to be trust-building and sustainability over time (Jagosh et al., 2015).

Quality appraisal typically means the scrutiny of methods used to produce findings to ensure the trustworthiness of the evidence. However, using realist-review methodology, we took a different approach to appraisal. Rather than critically appraising every method used in published CBPR literature, we examined the extent to which there was adequate description of participatory processes and contexts (often in introductions and discussion sections) suitable for realist synthesis. We also contacted authors by e-mail to solicit further information and subsequently interviewed key stakeholders in partnerships retained in the review for further theory validation. Evidence synthesis often requires a mind-set shift and can take time to undertake with confidence. We suggest conducting a realist project with someone with prior experience and triangulating data using a realist review and evaluation methods.

CONCLUSION

Choosing to use realist methodology can be a rewarding process with the potential of providing valuable guidance about how context affects the application of mechanisms corresponding to CBPR principles and practice, which in turn affect outcomes. With the many dimensions of heterogeneity, the assessment can be complex and time-consuming. The specific realist inquiry, however, of how, for whom, and under what circumstances can serve the CBPR agenda and assist in unpacking the complexity of partnership dynamics for improving research and health outcomes.

ACKNOWLEDGMENTS

The development of realist methodology for CBPR assessment has come from the sustained thinking during the PRAM review (2009–2013). I would like to acknowledge the following coinvestigators in building capacity in this area: Drs. Paula Bush, Margaret Cargo, Lawrence W. Green, Trish Greenhalgh, Carol Herbert, Ann Macaulay, Pierre Pluye, Jon Salsberg, and Geoff Wong.

NOTE

1. Funding by Canadian Institutes of Health Research Knowledge Synthesis Grant and further CIHR postdoctoral fellowship.

REFERENCES

Hawe, P., Shiell, A., & Riley, T. (2009). Theorising interventions as events in systems. *American Journal of Community Psychology, 43*(3–4), 267–276.

Jagosh, J., Bush, P. L., Macaulay, A., Salsberg, J., Greenhalgh, T., Wong, G., Cargo, M., Green, L. W., Herbert, C. P., & Pluye, P. (2015). A realist evaluation of community-based participatory research: Partnership synergy, trust building and related ripple effects. *BMC Public Health, 15*(725), 1–11.

Jagosh, J., Macaulay, A. C., Pluye, P., Salsberg, J., Bush, P. L., Henderson, J., Sirett, E., Wong, G., Cargo, M., Herbert, C. P., Seifer, S. D., Green, L. W., & Greenhalgh, T. (2012). Uncovering the benefits of participatory research: Implications of a realist review for health research and practice. *Milbank Quarterly, 90*(2), 311–346.

Jagosh, J., Pluye, P., Macaulay, A. C., Salsberg, J., Henderson, J., Sirett, E., Bush, P. L., Seller, R., Wong, G., Greenhalgh, T., Cargo, M., Herbert, C. P., Seifer, S. D., & Green, L. W. (2011). Assessing the outcomes of participatory research: Protocol for identifying, selecting, appraising, and synthesizing the literature for realist review. *Implementation Science, 6*(24).

Jagosh, J., Pluye, P., Wong, G., Cargo, M., Salsberg, J., Bush, P. L., Herbert, C. P., Green, L. W., Greenhalgh, T., & Macaulay, A. C. (2014). Critical reflections on realist review: Insights from customizing the methodology to the needs of participatory research assessment. *Research Synthesis Methods, 5*(2), 131–141.

Lasker, R. D., Weiss, E. S., & Miller, R. (2001). Partnership synergy: A practical framework for studying and strengthening the collaborative advantage. *The Millbank Quarterly, 79*(2), 179–205.

Macaulay, A. C., Jagosh, J., Pluye, P., Bush, P. L., & Salsberg, J. (2014). Quantitative methods in participatory research: Being sensitive to issues of scientific validity, community safety, and the academic-community relationship. *Nouvelles Pratiques Sociales, 25*(2), 159–172.

Macaulay, A. C., Jagosh, J., Seller, R., Henderson, J., Cargo, M., Greenhalgh, T., Wong, G., Salsberg, J., Green, L. W., Herbert, C. P., & Pluye, P. (2011). Assessing the benefits of participatory research: A rationale for a realist review. *Global Health Promotion, 18*(2), 45–48.

Pawson, R. (2013). *The science of evaluation: A realist manifesto*. London, UK: Sage.

Pawson, R., & Tilley, N. (1997). *Realistic evaluation*. London, UK: Sage.

Trickett, E. J., & Ryerson Espino, S. L. (2004). Collaboration and social inquiry: Multiple meanings of a construct and its role in creating useful and valid knowledge. *American Journal of Community Psychology, 34*(1), 1–69.

APPENDIX 7

PARTNERSHIP RIVER OF LIFE

CREATING A HISTORICAL TIME LINE

SHANNON SANCHEZ-YOUNGMAN AND NINA WALLERSTEIN

The River of Life is a reflective tool to describe the life journey for partnerships (or coalitions or organizations). Its purpose is to uncover the histories and influences that motivate individual and organizational partners to promote community empowerment, greater social participation in the research process, and community transformation for health equity. Building on the work of Paulo Freire, the exercise is premised on the process of dialogue and reflection wherein participants reflect and document the critical and significant moments of their partnership and empowerment work.

This exercise offers the opportunity for people committed to community organizing and change to construct a *communal narrative* about their origins, their histories of struggle, their successes, and their challenges. Through a process of co-creation, participants create conscious meanings of the ebbs and flows of their research and social justice work. As a critical reflection, it offers the opportunity for participants to give voice to the *collective narratives* that sustain their partnership. Through guided questions and by using the metaphor of a river, the exercise is designed to trigger community and academic partners to actively acknowledge, celebrate, critique, change, and sustain the processes, goals, and results of their health equity work.

Beyond reflecting on internal partnership dynamics, community and academic partners may also use the exercise to delve into the cultural, institutional, political, economic, and governmental context that enables or inhibits them to create effective collective action strategies.

From this external vantage point, the River of Life is a historical and contextual exercise in which participants are free to consider how past historical events, histories of community organizing, broader political-economic structures that influence social conditions, and the receipt of grant funding or the arrival or departure of partnership members create opportunities and challenges to advance multiple social justice agendas. For example, in the Research for Improved Health study (described in Chapters 6 and 17), one case study site used the narrative of the River of Life to identify how the legacy of the civil rights movement informed their current strategies to challenge governmental and health institutions for a more equitable distribution of resources to communities of color in an urban area.

By reflecting on the connections between external conditions and their impact on their partnerships or organizations, the River of Life also helps partnerships recognize and clarify multiple goals, successes, and opportunities for change. In sum, we have found that this exercise is a powerful tool for partnerships to learn from each other and to assess where the partnership came from, what progress has been made, and what directions people might begin to talk about for their future. As a caution, if partners find themselves in intense dialogue around longstanding conditions of powerlessness, discrimination, or historical trauma, then it may be important to follow up the exercise with personal support for individuals, as well as ongoing community building. The exercise itself, however, which brings people together to name and portray their partnership's strengths, has facilitated people as a team to identify their successes and therefore to find ways to support their own healing.

Though the exercise is presented here as a collective exercise, the University of New Mexico Center for Participatory Research has also used this tool successfully as an individual exercise for students, community members working together, or community groups to learn about each other's histories and values. If done as an individual exercise, the facilitator needs to remind people to take care of themselves and draw and present only issues or times in their lives that they will feel comfortable sharing.

PARTNERSHIP RIVER OF LIFE HISTORICAL TIME LINE EXERCISE

Objectives

To facilitate partnership (or organizational) reflection regarding the following:

1. The history and influences that motivate partners (as individuals or from organizations) to work together in their partnership or participatory research projects, coalitions, or organizations to promote community empowerment, social participation, and health equity
2. The goals, processes, and results of your partnership work

Time

Few minutes for individual team member reflection (step 1)

45 minutes for teamwork (steps 2 through 4)

15 minutes to reflect and report back (steps 5 and 6)

Materials

- Sheets of paper
- Plenty of colored markers
- Scissors, magazines, construction paper, and glue
- Flipchart or butcher paper

Procedure

Explain that a river is an important symbol in many cultures; it symbolizes life and change for many people, and it is stimulating to think about the river, nature, and what it represents. Every river has headwaters or springs (beginnings of the partnership or organization) and times or places where the river is flowing well (partners are working well together). Sometimes partnerships have a calm period where the river smooths out into a wide pool. Other times the partnership has obstacles or challenges, which can be represented by boulders, rapids, and waterfalls. There are times when bodies of water join through tributaries (new resources, mentors, or new members) or a stream branches off from the main river (members leave or new separate partnerships are formed).

Step 1. Each member of the partnership reflects independently about him- or herself and the partnership in terms of a river and answers these questions: How and why did you join? What is important to know about your community and how and why you started working together? What important events and changes have you seen?

Step 2. Lay out a long sheet of paper (or two flipcharts taped together) and other art supplies (markers, crayons, construction paper, glue) so that together you can draw your partnership river of life. Construction paper can also be used to cut out images (e.g., hearts to show positive moments or good river flow and boulders or rocks to show obstacles).

Step 3. Draw the river of life for your partnership. Discuss the beginnings, the influences, the obstacles, and the peaceful moments, because these are key aspects for the work and the commitment to change in the communities and across partnerships and coalitions. Start where you think it's important to start, which could be before the partnership began or historical moments that led to the formation of the partnership.

If it helps, write these instructions on a flipchart:

> Start where you think it is important to start, such as a historical moment before the partnership began, when you received funding, and so on.
>
> Draw important or influential stages.
>
> Draw key tributaries coming in, or tributaries leaving.
>
> What were factors that facilitated the work?
>
> What were obstacles that were challenging?
>
> Where are you headed?

Step 4. Make a historical time line with dates of months, years (or decades) below the river of life. Relate important historic events within the community, region, state, or nationally that might influence what is currently happening in your partnership (or coalition or organization), and consider whether this has had an impact on your partnership's life.

Step 5. Stand back and admire your River of Life and answer the following questions:

1. What stood out for you while doing this collective process? (Any general thoughts about what you learned or feelings this exercise raised?)
2. What were/are some of the facilitators you identified that were important for your partnership?
3. What were/are some of the challenges or obstacles you have faced in terms of moving forward in a good way with your partners?
4. Were there important external events that made a difference?
5. When do you think you could use the River of Life tool in your own work?

Step 6. If there are multiple teams or partnerships (or individuals) creating rivers at the same time, you will need enough time for the sharing of journeys and discussion of similarities and differences within different contexts and experiences. If time is limited, share specific rivers in groups of two to four (for ten minutes), and use the questions in step 5 for a larger group discussion of similarities and differences.

See facilitation guide and examples of Rivers of Life at: http://cpr.unm.edu/research-projects/cbpr-project/facilitation_tools.html

APPENDIX 8

PURPOSING A COMMUNITY-GROUNDED RESEARCH ETHICS TRAINING INITIATIVE

CYNTHIA PEARSON AND VICTORIA SÁNCHEZ

Historical unethical research practices have often generated community mistrust for research (discussed further in Chapters 14–16). To compound this history, academic research and institutional or ethical review boards (IRBs and ERBs) often lack familiarity with diverse community's specific risks and benefits, hampering the review of culturally ethical research protocols. As a result, practitioners of community-based participatory research (CBPR) and community-engaged research (CEnR) have raised questions about how well standard research ethics training fits with the principles and practices of CBPR and CEnR (Anderson et al., 2012). Specifically, the absence of culturally relevant human subject research education for community partners has been noted as an ongoing barrier to CBPR and CEnR. Currently, online ethics training for federally funded research has not been written for community research partners (Anderson et al., 2012), nor does it address research ethics issues unique to diverse cultural and environmental contexts.

The Collaborative IRB Training Initiative (CITI, 2000), the developer of online modules used most frequently to meet the NIH requirement for research ethics training, offers a potential gateway into ethical and respectful CBPR or CEnR partnerships. However, many community members and academics have identified CITI's critical gaps in ethical training pertinent to many stigmatized communities (e.g., men who sleep with men [MSM]) (Anderson et al., 2012; Pearson, Parker, Fisher, & Moreno, 2014) and ethnically and racially diverse (E-RD) communities. These gaps have included (1) ethics topics and examples relevant to stigmatized and E-RD populations; (2) clear, simple language; and (3) community-level oversight, risk, and benefit concerns (Cochran et al., 2008; Pearson et al., 2014).

IRBs have the authority to determine what constitutes sufficient training for those engaged in research (US Department of Health and Human Services, 2009) and thus can facilitate community-grounded, culturally centered human research ethics training that moves beyond meeting only institutional research requirements.

There has been increasing interest in the importance of culturally based ethical research. Nationally, several research conferences and academic institutes have hosted workshops on the conduct of ethical research in Indian country, and several IRB directors are seeking expertise and understanding in diverse community viewpoints for their boards. Internationally as well, leading organizations from Kenya (e.g., Kenya CDC, national ethical review boards, and the research policy council) are reaching out to develop a training that will highlight specific concerns when conducting HIV/AIDS research with MSM population in areas where human rights are constrained (i.e., when political and cultural norms outlaw same-sex relationships). All of which highlight a growing community and funder interest in obtaining relevant and community-specific ethical training materials.

This appendix presents the issues to consider in what would constitute an alternative ethics training, provides a short case study of the development of a new CITI module for Indigenous populations, and identifies resources of other academic and community institutions that use alternative research ethics training for community research partners.

In developing an alternative research ethics training for community partners, the key is to start with listening and learning from community partners to determine specific processes and content for translating research ethics content that reflects community history, experience, and culture. Essential to implementation of a culturally grounded ethic's training program is obtaining organizational commitment and leadership support in order to facilitate acceptability, credibility, and sustainability. As others have pointed out: "changing institutional culture starts with the leadership and commitment of top decision-makers" (Michener et al., 2012, p. 2). Researchers who have successfully implemented alternative research ethics training have worked in collaboration with their IRB leadership to implement their training. From a review of several of these modules as well as from the following case study, here we provide a summary of key considerations:

- *Content*. Although topics for any human subject research training will include the core ethical principles of respect for persons, beneficence, and justice, how these principles are applied will vary based on a culture's values and belief systems and likely change over time.
- *Risk and benefits*. The concept of individual risk and benefit may include community risk and benefit; understanding the balance between the two should be clearly articulated. Community-identified risk and benefits may vary greatly across communities.
- *Validity and acceptance*. To ensure validity as well as community and institutional acceptance, the training should be constructed with representatives from all three entities,

for example, community members or leaders, researchers, and the academic IRB. CEnR and CBPR researchers would help facilitate change within the university system and work with community research partners to determine specific processes and content for translating research ethics content that reflects community history, experience, and culture (Michener et al., 2012).

- *Training delivery.* Online training has been the norm; however, in-person training or a hybrid may enhance efficacy and feasibility for populations less connected to the Internet.
- *Literacy.* Originally trainings were developed specifically for members of the scientific community, written at a college level, and contained examples from laboratory settings with little or no direct relevance to CBPR or CEnR. The few training approaches developed specifically for community training in human subjects protections and research were often narrow in scope, focusing on responsibilities of project field staff members, techniques for primary data collection, and policy advocacy and missed the opportunity to develop research literacy in understanding human subjects protection. As the case study illustrates, complex regulations can be presented in lay terms, thus expanding reach for the understanding of the conduct of human subjects research for community members (Carroll-Scott et al., 2012; Goodman, Dias, & Stafford, 2010).
- *Assessing training outcomes.* Assessment may include group discussion or posttests. In some cases, the academic partner who conducts the training attests that the community partners completed the training, understood the material, and are able to apply the concepts to their research project.

CASE STUDY: ETHICAL TRAINING FOR HEALTH WITH INDIGENOUS COMMUNITIES

Pearson et al. (2014) used a CEnR process to adapt the CITI-certified human subjects training module on assessing risk and benefits from a Pacific Northwest AI/AN perspective. They prepared materials for panel review including mapping the modules' core components to the code of federal regulations. Three expert panels, one each of AI/AN community members, scientists, and ethicists (n=11), identified consent, risk and benefit, and confidentiality as primary areas needing adaptation to meet cultural perspectives and concerns.

The community panel decided to adapt the assessing risk and benefits module because it covered the area in which research has created the most harm and mistrust. A total of sixty-two changes in four categories: (1) "cultural relevance" included reference to AI/AN culture and laws (n=12); (2) "clarified concepts" included removing jargon, simplifying language, or expanding explanations (n= 22); (3) "human subjects relevance" addressed breaches of ethics that occur often, such as misuse of data or are more reflective of events in AI/AN communities versus a technologically advanced setting (n=11); and (4) "community protection," providing community-level risk and benefits to address a critical gap in ethical training pertinent to AI/AN communities (n=17).

After adapting the module in a two-arm randomized clinical trial, followed by debriefing interviews, they evaluated module acceptability and feasibility (i.e., relevance of materials, self-efficacy in applying concepts, and satisfaction) and understandability of module (test scores) among forty AI/AN reservation-based community members. Participants who took the adapted module as compared to those who took the standard module reported higher scores on relevance of the material (82.7 versus 65.8, t=3.06, p<0.01), overall satisfaction (81.4 versus 69.4, t=2.10, p<0.05), module mean quiz scores (75.7 versus 62.9, t=2.15, p<0.05), and a trend toward higher research self-efficacy (76.3 versus 68.1, t=1.71, p<0.10). CITI requires the quiz to be taken until a passing score is reached (˜80 percent). Pearson et al. (2014) calculated quiz scores based on first try and found that 65 percent of respondents in the adapted module group passed as compared to 35 percent in the control group (X^2=3.6, p=.058). In debriefing interviews (n=30), respondents reported that examples in the adapted module highlight potential risks for research that resonated with their lived experience, were interested in sharing the culturally adapted module with their tribe, and stressed the utility of the material in health care and social service settings outside of the research arena. One person said,"I'm ready to jump into research . . . I'm really glad I did this." One respondent also suggested the training would be good for academic researchers, "for non-Indians coming into a reservation, I thought it would be good for them to do this training. People coming out don't know about the sensitivity of elders and the damage they could be doing. Researchers are wanting to do something good, but could cause harm unintentionally."

Literacy, however, remained a concern. Although the adapted module was at a high school level, respondents expressed difficulty with the vocabulary, long sentences, and the time needed to understand the materials. This preliminary study demonstrates the acceptability of an adapted training, the feasibility of identifying core ethical concerns across diverse rural and urban tribal entities, the need to simplify language, and the utility of including community voice in adapting the CITI training materials and increasing potential for research partnerships with community members.

Following the pilot, community members spoke of the value a full certification curriculum would provide. Thus the investigators obtained funding from NIH for the Ethical Training for Health with Indigenous Communities (ETHICS). ETHICS expands the pilot to a national randomized control trial among five hundred American Indian and Alaska Natives. The national study will evaluate whether a culturally developed human subjects training curriculum (as compared to the CITI standard social behavioral curriculum) increases research ethics knowledge, research review efficacy, and trust in research and researchers. Findings from this study will be released in summer 2017, and the curriculum is scheduled for immediate dissemination through CITI as a full certification curriculum in their basic package at no additional charge to their more than six thousand subscribers. Moreover, the Department of Health and Human Services Administration for Children & Family Office of Planning, Research & Evaluation (OPRE) will soon provide open access to their national data on AI/AN children, their families, teachers, and providers. OPRE is proposing, prior to accessing the data, researchers take the ETHICS training. OPRE believes it will help sensitize researchers to the unique consideration when working with AI/AN communities.

This case study represents one alternative training mechanism that teaches concepts from the Belmont Report and the CFR 45SS on the conduct of ethical research with human subjects from a community's values. It offers an example of how to address ethical challenges in conducting research with stigmatized and E-RD populations who face health disparities by increasing informed IRB panels and academic partners and community involvement in research oversight, design, implementation, and dissemination.

Other academic institutions and community-based organizations have developed, tested, and implemented alternative research ethics training for community research members and partners including the University of Pittsburgh (Yonas et al., 2016); University of Colorado (Westfall et al., 2016); the University of North Carolina at Chapel Hill (http://research.unc.edu/offices/human-research-ethics/getting-started/training/ccm3_019063/); Harvard University (https://catalyst.harvard.edu/programs/regulatory/cenr.html); and the University of Michigan (Solomon & Piechowski, 2011). These curricula blend training in core ethical principles with community experiences with research through stories and case studies.

The significance of these initiatives lies in the potential to enhance IRB reviews, academic scholars' sensitivity in working with stigmatized and E-RD communities, and community participation in research through local or online community-driven research ethics training that highlights the cultural, policy, and environmental context of diverse communities.

These kinds of initiatives with community and academic partners will have a high impact by contributing to the development of CEnR capacity within national and international communities, facilitating more inclusive and ethical research aimed at reducing health disparities. From a CBPR or CEnR perspective, research ethics training with community research partners builds on a commitment to trust and respect, bidirectional learning, capacity building, and developing shared language and meaning. The extension of the research partnership into ethics training is a central ingredient to democratize knowledge and promote social justice within the research enterprise.

Examples of Online Resources

- Campus Community Partnerships for Health (CCPH). Reengaging Ethics: Ethical Issues in Engaged Research. https://ccph.memberclicks.net/research-ethics
- Training and Resources in Research Ethics Evaluation (TRREE) and regulation of health research involving human participant. TRREE focused primarily, but not exclusively, on the needs of African countries. http://elearning.trree.org/
- Family Health International (FHI). Designed and developed for an international audience of researchers and research ethics committee members. www.fhi360.org/sites/default/files/media/documents/Research%20Ethics%20Training%20Curricula.pdf
- Harvard Catalyst/Harvard CTSC. Provides resources for investigators, community partners, and IRB. https://catalyst.harvard.edu/programs/regulatory/cenr.html
- University of Michigan—Research Ethics Training for Community Research Partners. http://inventions.umich.edu/technologies/4768_research-ethics-training-for-community-research-partners
- University of Pittsburgh/CTCC—Introduction to Community Partnered Research Ethics Training (CPRET). www.ctsi.pitt.edu/cpret.shtml
- UNC Chapel Hill—Alternative Training for Special Circumstances. http://research.unc.edu/offices/human-research-ethics/getting-started/training/ccm3_019063/

REFERENCES

Anderson, E. E., Solomon, S., Heitman, E., DuBois, J. M., Fisher, C. B., Kost, R. G., . . . Ross, L. F. (2012). Research ethics education for community-engaged research: A review and research agenda. *Journal of Empirical Research on Human Research Ethics, 7*(2), 3–19. doi:10.1525/jer.2012.7.2.3

Carroll-Scott, A., Toy, P., Wyn, R., Zane, J. I., & Wallace, S. P. (2012). Results from the Data & Democracy initiative to enhance community-based organization data and research capacity. *American Journal of Public Health, 102*(7), 1384–1391.

CITI. (2000). Collaborative institutional training initiative: Social and behavioral sciences human subjects training. Miami, Florida. Retrieved from www.citiprogram.org/aboutus.asp?language=english

Cochran, P. A., Marshall, C. A., Garcia-Downing, C., Kendall, E., Cook, D., McCubbin, L., & Gover, R. M. (2008). Indigenous ways of knowing: Implications for participatory research and community. *American Journal of Public Health, 98*(1), 22–27.

Goodman, M. S., Dias, J. J., & Stafford, J. D. (2010). Increasing research literacy in minority communities: CARES fellows training program. *Journal of Empirical Research on Human Research Ethics, 5*(4), 33–41. doi:10.1525/jer.2010.5.4.33

Michener, M., Cook, J., Ahmed, S. M., Yonas, M. A., Coyne-Beasley, T., & Aguilar-Gaxiola, S. (2012). Aligning the goals of community-engaged research: Why and how academic health centers can successfully engage with communities to improve health. *Academic Medicine, 87*(3), 285–291.

Pearson, C. R., Parker, M., Fisher, C. B., & Moreno, C. (2014). Capacity building from the inside out: Development and evaluation of a CITI ethics certification training module for American Indian and Alaska Native community. *Journal of Empirical Research on Human Research Ethics (JERHRE), 9*(1), 46–57. doi:10.1525/jer.2014.9.1.46

Solomon, S., & Piechowski, P. J. (2011). Developing community partner training: Regulations and relationships. *Journal of Empirical Research on Human Research Ethics (JERHRE), 6*(2), 23–30. doi:https://doi.org/10.1525/jer.2011.6.2.23

US Department of Health and Human Services. (2009). Code of federal regulations, Title 45 Public Welfare, Part 46, Protection of Human Services, Subpart A Basic HHS Policy for Protection of Human Research Subjects. Rockville, MD: Author.

Westfall, J. M., Zittleman, L., Felzien, M., Ringel, M., Lakin, A., & Nease, D. (2016). Institutional review board training when patients and community members are engaged as researchers. *Family Practice, 10,* 1–4. doi:https://doi.org/10.1093/fampra/cmw112

Yonas, M. A., Jaime, M. C., Barone, J., Valenti, S., Documét, P., Ryan, C. M., & Miller, E. (2016). Community partnered research ethics training in practice: A collaborative approach to certification. *Journal of Empirical Research on Human Research Ethics (JERHRE), 11*(2), 97–105. doi:10.1177/1556264616650802

APPENDIX 9

PARTNERSHIP AGREEMENTS

A PRACTICAL GUIDE TO DEVELOPING DATA SHARING, OWNERSHIP, AND PUBLISHING AGREEMENTS

PATRICIA RODRÍGUEZ ESPINOSA AND AL RICHMOND

Advances in CBPR and community-engaged research are accompanied by a commitment to create processes and procedures that fully engage all partners, including community leaders and community-based organizations (CBOs) in the work, from concept design to dissemination. This appendix explores myriad opportunities to formalize partnership relationships and provides guidance that can facilitate meaningful and authentic engagement on the part of all partners. The information provided is not prescriptive but serves to capture the core values associated with partnership agreements and documents.

Although not all partnerships have formal agreements, and some partnerships may decide that shared guiding values are sufficient, at some point partnerships may want to consider signed agreements on specific issues such as data sharing and ownership. In the national Research for Improved Health study, use of formal agreements emerged as a promising practice in its association with greater resource sharing as well as power sharing in research (see Chapter 17). Whether or not partnerships choose to create a formal agreement, members of academic-community research partnerships have the opportunity and responsibility to work together collaboratively to protect, store, and share their data and disseminate findings in a way that is consistent with their partnership values and with the needs of their partners. The principles from

Community Campus Partnerships for Health might be useful starting points for partnerships to articulate their own values (https://ccph.memberclicks.net/principles-of-partnership).

This appendix provides suggested topics for agreements, that is, mission, partner responsibilities, data, addition of new investigators or students, and dissemination and coauthorship. As partnerships evolve, agreements can serve as a foundation for guiding decisions and can be revisited periodically. This appendix is not meant to be fully comprehensive of all possible sections; however, we hope to offer examples of major sections to consider and resources that can prompt partnership dialogue and decisions. Included are URLs intended to serve as more concrete examples.

PURPOSE

A purpose statement offers a partnership the opportunity to document the participants' commitment to working equitably and providing an introduction to sections that follow. It may define terms, such as *data,* meaning primary source information gathered in a project, or that "sharing or disseminating data" may take any forms, such as community or professional presentations, media communications, reports, grants, manuscripts, and information on websites.

AGREEMENT INTRODUCTION

This section underscores topics typically found in introductions of formal agreements along with some sample language.

Mission and Vision

Agreements oftentimes emphasize core missions of promoting health equity, social justice, and contributing to the knowledge and science of CBPR. Partnerships can benefit from dialogues and formal discussions regarding goals and values of the project.

Project Values and Principles

Agreements are often an expression of the principles of CBPR in the research. The data sharing, data storage, publication, and dissemination of the research results might follow generally accepted principles, which include but are not limited to the following:

- *Anonymity of individuals and partnerships.* The research results will be presented in an aggregated or grouped manner. Partnerships and communities have the right to decide if they want to be identified or not in the research results. Community and academic partners must agree to be identified.
- *Privacy and confidentiality.* All information collected from individual participants and partnerships will remain private and confidential.
- *Respect.* The cultural and intellectual integrity of any participating partnerships or projects must be respected in all publications and disseminations. Further discussion on what respect might mean for different partnerships is encouraged at the beginning of the conceptualization of agreements.

Respective Responsibilities

Many agreements include primary responsibilities for each partner or stakeholder group involved in the collaboration. Listing these responsibilities, in design, implementation of research or intervention, and data collection and analysis, can help organize efforts and reduce the risk of misunderstandings about deliverables or expectations. A key consideration is offering ample collaborative and equitable involvement of all partners in different phases of the project. Although some partners might be primarily responsible for certain areas (e.g., academic partners responsible for data analysis based on in-house expertise), it is important to encourage community partners to get involved throughout the research. Agreements can serve to formalize these efforts. Involving community partners in data interpretation and dissemination is key to translation and use of findings.

DATA-RELATED CHALLENGES

Ethical and other responsibilities involved in data collection and management make this a core section(s) in many agreements. For instance, who owns the data and what are the repercussions of that choice? If community partners own the data, can academic partners use it for publishing to support their promotion and tenure? Will data be aggregated or de-indentified, and who will have access to the raw de-identified data? How will data be shared with the community or the public? What are federal responsibilities?

Involvement in Data Collection

For formal research projects, data collection procedures must comply with institutional review boards (IRBs) (e.g., at the university, the community, or tribe). In addition to specifying who is involved in data collection efforts, it is useful to establish procedures for adding new team members, who need to comply with IRB guidelines.

Data Ownership and Data Sharing

Data ownership, sharing, and use agreements are especially important for partnerships with multiple teams (e.g., community, academic, tribes) in order to avoid potential conflicts. This becomes extremely important for small communities and for those who might face stigma or other negative consequences as a result of research participation or particular findings.

Case example: The Research for Improved Health study, in one of our tribal case studies, found that our agreement was insufficient for interview data. The university had assumed sharing of aggregated data, but after data collection, the tribe assumed the raw data would be stored with the tribe. The consent form, however, did not include sharing of individual raw data beyond the person interviewed. After multiple discussions, the team decided to re-consent the participants, with detailed data-sharing modifications, to allow sharing and storage of data with the tribe. Although this team was able to reach an agreement, ethical concerns such as this one are not uncommon.

Data Storage

For projects collecting identifiable data, agreements should detail guidelines for protecting participants' confidentially. For instance, will personally identifiable data be stored? What steps are taken to prevent loss of confidentiality (e.g., password protection or encryption)? Often, only few team members have access to identifiable data. Detailing their responsibilities, including sharing de-identified data, and communicating these processes to the larger team, would be in this section.

Procedures for Project Modifications

Given the fluid nature of CBPR projects, it is not uncommon for modifications to happen as the project develops. Partnerships can use agreements to establish processes for future modifications, such as new data collection efforts or new proposals based on findings. Establishing guidelines for modifications might include the creation of a subcommittee or appointing an individual who can oversee and approve the modifications, clarifying what needs to be submitted, and communicating clearly to the partnership these processes.

PUBLICATION, WRITING, AND GENERAL DISSEMINATION

Dissemination can be defined broadly, for example, as peer review venues as well as classroom or community presentations, media releases, monographs, policy briefs, white papers, and so on. Dissemination efforts can last many years and continue long after a research study has concluded data collection. Given the diversity of dissemination products, the long time frame, and different backgrounds of partners, this can be particularly difficult to navigate. Considerations should be made for (1) equitable or collaborative involvement of all partners and (2) honoring partnership and project values and goals when considering dissemination products. For a comprehensive example of dissemination, see Engage for Equity in "Examples of Agreements" at the end of this appendix.

General Dissemination

It can be useful to think about project goals and responsibilities (and to whom) when drafting this section. For instance, dissemination responsibilities may include funding agencies (e.g., NIH), communities involved in the research, and other stakeholders. After considering different responsibilities, it can be useful to clarify individual party responsibilities for developing needed products. Principal investigators are often responsible for facilitating these efforts, with many agreements including formal sections on the role of principal investigator.

Publications, Review Processes, and Opportunity for Collaborative Dissemination

This section can be used as starting points for discussion on publication and writing. We have found it helpful and transparent to create subcommittees, such as a publications committee. Although there are other options, we do encourage partnerships to establish a formal process for reviewing publications and for ensuring opportunities for all partners to participate and receive credit for their contributions.

Publications and Writing Teams The approval process needs to be consistent with relevant IRB, tribal government, NIH, or university policies and usual and customary academic standards pertaining to scholarly publications. Partnerships can discuss potential topics first. Or, the PI or publications committee could be designated to be approached by team members interested in potential topics and then can broker avoiding similar or overlapping papers, submitting papers to the same journal, or publishing articles in an illogical sequence.

The agreement can specify what should be submitted to the PI or publications committee (or both), that is, an abstract, desired journal (or other form of publication), lead authors and coauthors, list of information or data requested, and time line for completion. The approving body will return comments and a decision within a specified period of time. If the committee does not return a decision within the time frame, specify the responsibility of the lead author to follow up with the PI. It is helpful to establish a process by which all team members are informed of current opportunities to get involved in different dissemination efforts. For instance, a newsletter or a document with ongoing writing efforts can be circulated at regular time intervals to invite partners to join the writing teams.

Criteria for Authorship Consensus among the lead author and coauthors pertaining to roles and responsibilities should be obtained at the earliest planning stages of the manuscript. Agreements can detail the criteria required to qualify for authorship. For instance:

- Individuals who contribute substantially to the manuscript's concept, design, data analysis, or implications
- Individuals who provide essential expertise (e.g., academic, Indigenous knowledge, historical, cultural relevancy)
- Individuals who review or make substantive comments or edits on at least one draft

Authorship conditions can be included, such as modifications of author order based on actual work, approvals by all authors within a set time frame, and so on. Lead author responsibilities can be delineated with final draft to the PI(s) for review.

Student Authorship For students using project data to satisfy graduation requirements such as thesis or dissertations, further guidelines can be developed that take into consideration data sharing and dissemination of their work.

Planning and Development of a Manuscript When considering the selection, journals that pose the least difficulty for community access should be explored first. If a decision is made to publish in a journal with significant barriers to community access, the authors should identify ways to make the information accessible to community members.

Publication Guidelines Acknowledgment All those who contributed to the research project, but do not meet the authorship criteria, may be included in the acknowledgment section of the manuscript. Partnerships can write out an acknowledgment paragraph that might include advisory council members, core staff members, and so on, as well as funding sources.

RESOLVING GRIEVANCES

A process for acknowledging and resolving grievances is oftentimes included. Partnerships should consider nominating a person or group for arbitration. A process, with time lines, should take into account the ability of parties to engage in meaningful communication to resolve the dispute, followed by other steps, including potential termination of the agreement.

TERMINATION

Conditions for termination of the partnership can be included, such as approval by all parties, and stipulations regarding ongoing data sharing, ownership, and dissemination.

AGREEMENT PERIOD

It is useful to include dates under which the agreement will be in effect and can include review of the agreement once the initial approval period expires.

OTHER SECTIONS TO CONSIDER

An appendix listing those parties referred to in the agreement, subcommittee membership, and advisory boards may be helpful.

EXAMPLE AGREEMENTS

For comprehensive example, see Engage for Equity (E2):
http://cpr.unm.edu/common/new-engage-for-equity-data-publish-agreements-2017-.pdf
For comprehensive tribal examples, see the Indigenous Wellness Research Institute (IWRI):
http://health.iwri.org/tribal-colleges-universities-drug-and-alcohol-problems-and-solutions-study/
Community-Campus Partnerships for Health (Appendix E in the CBPR Curriculum) has an extensive list of agreements:
https://ccph.memberclicks.net/index.php?option=com_content&view=article&id=169:cbpr-curriculum-appendix-e&catid=31:cbpr-curriculum

Project Values and Principles

https://depts.washington.edu/ccph/pdf_files/MOU10.pdf
See Research for Improved Health: Project Code of Ethics and Integrity: http://cpr.unm.edu/research-projects/cbpr-project/RIH.html

Respective Responsibilities

http://catalyst.harvard.edu/pdf/chirp/Appendix%20F%20-%20Memorandum%20of%20Agreement.pdf

Data Related

www.ucdenver.edu/research/CCTSI/community-engagement/resources/Documents/DataSharingCreatingAgreements.pdf
health.iwri.org/wp-content/uploads/2016/02/Sample-Data-Sharing-Agmt.docx

www.reading.ac.uk/ssc/resource-packs/akf-surveypack/Session13-DataOwnership/FilesForCourseFolders/Template-DataOwnershipAgreement.pdf

Publication, Writing, and Dissemination

www.maine.edu/pdf/PublishingAgreementStandard.pdf
http://blogs.harvard.edu/infolaw/files/2009/05/authors_publishing_intro-tka1.pdf
www.copylaw.com/new_articles/collab.html
www.detroiturc.org/images/PDFs/URCDisseminationGuidelines.pdf

Student Involvement

http://health.iwri.org/wp-content/uploads/2016/01/NCAI-UNM-UW-NARCH-V-Research-for-Improved-Health-Protocol-for-Student-Involvement-in-the-Research-Team.pdf

Grievances

www.calpelra.org/pdf/von%20Kalinowski,%20Judy.pdf
http://ucnet.universityofcalifornia.edu/labor/bargaining-units/k8/docs/k8_2015–2016_23_grievance-procedure.pdf

Termination

https://seeingcollaborations.files.wordpress.com/2014/10/template-of-memorandum-of-understanding-for-mutual-aid-research-in-disasters-5–1–12.docx

APPENDIX 10

INSTRUMENTS AND MEASURES FOR EVALUATING COMMUNITY ENGAGEMENT AND PARTNERSHIPS

NINA WALLERSTEIN

As noted throughout this book, over the last decades, evaluation evidence has grown, showing that CBPR and community-engaged research (CEnR) partnerships have contributed to health and health equity improvements. Intervention studies, experimental and quasi-experimental design trials, case studies, CBPR policy analyses, as well as systematic reviews and meta-analyses have showcased engagement and collaborative practices that have contributed to a range of outcomes. These outcomes have included short-term increased partner synergy and culture-centered interventions; intermediate outcomes, such as increased community capacities, sustainability of projects and partnerships, health behavior changes, and shared power in research between community, agency, and academic stakeholders; as well as more long-term policy changes, transformed conditions, and health status outcomes.

Although partnerships have often focused on evaluating outcomes of their research project aims, increasingly they are adopting qualitative and quantitative evaluation methods to assess their partnership or engagement practices. This appendix identifies measurement tools and instruments that have been published or available on public websites that may prove useful to partnerships to strengthen capacity and practices in evaluation and collective reflection. Because of the vast diversity of individual evaluation tools for specific projects, it is not meant to be comprehensive but identifies various resources in the field.

A few early reviews of literature on collaboration deserve special mention. Granner and Sharpe (2004) published the first summary of measurement tools on coalitions. This summary identified 26 articles and 146 measurement scales in multiple categories, including member and organizational characteristics, group processes and functioning, and impacts. The *American Journal of Preventive Medicine* published a supplement in 2008, led by Daniel Stokols and colleagues, which included articles on measures of team science as a result of the National Cancer Institute (NCI) investment in transdisciplinary research centers (Hall et al., 2008; Mâsse et al., 2008). This further led to an NCI-hosted team science tool kit on the web that includes collaboration measures (www.teamsciencetoolkit.cancer.gov/Public/searchAdvResult.aspx?st=a&sid=2).

The Research for Improved Health (RIH) study (discussed in Chapters 6 and 17) conducted a literature review from 2002 to 2008 of measures of coalitions, inter-agency partnerships, community-academic partnerships, CBPR, and other community-engaged research. Forty-six instruments were identified with 224 individual measures, which tracked along constructs from the CBPR conceptual model (Sandoval et al., 2011). Partnering processes had the largest number of identified measures, including instruments such as the widely used Wilder Collaboration tool (http://wilderresearch.org/tools/cfi/index.php; Mattessich, Murray-Close, & Monsey, 2001).

This RIH study then went on to integrate some of these published measures (such as Khodyakov et al., 2011; Lasker, Weiss, & Miller, 2001) with newly created ones, such as alignment with CBPR engagement principles, to assess partnering practices and outcomes in two Internet surveys of two hundred federally funded research partnerships in 2009 (see Chapter 17). Scales from these survey instruments have been validated (Oetzel et al., 2015; Wallerstein et al., under review; Chapter 5). The measures themselves are provided in Excel spreadsheets and in pdf form on the Center for Participatory Research, University of New Mexico (UNM-CPR), website (http://cpr.unm.edu/research-projects/cbpr-project/research-for-improved-health.html) for partnerships to use or adapt for their own needs. The matrix of the variables used in these scales was published by CES4Health (Pearson et al., 2014).

In addition, the RIH study included a number of qualitative evaluation and reflection tools including historical time lines and Rivers of Life (Appendix 7), and open-ended focus group and interview guides for in-depth case studies are also available at UNM-CPR (see http://cpr.unm.edu/research-projects/cbpr-project/index.html). Realist methodology has contributed important analytic methodologies for theorizing from the data (see Appendix 6).

A follow-up UNM-CPR Engage for Equity study (2015–2020), with five other university and community partners and a think tank of CBPR practitioners, has refined these instruments (also translating them into Spanish). A new Internet survey has been conducted with close to two hundred federally funded partnerships in 2015 to provide additional validation and understanding of promising practices contributing to multiple outcomes. The CBPR model is being used as a reflection tool for visioning and assessing where partnerships have been and where they're headed. See http://cpr.unm.edu/research-projects/cbpr-project/facilitation_tools.html for facilitation planning and evaluation visioning guides, among other tools.

Some constructs, such as trust, have received much attention because of the importance of relationships in CBPR. Trust, however, has been difficult to measure because of its dynamic nature and its history of being seen as a binary construct. The Centers for Disease Control published one of the first trust tool surveys (www.cdc.gov/prc/pdf/partnershiptrusttoolsurvey.pdf).

Lucero and colleagues in the Research for Improved Health study have tested a new trust typology measure with qualitative and quantitative evidence (Lucero et al., 2016; see Chapter 5). Jagosh and colleagues, using a qualitative approach of realist evaluation, have identified trust and synergy as important pathways within CBPR (see Appendix 6).

Over the course of the last several decades, many established CBPR centers have developed their own qualitative and quantitative methods and instruments, including the well-regarded and long-standing Detroit Community-Academic Urban Research Center (www.detroiturc.org/resources/urc-cbpr-tools.html; Israel, Eng, Schulz, & Parker, 2013). The University of Kansas Community Tool Box (Appendix 11) has provided substantial evaluation expertise to collaboratives with innovative tracking tools to enable communities to conduct self-evaluations. Green and colleagues first published in 1995 (and later amended) their reliability-tested guidelines for funders, evaluators, and partnerships to assess the extent projects were using participatory criteria at all stages of the research process (Mercer et al., 2008; http://lgreen.net/guidelines.html).

Colleagues at the University of California, Los Angeles, the RAND Corporation, and Healthy African American Families and others have developed strategies and measures to assess the added value of participation in mental health services research (Khodyakov et al., 2011, 2013; Ngo et al., 2016; see Chapters 10 and 17). The core practice of alignment with CBPR or community engagement principles has been assessed by multiple teams (Braun et al, 2012; Goodman et al., 2017; Oetzel et al., 2015).

The network of Clinical Translational Science Awardees (CTSAs) since 2006 has supported greater interest in community engagement across academic health centers. The CTSA Community Engagement Key Functions Committee first produced a community engagement infrastructure logic model, with a call to identify measures that could be shared across sites (Eder et al., 2013). In 2016, NIH's National Center for Advancing Translational Science, which currently supports the CTSAs, charged their more recently formed Collaboration and Engagement Domain Task Force to identify existing measures of collaboration and team science quality and collaboration outcomes, including measures of community engagement and team science, to share across academic health centers. The work group[1] that formed started with a review of the literature and found, similar to Granner and Sharpe (2004) and Sandoval et al. (2011), a greater focus on group dynamics, with only some measures having rigorous validity or reliability data. Social network analyses also have been growing as a newer measure of engagement processes and outcomes (Franco et al., 2015).

The NCI has continued their interest in measures with their interactive Grid-Enabled Measures (GEM) website (www.gem-beta.org/Public/Home.aspx), a "collaborative tool containing behavioral, social science, and other relevant scientific measures" that includes measures and constructs on dissemination and implementation, community collaboration, CBPR, and CEnR. Ongoing "Research to Reality" NCI-sponsored webinars continue to share community engagement methods and measures (Glasgow & Stange, 2017). While distinct, measures from the Consolidated Framework for Implementation Research may also be useful (see http://www.cfirguide.org/quant.html; Lewis et al, 2015).

In summary, there are a number of approaches for evaluation in CBPR contexts, processes, impact on research, and outcomes. Previous evaluation tools tended to be locally developed and thus lacked some psychometric validation because sample sizes were small by design. More recent tools have been developed with large samples of partnerships and have strong measurement validity. In addition, recent tools have also moved beyond a focus on group dynamics to other domains in the CBPR conceptual model, including contextual issues and strategies that affect intervention and research design, such as level of community involvement in research steps, intervention fit to culture, and partnership synergy in working together. A broader array of outcomes is also being collected in addition to specific research outcomes. Intermediate capacity, policy changes, and sustainability outcomes are being seen as important, as are the larger outcomes of community transformations to improve health and health equity.

Finally, qualitative methods are being recognized as equally important to triangulate with the quantitative data. Mixed methods are needed to produce a rich picture and understandings of the depth and breadth of partnering and engagement processes that contribute to outcomes. Probably most importantly, however, is the recognition that participatory processes are dynamic and ever-changing, and partnerships need to identify what practices may be most important for them to assess and strengthen as they move forward toward their own outcomes and goals of promoting health equity (Brennan Ramirez, Baker & Metzler, 2008, pg. 82). All these developments are welcome for advancing our understanding and practice of CBPR.

NOTE

1. With findings to be published by Developing Measures of Collaboration Workgroup led by Beth Tigges, PhD (University of New Mexico), Usha Menon, PhD (University of Arizona), and Doriane Miller, MD (University of Chicago). See Collaboration/Engagement Domain Task Force for other resources: https://ctsacentral.org/articles/?article=Collaboration%20Engagement.

REFERENCES

Braun, K. L., Nguyen, T. T., Tanjasiri, S. P., Campbell, J., Heiney, S. P., Brandt, H. M., Smith, S. A., Blumenthal, D. S., Hargreaves, M., Coe, K., Ma, G. X., Kenerson, D., Patel, K., Tsark, J., & Hébert, J. R. (2012). Operationalization of community-based participatory research principles: Assessment of the National Cancer Institute's community network programs. *American Journal of Public Health, 102*(6), 1195–1203.

Brennan Ramirez, L. K., Baker, E. A., & Metzler, M. (2008). *Promoting health equity: A resource to help communities address social determinants of health*. Atlanta: US Department of Health and Human Services, Centers for Disease Control and Prevention. https://www.cdc.gov/nccdphp/dch/programs/healthycommunitiesprogram/tools/pdf/sdoh-workbook.pdf, Accessed, June, 2017.

Eder, M., Carter-Edwards, L., Hurd, T. C., Rumala, B. B., & Wallerstein, N. (2103). A logic model for community engagement within the CTSA Consortium: Can we measure what we model? *Academic Medicine, 88*(9), 1430–1436.

Franco, Z. E., Ahmed, S. M., Maurana, C. A., DeFino, M. C., & Brewer, D. D. (2015). A social network analysis of 140 community-academic partnerships for health: Examining the healthier Wisconsin partnership program. *Clinical and Translational Science, 8*, 311–319. doi:10.1111/cts.12288

Glasgow, R. E., & Stange, K. C. (2107, May). How engaged are we? Measuring community engagement and partnership. Research to Reality. Retrieved from https://researchtoreality.cancer.gov/discussions/how-engaged-are-we-measuring-community-engagement-and-partnership

Goodman, M., Sanders Thompson, V., Johnson, C. A., Gennarelli, R., Drake, B. F., Bajwa, P., Witherspoon, M., & Bowen, D. (2017). Evaluating community engagement in research: Quantitative measure development. *Journal of Community Psychology, 45*(1),17–32.

Granner, M. L., & Sharpe, P. A. (2004). Evaluating community coalition characteristics and functioning: A summary of measurement tools. *Health Education Research, 19*, 514–532.

Hall, K. L., Stokols, D., Moser, R. P., Taylor, B. K., Thornquist, M. D., Nebeling, L. C., . . . Jeffery, R. W. (2008). The collaboration readiness of transdisciplinary research teams and centers: Findings from the National Cancer Institute's TREC year-one evaluation study. *American Journal of Preventive Medicine, 35*(2S), S161–S172. doi:10.1016/j.amepre.2008.03.035

Israel, B. A., Eng, E., Schulz, A. J., & Parker, E. A. (Eds.). (2013). *Methods in community-based participatory research for health: From processes to outcomes* (2nd ed.). San Francisco, CA: Jossey-Bass.

Jagosh, J., Bush, P. L., Macaulay, A., Salsberg, J., Greenhalgh, T., Wong, G., Cargo, M., Green, L. W., Herbert, C. P., & Pluye, P. (2015). A realist evaluation of community-based participatory research: Partnership synergy, trust building and related ripple effects. *BMC Public Health, 15*(725), 1–11.

Khodyakov, D., Stockdale, S., Jones, A., Mango, J., Jones, F., & Lizaola, E. (2013). On measuring community participation in research. *Health Education Behavior, 40*(3), 346–354.

Khodyakov, D., Stockdale, S., Jones, F., Ohito, E., Jones, A., Lizaola, E., et al. (2011). An exploration of the effect of community engagement in research on perceived outcomes of partnered mental health services projects. *Society and Mental Health, 1*(3), 185–199.

Lasker, R., Weiss, E., & Miller, R. (2001). Partnership synergy: A practical framework for studying and strengthening the collaborative advantage. *The Milbank Quarterly, 79,* 179–205.

Lewis, C. C., Fischer, S., Weiner, B., Stanick, C., Kim, M., & Martinez, R. (2015). Outcomes for implementation science: An enhanced systematic review of instruments using evidence-based rating criteria, *Implementation Science*, 10:155, DOI: 10.1186/s13012-015-0342-x

Lucero, J., Wallerstein, N., Duran, B., Alegria, M., Greene-Moton, E., Israel, B., Kastelic, S., Magarati, M., Oetzel, J., Pearson, C., Schulz, A., Villegas, M., & White Hat, E. (2016). Development of a mixed methods investigation of process and outcomes of community based participatory research. *Journal of Mixed Methods*. doi:10.1177/1558689816633309

Mâsse, L. C., Moser, R. P., Stokols, D., Taylor, B. K., Marcus, S. E., Morgan, G. D., . . . Trochim, W. M. (2008). Measuring collaboration and transdisciplinary integration in team science. *American Journal of Preventive Medicine, 35*(2S), S151–S160. doi:10.1016/j.amepre.2008.05.020

Mattessich, P., Murray-Close, M., & Monsey, B. (2001). *Wilder collaboration factors inventory*. St. Paul, MN: Wilder Research.

Mercer, S., Green, L. W., Cargo, M., Potter, M., Daniel, M., Olds, R. S., & Reed-Gross, E. (2008). Appendix C: Reliability-tested guidelines for assessing participatory research projects. In W. Minkler & N. Wallerstein (Eds.), *Community-based participatory research for health: From processes to outcomes* (2nd ed.). San Francisco, CA: Jossey-Bass.

Ngo, V. K., Sherbourne, C., Chung, B., Tang, L., Wright, A. L., Whittington, Y., Wells, K., & Miranda, J. (2016). Community engagement compared with technical assistance to disseminate depression care among low-income, minority women: A randomized controlled effectiveness study. *American Journal of Public Health, 106*(10), 1833–1841.

Oetzel, J. G., Zhou, C., Duran, B., Pearson, C., Magarati, M., Lucero, J., Wallerstein, N., & Villegas, M. (2015). Establishing the psychometric properties of constructs in a community-based participatory research conceptual model. *American Journal of Health Promotion, 29,* e188–e202.

Pearson, C., Duran, B., Martin, D., Lucero, J., Sandoval, J., Oetzel, J., Tafoya, G., Belone, L., Avila, M., Wallerstein, N., & Hicks, S. (2014, December). CBPR variable matrix: Research for improved health in academic-community partnerships. CES4Health.info. Retrieved from http://ces4health.info/find-products/view-product.aspx?code=FWYC2L2T

Sandoval, J. A., Lucero, J., Oetzel, J., Avila, M., Belone, L., Mau, M., Pearson, C., Tafoya, G., Duran, B., Rios, L. I., & Wallerstein, N. (2011). Process and outcome constructs for evaluating community-based participatory research projects: A matrix of existing measures. *Health Education Research, 27,* 680–690. doi:10.1093/her/cyr087

Stokols, D., Hall, K. L., Taylor, B. K., & Moser, R. P. (2008). The science of team science: Overview of the field and introduction to the supplement. *American Journal of Preventive Medicine, 35*(2S), S77–S89.

Wallerstein, N., Oetzel, J., Duran, B., Magarati, M., Pearson, C., Belone, L., Davis, J., Dewindt, L., Lucero, J., Ruddock, C., Sutter, E., Villegas, M., & Dutta, M. (under review). Conceptualizing and measuring the culture-centered approach in community based participatory research. *Social Science & Medicine.*

APPENDIX 11

PARTICIPATORY MONITORING AND EVALUATION OF COMMUNITY HEALTH INITIATIVES USING THE COMMUNITY CHECK BOX EVALUATION SYSTEM

STEPHEN FAWCETT, JERRY SCHULTZ, VICKI COLLIE-AKERS, CHRISTINA HOLT, JOMELLA WATSON-THOMPSON, AND VINCENT FRANCISCO

How do we see and reflect on what community health initiatives are accomplishing and use the information to enhance progress?

Comprehensive community health initiatives are challenging to evaluate; they are complex, dynamic, unfolding, with their effects on outcomes often delayed. For an evaluation approach to be useful and used, it needs to be able to document the unfolding of key activities (the intervention) over time, characterize and report the information in meaningful ways, and examine possible associations between activities and indicators of success. Consistent with principles of community-based participatory research (CBPR) (Fawcett, Collie-Akers, Schultz, & Cupertino, 2013; Minkler & Wallerstein, 2008), a participatory evaluation system should make it easier for community and evaluation partners to (1) document activities and indicators of success, (2) reflect on patterns in the data (e.g., factors related to a marked increase in community or systems changes), and (3) use the information for decision making and adjustments.

BACKGROUND AND TECHNICAL SUPPORTS FOR MONITORING AND EVALUATION

Since the early 1990s, the Work Group for Community Health and Development at the University of Kansas (http://communityhealth.ku.edu) has developed and implemented supports for participatory evaluation using the Community Check Box Evaluation System, an online documentation and support system (Fawcett & Schultz, 2008). This evaluation system has been used with a variety of community health initiatives, including those to prevent chronic diseases, communicable diseases, adolescent pregnancy, substance abuse, violence, child abuse, and limited access to health care (e.g., Collie-Akers et al., 2013; Fawcett et al., 1997, 2013, 2015; Paine-Andrews et al., 2002; Watson-Thompson et al., 2013).

Each customized Community Check Box integrates tools for participatory evaluation with supports for systematic reflection and making adjustments. It includes tools to make the following easier:

- Documenting activities and importing of indicators of success
- Graphing key measures (e.g., development activities, resources generated, services provided, community and systems change, indicators of population-level outcomes)
- Shared sensemaking (i.e., using embedded questions to reflect on the data—what are we seeing and what does it mean, e.g., in patterns of activity over time, distribution of activities by goal area)
- Reporting to stakeholders (e.g., about activities, outcomes, factors affecting success, lessons learned)

The Community Check Box also features integrated supports for reflection and action curated from the content of the Community Tool Box (CTB) (http://ctb.ku.edu). For instance, if review of data for an initiative suggests that "there is not enough improvement in outcomes," the Check Box user is prompted to ask questions of the situation (e.g., "Are changes in place long enough to make a difference?"). Links are also provided to Tool Box resources to support improvement (e.g., tool kits and troubleshooting guides for evaluation and sustainability). Selected supports are curated from the Community Tool Box's more than seven thousand pages of free resources for building healthy communities. Reaching more than 5 million unique users annually, these include CTB open source content for (1) learning skills (e.g., conducting listening sessions), (2) doing the work (e.g., assessing needs and resources), (3) solving problems (e.g., not enough participation), and (4) implementing processes for change (e.g., implementing effective interventions).

This report outlines a protocol for participatory monitoring and evaluation, sensemaking, and adjustments made easier by the Community Check Box Evaluation System.

PROTOCOL FOR PARTICIPATORY MONITORING AND EVALUATION

As depicted in Figure A11.1, the Community Check Box Evaluation System enables a four-step process to do the following:

1. *Capture* instances of key activities implemented in the effort. Methods used include reporting of activities by implementers, interviews with key informants (i.e., people knowledgeable about the initiative), and review of documents (e.g., progress reports). This results in identified instances of activities and relevant details (i.e., what was done, when, by whom, toward what goal).
2. *Code* by type of activity using definitions and scoring instructions to ensure consistency of entries. For instance, typical initiative activities and outputs may include development activities (e.g., action plans), services provided (e.g., delivery of programs), resources generated (e.g., new grants), and community or systems changes (e.g., new or expanded programs, policies, environmental changes).

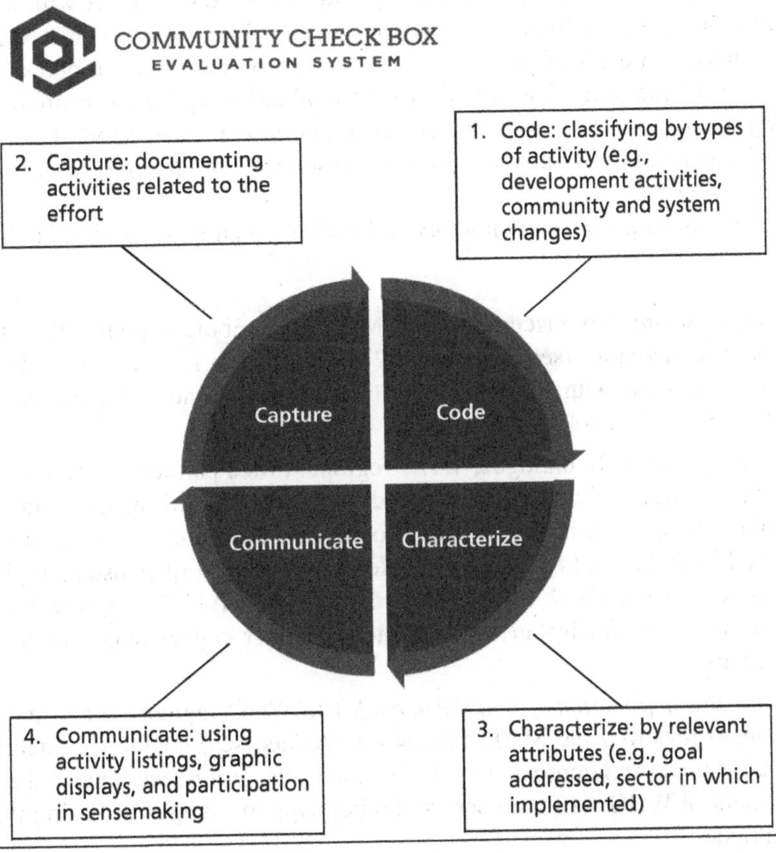

FIGURE A11.1 *Protocol for Participatory Monitoring and Evaluation Using the Community Check Box Evaluation System*

3. *Characterize* the activity by attributes important-to-understanding implementation. For instance, documented community or system changes may be characterized by (a) goal addressed (e.g., infant mortality, poverty, and jobs); (b) strategy used (e.g., modifying access, policy change); (c) estimated reach (e.g., low—less than 5 percent of population); (d) duration (e.g., one-time event, ongoing); (e) target group (e.g., children, marginalized group); (f) sector in which implemented (e.g., schools, government); and other attributes.
4. *Communicate* and dialogue about progress. For instance, community and evaluation partners can use summary activity listings, online graphs, and reflection questions to report, critically review, and make sense of the data (see Figure A11.2).

PARTICIPATORY SENSEMAKING AND ADJUSTMENTS

A hallmark of CBPR and other participatory approaches is that community and research partners have shared roles in collecting and analyzing data. As an example, we used the check box in a participatory monitoring and evaluation (M&E) project with partners at the World Health Organization Regional Office for Africa. They were interested in examining the implementation and effects of Ebola response activities in an outbreak area in Liberia. We used the Community Check Box (CCB) Evaluation System to support participatory sensemaking by pairing (1) graphs of activities and outcomes (see the graph at the left in Figure A11.2) with (2) CCB questions to guide systematic reflection (see the text box at the right of Figure A11.2).

Shared sensemaking among community and evaluation partners focused on three reflection questions:

1. *What are we seeing*? For instance, for this M&E of the Ebola response effort, the line graph of cumulative activities (see Figure A11.2) showed a marked increase in Ebola response activities over time, with an acceleration (steeper curve) and sustained activity from late June 2014 through October 2014.
2. *What does it mean?* In dialogue, WHO regional office partners noted that this increase in Ebola response activity was associated with a bending of the curve in the incidence of Ebola virus disease in this affected county (by mid-August 2014) and in achieving zero (by November 2014). Marked acceleration in Ebola response activities (late June 2014) was associated with several factors (see Figure A11.2, boxes with arrows showing date of onset), for instance, WHO staff member engagement and development of action plans.
3. *What are the implications for adjustment*? The WHO regional office for Africa leadership team reviewed the M&E data and associated sensemaking to identify areas for future adjustment and improvement. For instance, the group recommended ensuring early deployment of WHO staff members and other supports suggested during the sensemaking dialogue.

Using Community Check Box Reflection Questions (What are we seeing? Meaning? Adjustments?) to dialogue with partners about key events [in boxes] that are associated with increased or decreased implementation activity and related improvement or worsening of outcomes.

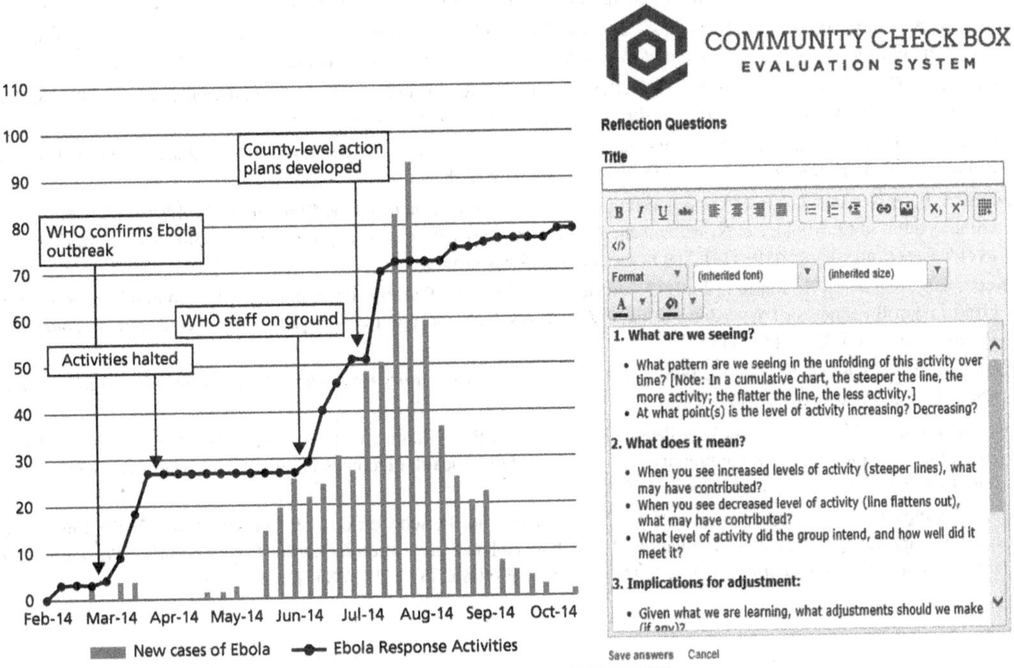

FIGURE A11.2 *Participatory Sensemaking*

CONCLUSION

Adherence to CBPR principles—especially fostering co-learning and capacity building among all partners—is a particular strength of this approach. In supporting participatory sensemaking, this evaluation approach strengthens the capabilities of community and research partners to systematically reflect on what is happening—what we are seeing, its meaning, and implications for adjustment. By making documentation and reporting easier and more transparent, this evaluation system creates opportunities for shared learning, communication, and accountability. Through coding of key implementation activities and outcomes, it enables attention to core evaluation questions such as whether the initiative is bringing about community and environmental change and whether these changes are associated with improvements in indicators of population health and health equity.

By enabling characterization of activities by key attributes, we can more effectively estimate the dose of comprehensive community initiatives (i.e., the amount and type of interventions implemented) and their contribution to population health improvement (Fawcett, Collie-Akers, Schultz, & Kelley, 2015). Our hope is that such participatory evaluation approaches can strengthen the capacity of community and research partners to understand and improve efforts to build healthier and more just communities.

REFERENCES

Collie-Akers, V. L., Fawcett, S. B., & Schultz, J. A. (2013). Measuring progress of collaborative action in a community health effort. *Revista Panamericana de Salud Pública/Pan American Journal of Public Health, 34*(6), 422–428.

Fawcett, S. B., Collie-Akers, V., Schultz, J. A., & Cupertino, P. (2013). Community-based participatory research within the Latino Health for All Coalition. *Journal of Prevention and Intervention in the Community, 41*(3), 142–154.

Fawcett, S. B., Collie-Akers, V., Schultz, J., & Kelley, M. (2015). Measuring community programs and policies in the Healthy Communities Study. *American Journal of Preventive Medicine, 49*(4), 636–641.

Fawcett, S. B., Lewis, R. K., et al. (1997). Evaluating community coalitions for the prevention of substance abuse: The case of Project Freedom. *Health Education and Behavior, 26*(6), 812–828.

Fawcett, S. B., & Schultz, J. A. (2008). Supporting participatory evaluation using the Community Tool Box online documentation system. In M. Minkler & N. Wallerstein (Eds.), *Community-based participatory research for health: From process to outcomes* (2nd ed., pp. 419–424). San Francisco, CA: Jossey-Bass.

Fawcett, S. B., Sepers, C. E., Jones, J., Jones, L., & McKain, W. (2015). Participatory evaluation of a community mobilization effort to enroll residents of Wyandotte County, Kansas residents through the Affordable Care Act. *American Journal of Public Health, 105*(S3), S433–S437.

Minkler, M., & Wallerstein, N. (Eds.). (2008). *Community-based participatory research for health: From process to outcomes* (2nd ed.). San Francisco, CA: Jossey-Bass.

Paine-Andrews, A., Fisher, J. L., Berkley-Patton, J., Fawcett, S. B., Williams, E. L., Lewis, R. K., & Harris, K. J. (2002). Analyzing the contribution of community change to population health outcomes in an adolescent pregnancy prevention initiative. *Health Education and Behavior, 29*(2), 183–193.

Watson-Thompson, J., Jones, M. D., Colvin, J. D., McClendon-Cole, T., Schober, D. J., & Johnson, A. M. (2013). Supporting a community-based participatory evaluation approach to violence prevention in Kansas City. *Journal of Prevention and Intervention in the Community, 41*(3), 155–166. doi:10.1080/10852352.2013.788342

APPENDIX 12

POWER MAPPING

A USEFUL TOOL FOR UNDERSTANDING THE POLICY ENVIRONMENT AND ITS APPLICATION TO A LOCAL SODA TAX INITIATIVE

JENNIFER FALBE, MEREDITH MINKLER, ROBIN DEAN, AND JANA CORDEIERO

Power mapping is increasingly used by CBPR partnerships and community-based organizations to better understand local or regional policy environments for a particular issue or legislation they hope to see passed (or defeated). Best used in small groups of five or six members, this power-mapping exercise is helpful for identifying key organizational, community, and individual players; their stance on the issue; and their relative strength and influence (Ritas, Ni, Halpin, & Minkler, 2008).

Policy mapping is particularly useful in cases of "strange bedfellows," for example, when an organization that has historically favored measures promoting public health takes an uncharacteristic opposing stand on a health-promoting measure. As illustrated in the following, the acceptance of donations or other support from an industry or group opposing the measure may be behind such unexpected reversals.

After briefly describing how to make and use a power map, we turn to a case study of a coalition's efforts to pass a soda tax ballot measure in San Francisco in 2014 and again in 2016. We demonstrate how understanding where key community, organizational, and government and other actors stood helped partially explain the measure's initial failure, as well as how changes in the initiative and its support strategies may have helped a subsequent measure succeed.

MAKING AND USING A POWER MAP

First, select the *specific policy measure* your group wants to help pass or defeat, for example, a state legislative initiative to increase the smoking age from eighteen to twenty-one or a city council proposal to ban the shipping of coal from its port.

As a group, do the following:

1. Identify the policy *target(s):* the individuals and organizations with the power to make a particular change happen
2. Identify the other *key players* in this situation: the individuals, organizations, or communities that may be affected by the problem or policy or that have the potential to influence the situation. Keep in mind that as change becomes imminent, many people will be drawn into the issue who did not know or care about it before. Try to anticipate who this will be.
3. On a sheet of paper, write your *policy objective* at the top. Label the left side *supporters,* the middle *undecided* (or divided), and the right side *opposition.* Indicate on this page your *targets* (depicted as circles) and *key players* (squares), according to where they fall along the spectrum. As illustrated in Figure A12.1, for visual reference use *larger* squares and circles to indicate more powerful targets and players, or those with more at stake, and *smaller* ones to indicate those who are weaker or less affected by the outcome.

   In your mapping, remember that many considerations go into decisions about relative power (depicted in the size of the squares or circles), among them the target's or player's

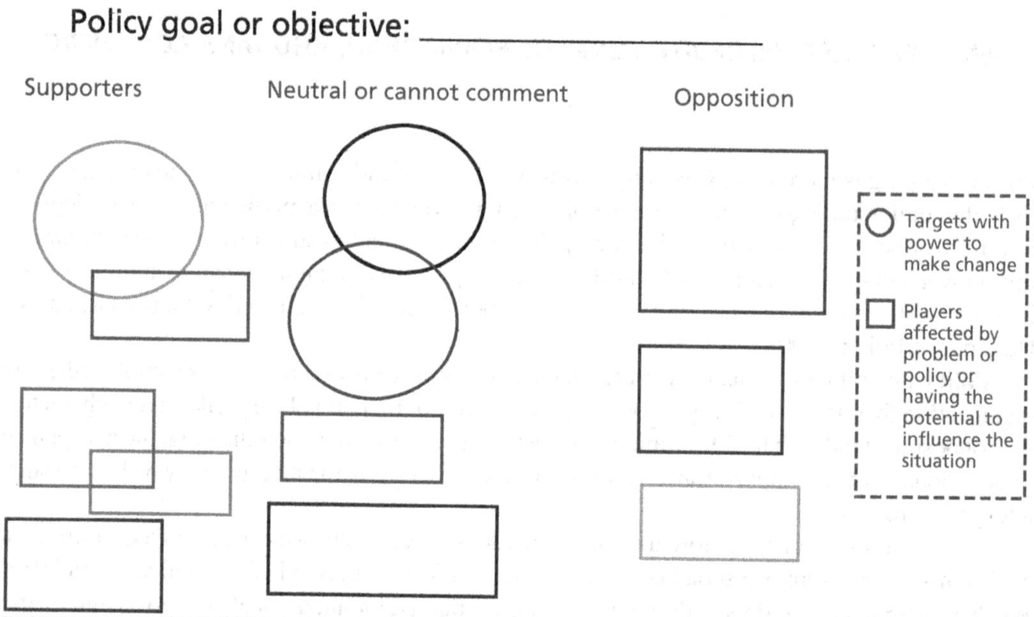

FIGURE A12.1 *Creating a Power Map*
Source: Reprinted from Ritas, Ni, Halpin, and Minkler (2008).

scope (size), *resources* (staff, money, lobbyists), *skills,* and *access,* as well as *how intensely the issue affects each target or player* (e.g., is it a burning or tangential issue?). A small group that cares deeply about an issue and has great resources and organization may be more effective than a larger group with few resources or poor organization or one that feels less strongly (Ritas et al., 2008). When possible, allow the circles and squares to overlap where interests overlap. However, because some supporters may share interests with those opposed to your policy, finding areas of (sometimes unspoken) overlap between supporters may not always be possible (Ritas et al., 2008).

4. Particularly important in an election or decision year is to find out what campaign contributions, donations, or perks may have been received in current or recent years and by which player(s) in a position of influence. This step typically is not included in an initial power map and often takes place subsequently because there is usually a time lag between when campaign contributions are made and when they are publicly disclosed. However, when available, campaign contribution information may be useful in updating the map and considering strategic choices. Such information may serve as an important reality check or point of leverage in your group's efforts.
5. Given your current knowledge base, choose the three most important individuals and organizations to influence. Consider the following:
   - Is it more important now to strengthen your allies, persuade those who are neutral, or weaken the opposition?
   - Is it time to approach a target or to work with key players?
   - Can we get more information to increase the map's accuracy? If so, where, when, and how?

Questions for reflection: For the policy you have chosen, was it easier to identify supporters or sources of opposition? Why or why not? Were there surprises when considering potential overlapping interests? If your group decided the time was right to approach a key target or player, what are useful *next steps*?

ILLUSTRATION OF POLICY MAPPING REGARDING A LOCAL SODA TAX INITIATIVE

Reducing consumption of sugar-sweetened beverages (SSBs) is a major public health priority because its consumption increases the risk of obesity, diabetes, and heart disease (Hu, 2013). Based on the success of tobacco taxation in reducing smoking, public health experts have called for SSB taxes (so-called soda taxes) to reduce consumption and raise revenues for public health programs (Brownell et al., 2009). Mexico implemented a soda tax in 2014, and in the wake of dozens of unsuccessful attempts in the United States, Berkeley, California, became the first US jurisdiction to pass a soda tax in 2014. Berkeley's successful passage has since been followed by Philadelphia, Oakland, San Francisco, Albany, Boulder, and Cook County in 2016. A comprehensive junk food and soda tax passed the Navajo Nation Council in 2015, after three years of education and organizing campaigns. As predicted from economic models, Mexico's and Berkeley's soda taxes resulted in reduced consumption of SSBs (Colchero, Popkin, Rivera, & Ng, 2016; Falbe et al., 2016), especially in lower-income households, which bear the brunt of diet-related chronic disease.

In November 2014, at the same time that Berkeley passed a soda tax, San Francisco residents took to the polls for a vote on a two-cent-per-ounce tax on the distributors of sugary drink. Tax revenues were to be allocated to physical activity and nutrition programs, child dental care, and healthy food and drinks access for those most at risk for chronic diseases. Three city supervisors who crafted the measure did so by consulting with advocates, academics, and experts. Because the measure designated specific revenue allocations, it needed a two-thirds majority to pass under California tax law, unlike Berkeley's general soda tax, which required only a simple majority.

One group of soda tax advocates' assessment of support, opposition, and neutrality vis-à-vis the tax informed the power map shown in Figure A12.2. These power dynamics are based on advocates' knowledge and information gleaned from policy makers, news media, public health research, and advocacy and philanthropic organizations.

Before the initiative was on the ballot, advocates had a good understanding of its key supporters, opponents, and neutral players and had learned from soda tax attempts in other cities that the beverage industry would use tremendous financial and political resources to fight the measure. However, the pro-tax advocates were unsure which organizations the industry could sway. San Francisco's first Chinese American mayor, who was extremely popular in the Chinese community, was neutral from the start of the campaign. Advocates were unsure if his silence was the result of the city previously having received funds from the beverage industry, his close relationship with the business community, or competing political priorities. Without the mayor's support and significant resources, advocates knew they needed to gain support and build their power base through endorsements from the city's many education, health, youth-serving, and political Democratic groups that publish voter guides. Throughout the campaign, the mayor remained neutral, likely resulting in failure to garner support from Chinese voters. Further, opposition funding appeared to sway the positions of some other key players.

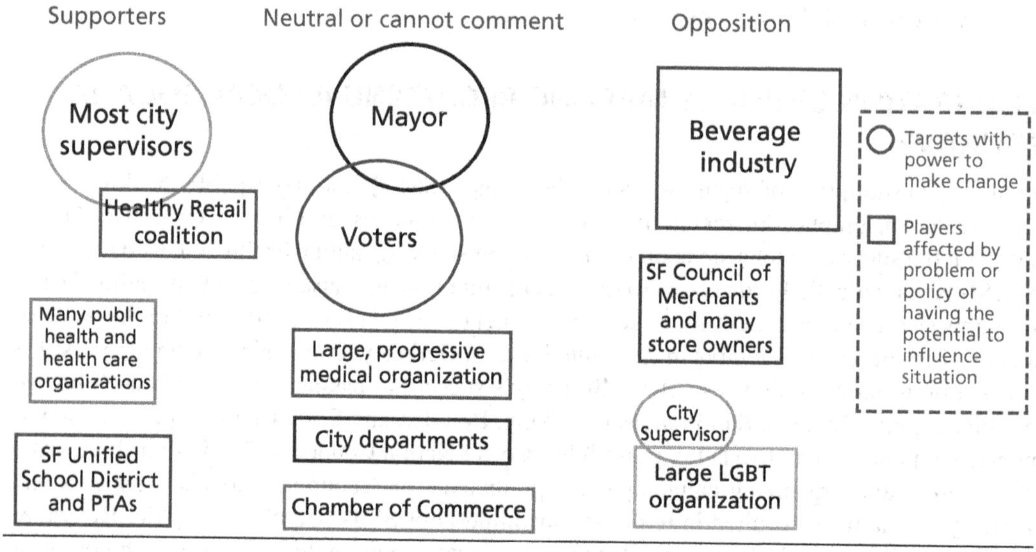

FIGURE A12.2 *Power Map for San Francisco Soda Tax 2014*

At the start of the campaign, a city supervisor's vote to place the initiative on the ballot suggested he was a supporter. However, when his comments at a board of supervisor's meeting mirrored arguments from the No campaign, advocates were unsure where to place him. This supervisor was strongly supported by a progressive LGBT group, which was actively campaigning for his election to a higher office. That group had received $70,000 early in the election year from the American Beverage Association (ABA)–funded opposition. ABA support was evident from the many mailers advocating for this candidate and against the soda tax measure. This infusion of campaign funds, and its apparent influence, led advocates to move the supervisor from "supporter" to "opponent" on the power map.

Although two other city supervisors and some Democratic clubs also received ABA funds, because of their perceived minimal influence, they were not included on the map.

The inability of some likely and potentially powerful supporters to take a stand on the tax also may have hurt the measure's chances. For example, the SF Health Commission—the governing policy body of the San Francisco Department of Public Health (SFDPH) whose members are appointed by the mayor—passed a resolution supporting public health efforts to reduce soda consumption (SFDPH, 2014). By law, however (and unlike elected officials), city and state employees are not permitted to advocate for ballot initiatives, so they could not mention the soda tax initiative in their resolution. Experts from a well-respected public university, who also are state employees, were largely silent and had indeed received warnings from the university prohibiting activity in political campaigns.

Yet even nongovernmental employees sometimes failed to take a stand. The heads of some community-based organizations with city contracts thus were concerned that those contracts might be at risk if they supported the soda tax given the mayor's neutrality. Finally, a large and progressive medical organization, whose support could have provided credibility to help sway voters, also remained silent for reasons that are unclear.

The 2014 San Francisco soda tax measure never had unanimous support from key political leaders, and this case illustrates how the opposition's money eroded some of the political support it did have. Creating and periodically updating a power map can track this support, help explain why an initiative is succeeding or failing, and inform course corrections.

However, power mapping also has limitations. Even with periodic updates, it cannot account for all factors operative in the success or failure of political campaigns. Along with the money-influenced shifting power dynamics, several other factors influenced the SF soda tax measure's initial failure. These included lack of funds to fight an opponent with seemingly unlimited resources (soda tax advocates were outspent thirty-one to one), the two-thirds vote threshold for passage, and a coalition that was narrower and less diverse than desirable. Finally, the ABA-funded opposition harnessed one of the city's most urgent concerns—cost of living—in campaign materials. By contrast, Philadelphia's passage of a soda tax in June 2016 was helped, in part, by strong leadership from the mayor but also by its focus on connecting tax-generated revenue to an issue of great local concern: early childhood education. Further, it required passage by only the city council.

MOVING TO VICTORY THE SECOND TIME AROUND

As San Francisco supporters embarked on a subsequent soda tax measure for November 2016, they pushed to get and retain mayoral support and endorsements from a wide range of education, health, civic, and political groups and individuals, which helped balance the power and resources of the beverage industry. The ultimate victory of the 2016 soda tax measure by 62 percent of the vote (www.sfelections.org/results/20161108/) also had to do with ordinance revisions proposing a general tax (requiring only a simple majority to pass in California), coupled with the establishment of an advisory committee to make recommendations to the city on funding of programs to reduce the consumption of sugary drinks. This echoed the structure of Berkeley's successful Measure D. Thus far, the Berkeley city council has acted on its advisory commission's recommendations to fund school, community, and city programs focused on nutrition and health promotion (www.takepart.com/article/2016/04/25/soda-public-health).

Despite the soda tax's passage, the overwhelming opposition and resources of the ABA illustrate the incredibly difficult odds soda tax supporters faced. Indeed, the industry spent over $28 million to defeat 2016 soda taxes in three Bay Area (https://cspinet.org/resource/big-sodas-spending-spree-fight-public-health-measures)!

CONCLUSION

As illustrated by the soda tax case study, power mapping is a useful tool for CBPR partnerships and advocacy groups wishing to better understand the political lay of the land on particular legislation. Periodic mapping updates, and the inclusion of diverse mapping partners with unique knowledge, can broaden and deepen the evolving story. Meanwhile, supplementing mapping with ongoing analysis of other make-or-break factors for passage of a new measure, ideally with the help of policy mentors and other knowledgeable insiders and community leaders, may provide the most realistic knowledge base for informing subsequent action.

REFERENCES

Brownell, K. D., Farley, T., Willett, W. C., et al. (2009). The public health and economic benefits of taxing sugar-sweetened beverages. *New England Journal of Medicine, 361*(16), 1599–1605.

Colchero, M. A., Popkin, B. M., Rivera, J. A., & Ng, S. W. (2016). Beverage purchases from stores in Mexico under the excise tax on sugar sweetened beverages: Observational study. *BMJ, 352,* h6704.

Falbe, J., Thompson, H. R., Becker, C. M., Rojas, N., McCulloch, C. E., & Madsen, K. A. Impact of the Berkeley excise tax on sugar-sweetened beverage consumption. *American Journal of Public Health, 106*(10), 1865–1871.

Hu, F. B. (2013). Resolved: There is sufficient scientific evidence that decreasing sugar-sweetened beverage consumption will reduce the prevalence of obesity and obesity-related diseases. *Obesity Review, 14*(8), 606–619.

Ritas, C., Ni, A., Halpin, H., & Minkler, M. (2008). Using CBPR to promote policy change. In M. Minkler & N. Wallerstein (Eds.), *Community-based participatory research for health: From process to outcomes* (2nd ed., p. 461). San Francisco, CA: Jossey-Bass.

San Francisco Department of Public Health (SFDPH). (2014). Health Commission Resolution 11–2. Retrieved from www.sfdph.org/dph/files/hc/HCRes/Resolutions/2014/Sugar%20Beverages%20Jan%202014rev.pdf

APPENDIX 13

CBPR INTERACTIVE ROLE-PLAYS

THREE SCENARIOS

MICHELE POLACSEK AND GAIL DANA-SACCO

An interactive online teaching tool provides an ideal environment within which to develop a virtual community where students and faculty members can define problems through dialogue, practice solutions, and engage in disciplined self-reflection and critical thinking. This digital learning space provides real-life-like opportunities to apply knowledge gained though other CBPR course materials. Short ten- to fifteen-minute interactive scenarios paused for discussion and replay or longer improvised scenarios lasting up to thirty minutes or more could be used in a classroom setting or as a synchronous or asynchronous online teaching tool. This tool is particularly suited to digitally inclined students, who may have little opportunity or time to practice interacting with community research projects or when faculty members are reticent to overburden a community with student learners.

We envision a game with five CBPR modules (community-based practice, defining the issue, partnering with the community, the research process and its transformative power, and action planning), each of which can stand alone or be presented in sequence. Each module will provide students with opportunities to attain cross-cutting and module-specific learning objectives.

The use of interchangeable avatars or digital characters (e.g., minority population, majority population, gender identity, race, SES) enables students to take on and personally experience diverse characters, promoting cultural competence, cultural humility, and empathy. Faculty members, acting as "provocateur," facilitate the problem-based learning by establishing parameters, posing questions, and actively participating with students in the learning environment.

Further development of this approach will require substantial investments. If you are interested in partnering in this venture please contact Giant Otter at http://giantotter.com or Michele Polacsek at the University of New England, 716 Stevens Avenue, Portland, ME 04103. One screenshot of the game with sample characters and dialogue is included.

SAMPLE MODULE 1: CONDUCTING CBPR RESEARCH ON INTIMATE PARTNER VIOLENCE IN A HIGH SCHOOL WITH A SIGNIFICANT NEW IMMIGRANT POPULATION

The following is an example of a situation in which community and academic partners are called to action to address a public health issue. The flexible format in which multiple characters and roles can be created encourages reflection and discussion. Background, sample roles, and instructions are included.

Background for Module 1

Urban high school officials have determined that there is a high reported rate of intimate partner violence (IPV) among the local high school students as reported on a recent Youth Behavioral Risk Factor Survey (YBRFS). There appears to be a higher prevalence in schools with higher new immigrant populations. This high school serves a population composed of a significant number of new immigrant families as well as a well-established working class white majority. Because of the preliminary YBRFS findings and recent influx of new immigrants, school officials are open to an invitation from a well-established community service organization to partner with a local university to develop and provide health education materials for an IPV-prevention campaign.

Sample Roles, Characteristics, and Cue Card Instructions for Module 1

1. University faculty member (second-generation East Indian female)—You are working with a limited time frame because students are available for one semester only. You're eager to move the project forward. You have experience studying IPV but no experience with the new immigrant population. You have partnered with this community service organization once before.
2. Community service organization staff member (Hispanic female)—You are a long-standing community activist with deep experience in IPV and extensive knowledge of the transitions this community has experienced over the last thirty years or so.
3. School guidance counselor (white female)—You are very familiar with the IPV issues that have surfaced. They confirm what you know anecdotally, and you're eager to find solutions.
4. School principal (white male)—You recognize that IPV is a problem, but you're concerned that findings don't reflect well on the school and that racial stereotyping will fuel tensions.

5. High school student 1 (white male)—You've been an active student leader and are looking to end your senior year with several commitments including a social service project. Although not known to others, your family currently experiences IPV.
6. High school student 2 (new immigrant female)—You understand the stresses experienced by new immigrant families, including reluctance to access public safety resources because of fear of deportation.
7. University student 1 (mixed-race female)—You have personal experience with family issues involving substance use and IPV. You have completed two internships addressing these issues. You're convinced that substance abuse is most often a driver of IPV. You come from a well-resourced family and have had many opportunities throughout your life to further your education and have traveled extensively outside the United States.
8. University student 2 (white female)—You've organized a get-out-the-vote campaign among your peers in your home community. You are sensitive to the potential challenges of working with this issue within the new immigrant population. You come from a modest working-class background and have no international experience.
9. Parent or school board member (white female)—You are a long-standing member of the school board and your children grew up in the district and attended the school here. You're not sure that the finding of greater substance use among white students is accurate.

Instructions for Students

As you participate, ensure that you attend to relevant CBPR principles. For successful CBPR, reflective practice is essential. Think critically about your role as a researcher and the implications of your experience and your social status and relative positions of power and privilege in these interactions (as indicated in the introductory chapters of this book).

Scenario 1: Developing Consensus on a Research Agenda

Setting for Scenario 1

High school classroom

Learning Objectives for Scenario 1

1. Identify key challenges of race-ethnicity and social privilege in the research process.
2. Name the essential elements of conflict management in meetings.
3. Describe the benefits of an inclusive approach to stakeholder participation in CBPR.

Background for Scenario 1

A university faculty member is visiting the school to discuss the YBRFS findings and decide next steps with the school principal, the guidance counselor, and a community service organization staff member. She proposes a pilot project in this high school to further investigate factors associated with IPV among high school students in order to understand how best to intervene. A peer leader group in the high school, represented by a student in the meeting, will inform the process and perhaps participate in the research. The group discusses how best to proceed.

(*Continued*)

Scenario 1 (CONTINUED)

Characters in Scenario 1

University faculty member, community service organization staff member, school guidance counselor, school principal, high school student 1, and high school student 2

Discussion Questions for Scenario 1

1. What steps does the research team take next?
2. How are the important stakeholders identified and involved in this process?
3. What are the challenges that the research team faces?
4. What challenges do the community members face?
5. What challenges do the students face?
6. What decision-making process should be used to establish the research agenda?

Scenario 2: Research Team Meeting

Setting for Scenario 2

At a café or restaurant

Learning Objectives for Scenario 2

1. Name key elements of successful community partnerships in CBPR.
2. Recognize and name own social privilege.
3. Describe how social privilege can bias research processes and outcomes.
4. Demonstrate understanding of complexities of race-ethnicity and social privilege in the research process.
5. Demonstrate effective group or meeting process in CBPR.

Background for Scenario 2

The faculty member reports back preliminary plans and concerns about the project and any next steps that have already been decided in an initial meeting at the high school. The research team comes up with two aims: to conduct more research among students to compare factors associated with IPV in the established and new immigrant populations and to develop recommendations for interventions based on YBRFS and formative research data. The team develops a formative research strategy. A short survey with ten questions is developed. An equal number of respondents will be drawn from volunteers in eleventh- and twelfth-grade health classes.

Characters in Scenario 2

University faculty member, university student 1, and university student 2

Discussion Questions for Scenario 2

1. How does the research team make decisions that are responsive to community concerns?
2. What considerations does the research team need to take into account with regard to developing community partnerships?
3. What does the research team need to keep in mind to maximize community partner engagement?

Scenario 3: Research Team Prepares for a Community Meeting

Setting for Scenario 3

School cafeteria

Learning Objectives for Scenario 3

1. Demonstrate understanding of the role of researcher in the CBPR process.
2. Name structural considerations important to a successful CBPR process.
3. Describe ethical considerations working with sensitive information.

Scenario 3 (After the formative research process has taken place)

The research team, at the invitation of the school, plans to attend a community meeting in the school to report the results of the study. The study does not confirm earlier indicators of a higher incidence of IPV in the new immigrant community. The research also demonstrates differing associations with IPV in the two populations studied. Among whites, substance use is associated with IPV. Among new immigrants, IPV seems to be more associated with economic status of the family. There is a reluctance to report incidence of IPV within both populations but for different reasons.

Characters in Scenario 3

University faculty member, community service organization staff members, school guidance counselor, high school student 1 and high school student 2, university student 1 and university student 2, parent or school board member.

In the following screen shot, the two university students are discussing strategy for the upcoming community meeting.

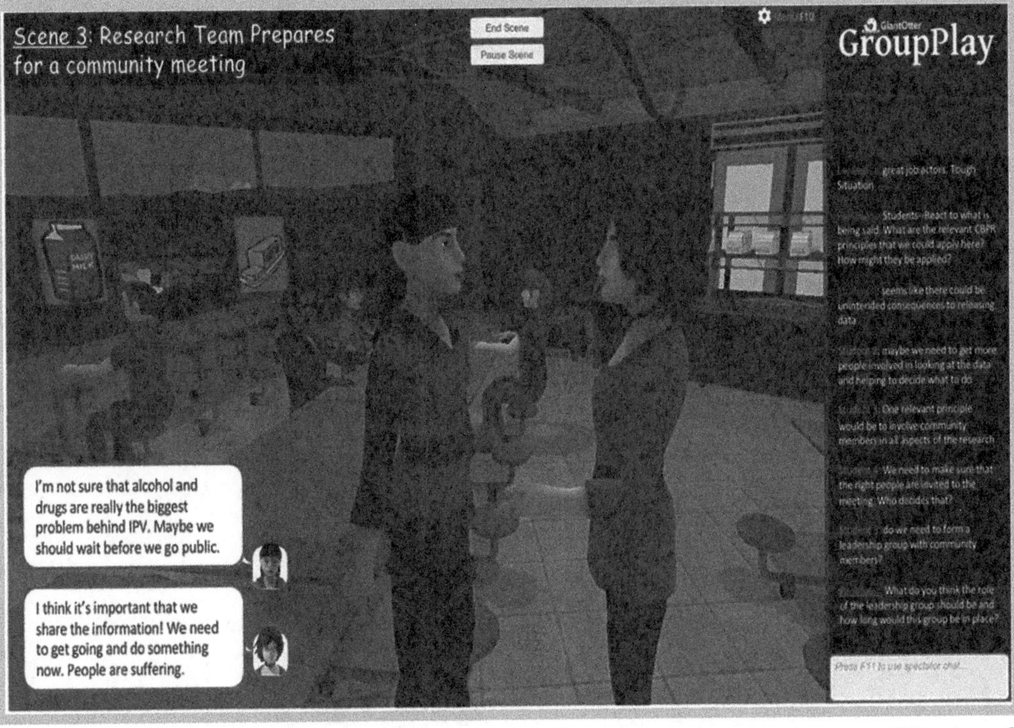

(Continued)

Scenario3 (CONTINUED)

Discussion Questions for Scenario 3

1. How should the research team interact with people at the community meeting?
2. Is the group meeting too fast? Are there other steps that need to be taken before the community meeting?
3. How does the research team develop the recommendations using a CBPR approach?
4. What steps should the team take to involve the appropriate stakeholders in interpreting the research results and developing an action plan?

Avatar interaction continues as long as the facilitator deems useful. Faculty members and students have the opportunity to participate as characters or facilitators. Avatar interaction may be halted at any time to allow for group discussion and recommendations for improvement.

This virtual reality approach provides an innovative pedagogical tool to practice CBPR in a dynamic, interactive environment, which can be used in a wide variety of settings.

AFTERWORD

BUDD HALL AND RAJESH TANDON

What a pleasure to be able to share a few thoughts on reading this third edition of *Community-Based Participatory Research for Health*. It is a joy to see that Nina Wallerstein and Meredith Minkler are continuing their productive, insightful, and inspirational leadership in this critically important role of understanding health and justice within a framework of knowledge democracy. That framework, and this book, are inclusive of each and all of our bodies and diversities, including the diversities of the knowledge of the earth and the rest of nature. It makes us happy that Nina and Meredith have found Bonnie Duran and John G. Oetzel with whom to curate this important new edition. Perhaps most impressive is the fact that this book continues a passionate call for justice, inclusion, change, and democracy. The editors and contributors emphatically reject the idea that the highest standards in health research can be reached only when detached from the bias of community, our bodies, inequality, racism, or poverty. In some places, they even challenge the domination of the Western canon of white-male scientific knowledge, providing examples from women's knowledge, Indigenous knowledge, knowledge of the street-involved, and others.

The two of us met in the mid-1970s. Budd had been working in Tanzania in the field of adult education. He met Paulo Freire there in 1971 and continued a friendship with him over a lifetime. But it was the group of Tanzanian and expatriate researchers working together at the time to explore what they were calling *non-colonial research methods* who first articulated the concept of participatory research (Hall,1975, 2005). Rajesh fell into what we both began calling *participatory research* during the course of doing his fieldwork with Indigenous farmers in southern Rajasthan, also in the mid-1970s. He discovered that in spite of his elite level of education at the best universities in India and the United States, the women and men of the villages in Rajasthan were vastly more knowledgeable in every aspect of rural agricultural life than he was.

The two of us found others in Latin America, Europe, North America, and Asia who were challenging the dominant research paradigms of the time, including Nina Wallerstein, Barbara Israel, and Meredith Minkler from the health field and John Gaventa, Peter Park, and John Hurst from social movement fields in the United States. We were fortunate to have the organizational structure of the International Council for Adult Education to provide a home for the first International Participatory Research Network, a network that Rajesh coordinated for most of the years between 1978 and 1992.

Why do we mention this? We mention this because in those days, nearly all of the support for CBPR (and its many other names) came from outside the academy. The idea that knowledge of persons living with HIV/AIDS, of women's movements, of Indigenous peoples, of peasant farmers in Brazil, and of the homeless could be recognized, valued, or drawn on to make improvements in the lives of people was heretical. CBPR was not taught in universities back then. When many of us were invited in those early days to give talks about these kinds of ideas we were even shouted down. Our ideas were shared excitedly in the democracy movements in the Philippines, South Africa, Nicaragua, and the Black and Latino communities in the United States, but a book on CBPR for health could not have been published at the time.

That was forty years ago. As a result of a refusal to separate the ideas of knowledge and justice, evidence and passion, and the body and the world, particularly in the field of public health and health care, we have a third edition of a book that takes our collective hopes that much further ahead. This book is a wonderful addition to the state of the field largely in the United States, although there are some global chapters. Yet, the knowledge democracy movement is exploding around the world in ways that we could never have imagined forty years ago. Our jointly shared UNESCO chair was created in 2012 to support the building of capacity of CBPR in the Global South and the excluded North. We work with many global networks of higher education institutions on issues of community-university engagement, decolonization of higher education, knowledge democracy, and the question of how to facilitate learning for a new generation of CBPR workers (Hall, Tandon, & Tremblay, 2015).

Challenges remain, many of which are touched on in the chapters of this book. Inequality in the United States and in other parts of the world has grown dramatically over the past forty years. This results in more health inequities for many more people. Violence against women is a global threat ranging from the rape stories in India to the campuses of elite universities of the United States and Canada. Indigenous peoples' land continues to be pillaged for resource extraction that benefits only the very richest. Black Lives Matter in the United States, Idle No More in Canada, the Latin American African Descendants movement, and others illustrate the continued use of race to exclude and marginalize. Sixty million people have been forced from their homes because of war and violence and live precarious lives as refugees and outsiders.

We draw these matters to readers' attention to underscore the importance of not only multiplying and carrying on the kinds of work in CBPR shared in this book but also to continue to deepen our understanding of how knowledge, organizing, speaking out, and co-learning can contribute to healthy, just, sustainable, and joyful lives for each person in this glorious, troubled, and perplexing world.

REFERENCES

Hall, B. L. (1975). Participatory research: An approach for change. *Convergence, 8*(2), 24–31.

Hall, B. L. (2005). From the cold? Reflections on participatory research 1970–2005. *Convergence, 38*(1), 5–24.

Hall, B. L., Tandon, R., & Tremblay, C. (Eds.). (2015). *Strengthening community-university research partnerships: Global perspectives.* Victoria, BC, Canada: University of Victoria.

INDEX

Page numbers in *italics* refer to illustrations.

N

O

P

Q

R

T

Y

COMMUNITY-BASED PARTICIPATORY RESEARCH FOR HEALTH